Advances in Neurology

Volume 94

INTERNATIONAL ADVISORY BOARD

ADVANCES IN NEUROLOGY

Volume 94

Dystonia 4

Editors

Stanley Fahn, M.D.
H. Houston Merritt Professor
Department of Neurology
Columbia Presbyterian Medical Center
New York, New York, USA

Mark Hallett, M.D.
Chief, Human Motor Control Section
National Institute of Neurological Disorders and Stroke
National Institutes of Health
Bethesda, Maryland, USA

Mahlon R. DeLong, M.D.
Professor and Chairman
Department of Neurology
Emory University School of Medicine and Neurology
Section Chief, The Emory Clinic
Atlanta, Georgia, USA

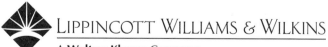
LIPPINCOTT WILLIAMS & WILKINS
A **Wolters Kluwer** Company
Philadelphia • Baltimore • New York • London
Buenos Aires • Hong Kong • Sydney • Tokyo

Acquisitions Editor: Anne M. Sydor
Developmental Editor: Alyson Forbes
Production Editor: Emmeline Parker
Manufacturing Manager: Benjamin Rivera
Cover Designer: Patricia Gast
Compositor: Lippincott Williams & Wilkins Desktop Division
Printer: Edwards Brothers

Library of Congress Cataloging-in-Publication Data
ISBN: 0-7817-4600-0
ISSN: 0091-3952

Care has been taken to confirm the accuracy of the information presented and to describe generally accepted practices. However, the authors, editors, and publisher are not responsible for errors or omissions or for any consequences from application of the information in this book and make no warranty, expressed or implied, with respect to the currency, completeness, or accuracy of the contents of the publication. Application of this information in a particular situation remains the professional responsibility of the practitioner.

The authors, editors, and publisher have exerted every effort to ensure that drug selection and dosage set forth in this text are in accordance with current recommendations and practice at the time of publication. However, in view of ongoing research, changes in government regulations, and the constant flow of information relating to drug therapy and drug reactions, the reader is urged to check the package insert for each drug for any change in indications and dosage and for added warnings and precautions. This is particularly important when the recommended agent is a new or infrequently employed drug.

Some drugs and medical devices presented in this publication have Food and Drug Administration (FDA) clearance for limited use in restricted research settings. It is the responsibility of the health care provider to ascertain the FDA status of each drug or device planned for use in their clinical practice.

10 9 8 7 6 5 4 3 2 1

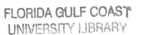

Advances in Neurology Series

Contents

I: Pathophysiology

II: Oppenheim's Dystonia

Contributing Authors

Aviva Abosch, M.D., Ph.D. *Associate Professor, Department of Neurosurgery, Emory University; Attending Physician, Department of Neurosurgery, Emory University Hospital, Atlanta, Georgia, USA*

Charles Adler*, M.D., Ph.D. *Assistant Professor, Department of Neurology and Neuroscience, Weill Medical College of Cornell University, New York, New York, USA*

Alberto Albanese, M.D. *Head, First Department of Neurology, National Neurological Institute; Professor, Department of Neurology, Catholic University, Milan, Italy*

David S. Albers, Ph.D. *Assistant Professor, Department of Neurology and Neuroscience, Weill Medical College of Cornell University, New York, New York, USA*

Eckart Altenmüller, M.D., M.A. *Neurologist, Chair, and Director, Institute of Music Physiology and Musicians' Medicine, University of Music and Drama, Hanover, Germany*

Kotaro Asanuma, M.D., Ph.D. *Foreign Researcher, Functional Brain Imaging Lab, North Shore University Hospital, Manhasset, New York, USA*

Friedrich Asmus, M.D. *Department of Neurodegenerative Disorders, Hertie-Institute for Clinical Brain Research, University of Tübingen, Tübingen, Germany*

Sarah J. Augood, Ph.D. *Assistant Professor, Department of Neurology Research, Center for Aging, Genetics, and Neurodegeneration, Massachusetts General Hospital, Charlestown, Massachusetts, USA*

Huriye Aydin, M.D. *Neurologist, Department of Neurology, Dokuz Eylül University, Izmir, Turkey*

Melisa J. Baptista, Ph.D. *Cell Biology and Gene Expression Section, Laboratory of Neurogenetics, National Institute on Aging, National Institutes of Health, Bethesda, Maryland, USA*

Sergio Barbieri, M.D., Ph.D. *Neurophysiology Unit, Department of Neurological Sciences, IRCCS—Ospedale Maggiore Milano; Professor, Department of Neurological Sciences, University of Milan, Milan, Italy*

Michael P. Barnes, M.D., F.R.C.P. *Professor, Department of Neurological Rehabilitation, University of Newcastle, Hunters Moor Rehabilitation Centre, Newcastle-upon-Tyne, United Kingdom*

Alim-Louis Benabid, M.D., Ph.D. *Professor, Departments of Biophysics and Neurosurgery, Joseph Fourier University, and INSERM; Head, Department of Neurosurgery, University Hospital, Grenoble, France*

Reiner Benecke, M.D. *Director, Department of Neurology, Rostock University, Rostock, Germany*

Anna Rita Bentivoglio, M.D., Ph.D. *Institute of Neurology, Catholic University and A. Gemelli Hospital, Rome, Italy*

Kailash P. Bhatia, M.D., D.M., F.R.C.P. *Reader in Clinical Neurology, Sobell Department of Motor Neuroscience and Movement Disorders, Institute of Neurology; Consultant Neurologist, Department of Clinical Neurology, National Hospital for Neurology and Neurosurgery, London, United Kingdom*

John L. Bradshaw, Ph.D., D.Sc. *Professor Emeritus, Department of Psychology, Monash University, Clayton, Australia*

D. Cristopher Bragg, Ph.D. *Molecular Neurogenetics Unit, Department of Neurology, Massachusetts General Hospital; Program in Neuroscience, Harvard Medical School, Boston, Massachusetts, USA*

Melanie Brandabur* *Neuropsychiatric Institute, Chicago, Illinois, USA*

Alice G. Brandfonbrener, M.D. *Director, Medical Program for Performing Artists, Rehabilitation Institute of Chicago, Chicago, Illinois, USA*

Allison Brashear*, M.D. *Department of Neurology, Indianapolis, Indiana, USA*

Xandra O. Breakefield, Ph.D. *Molecular Neurogenetics Unit, Department of Neurology, Massachusetts General Hospital; Program in Neuroscience, Harvard Medical School, Boston, Massachusetts, USA*

Susan B. Bressman, M.D. *Chair, Department of Neurology, Beth Israel Medical Center, New York; Professor of Neurology, Albert Einstein College of Medicine, Bronx, New York, USA*

Anthony G. Butler, Ph.D., M.B.A. *Dystonia Epidemiologist, Bath Cottage, Dinsdale Park, Middleton St. George, County Durham, United Kingdom*

Nancy Byl, P.T., M.P.H., Ph.D., F.A.P.T.A. *Professor and Chair, Department of Physical Therapy and Rehabilitation Science, School of Medicine, University of California, San Francisco, California, USA*

Raif Cakmur, M.D. *Professor, Department of Neurology, Dokuz Eylül University, Izmir, Turkey*

Guy A. Caldwell, Ph.D. *Assistant Professor, Department of Biological Sciences, The University of Alabama, Tuscaloosa, Alabama, USA*

Kim A. Caldwell, Ph.D. *Adjunct Assistant Professor of Biological Sciences, Department of Biological Sciences, The University of Alabama, Tuscaloosa, Alabama, USA*

Songsong Cao, B.S. *Graduate Program, Department of Biological Sciences, The University of Alabama, Tuscaloosa, Alabama, USA*

Maren Carbon, M.D. *Assistant Investigator, Center for Neurosciences, North Shore-Long Island Jewish Research Institute, Manhasset, New York, USA*

Stéphan Chabardes, M.D. *Department of Neurosurgery, University Hospital; Department of Biological and Clinical Neurosciences, Joseph Fourier University, Grenoble, France*

Michael E. Charness, M.D. *Associate Professor, Department of Neurology, Faculty Associate Dean, Harvard Medical School; Assistant Dean, Boston University School of Medicine, Performing Arts Clinic, Department of Neurology, Brigham and Women's Hospital; Chief of Staff, Veterans Affairs Boston Healthcare System, Boston, Massachusetts, USA*

Robert Chen* *University of Toronto, Toronto, Ontario, Canada*

Marie-Françoise Chesselet, M.D., Ph.D. *Charles H. Markham Professor of Neurology and Chair, Departments of Neurology and Neurobiology, David Geffen School of Medicine at the University of California at Los Angeles, Los Angeles, California, USA*

T. Chumra* *Rush Presbyterian–St. Luke's Medical Center, Chicago, Illinois, USA*

Cynthia Comella*, M.D. (corresponding author) *Associate Professor, Department of Neurological Sciences, Rush-Presbyterian St. Lukes Medical Center; Attending Physician, Department of Neurology, Rush Medical Center, Chicago, Illinois, USA*

Mark R. Cookson, Ph.D. *Chief, Cell Biology and Gene Expression Section, Laboratory of Neurogenetics, National Institute on Aging, National Institutes of Health, Bethesda, Maryland, USA*

Carla Cordivari, M.D. *Consultant, Department of Clinical Neurophysiology, The National Hospital for Neurology and Neurosurgery; Senior Research Fellow, Department of Neurophysiology, Institute of Neurology, Queen Square, London, United Kingdom*

William Dauer, M.D. *Assistant Professor, Departments of Neurology and Pharmacology, Columbia University; Assistant Attending Physician, Department of Neurology, New York Presbyterian Hospital, New York, New York, USA*

Olivier Detante, M.D. *President, Department of Neurology, Grenoble Hospital, Grenoble, France*

Berril Donmez, M.D. *Neurologist, Department of Neurology, Dokuz Eylül University, Izmir, Turkey*

Dirk Dressler, M.D. *Head, Movement Disorders Section, Department of Neurology, Rostock University, Rostock, Germany*

Drake D. Duane, M.D. *Director, Arizona Dystonia Institute, Scottsdale; Professor, Department of Speech and Hearing Sciences, Arizona State University, Tempe, Arizona, USA*

Philip O. F. Duffey, M.B., B.S., M.R.C.P. *Consultant Neurologist, York District Hospital, York, United Kingdom*

The Dystonia Study Group *Rush Medical Center, Chicago Illinois, USA*

David Eidelberg*, M.D. *Director, Center for Neurosciences, North Shore-Long Island Jewish Research Institute, Manhasset; Professor, Department of Neurology and Neurosurgery, New York University School of Medicine, New York, New York, USA*

Antonio E. Elia, M.D. *Resident, Institute of Neurology, Catholic University and Policlinico Gemelli Hospital, Rome, Italy*

Marian L. Evatt* *Emory University, Atlanta, Georgia, USA*

Stewart A. Factor,* D.O. *Albany Medical Center, Albany, New York, USA*

Alfonso Fasano*, M.D. *Resident, Department of Neurology, Catholic University; Post-Doctoral Fellow, Department of Neurology, Policlinico Gemelli Hospital, Rome, Italy*

Graziella Filippini*, M.D. *Chief, Deparment of Neuroepidemiology, National Neurological Institute "Carlo Besta," Milan, Italy*

Saša R. Filipović, M.D., Ph.D. *Senior Research Fellow, Burden Neurological Institute; Clinical Research Fellow, Department of Neurology, Frenchay Hospital, Bristol, United Kingdom*

Blair Ford*, M.D. , F.R.C.P. *Associate Professor, Department of Neurology; Attending Neurologist, Department of Neurology, Neurological Institute, Columbia University, New York, New York, USA*

Richard S. J. Frackowiak* *Professor, Wellcome Department of Imaging Neuroscience, Institute of Neurology, University College London, London, United Kingdom*

Jennifer Friedman*, M.D. *Boston Medical Center, Boston, Massachusetts, USA*

Steven J. Frucht*, M.D. *Assistant Professor, Department of Neurology, Columbia University, New York, New York, USA*

Rebecca Fuller* *Maryland Psychiatric Research Center, Outpatient Research Program, University of Maryland, Baltimore, Maryland, USA*

Yoshiaki Furukawa*, M.D. *Director, Movement Disorders Research Laboratory, Centre for Addiction and Mental Health Clarke Division, Toronto, Ontario, Canada*

Nestor Galvez-Jimenez*, M.D., F.A.C.P. *Associate Professor and Chief, Department of Movement Disorders and Director, Neurology Residency Training Program, Department of Neurology, The Cleveland Clinic Florida, Weston, Florida, USA*

Thomas Gasser* *Department of Neurodegenerative Disorders, Hertie-Institute for Clinical Brain Research, University of Tübingen, Tübingen, Germany*

Christopher C. Gelwix*, B.S. *Graduate Program, Department of Biological Sciences, The University of Alabama, Tuscaloosa, Alabama, USA*

Willibald Gerschlager* *Sobell Department of Motor Neuroscience and Movement, Disorders, Institute of Neurology, London, United Kingdom; Department of Neurology, University of Vienna, Vienna, Austria*

Marie Felice Ghilardi*, M.D. *Center for Neurobiology and Behavior, Columbia College of Physicians and Surgeons, New York, New York, USA; INB-CNR, Milano, Italy*

Rose Goodchild*, Ph.D. *Postdoctoral Fellow, Department of Neurology, Columbia University, New York, New York, USA*

Mark Forrest Gordon*, M.D. *Long Island Jewish Medical Center, New Hyde Park, New York, USA*

Robert G. Grossman*, M.D. *Professor and Chairman, Department of Neurosurgery, Baylor College of Medicine; Chief, Department of Neurosurgery, The Methodist Hospital, Houston, Texas, USA*

Stephen Hague*, Ph.D. *Molecular Genetics Section, Laboratory of Neurogenetics, National Institute on Aging, National Institutes of Health, Bethesda, Maryland, USA*

Mark Hallett*, M.D. *Chief, Human Motor Control Section, National Institute of Neurological Disorders and Stroke, National Institutes of Health, Bethesda, Maryland, USA*

Winifred J. Hamilton, Ph.D., S.M. *Assistant Professor, Departments of Neurosurgery and Medicine, Baylor College of Medicine, Houston, Texas, USA*

Maurice R. Hanson, M.D. *Chairman, Department of Medicine, The Cleveland Clinic Florida, Weston, Florida, USA*

Melanie J. A. Hargreave, R.N. *Movement Disorders Program, Department of Neurology, The Cleveland Clinic Florida, Weston, Florida, USA*

Maurice R. Hawthorne, B.S., F.R.C.S. *Consultant Otolaryngeal Surgeon, The North Riding Infirmary, Middlesbrough, United Kingdom*

Dena Hernandez, B.S. *Molecular Genetics Section, Laboratory of Neurogenetics, National Institute on Aging, National Institutes of Health, Bethesda, Maryland, USA*

Peter Heywood, M.D., F.R.C.P. *Department of Neurology, Frenchay Hospital, Bristol, United Kingdom*

Z. Hollingsworth, M.P.H.   *Department of Neurological Sciences, Rush-Presbyterian St. Luke's Medical Center, Chicago, Illinois, USA*

Hans-Christian Jabusch, M.D.   *Dipl. Mus. Postdoctoral Fellow, Assistant Director, Institute of Music Physiology and Musicians' Medicine, University of Music and Drama, Hanover, Germany*

Marjan Jahanshahi, Ph.D.   *Reader in Cognitive Neuroscience, Sobell Department of Motor Neurosciences and Movement Disorders, Institute of Neurology, Queen Square, London, United Kingdom*

Joseph Jankovic, M.D.   *Professor, Department of Neurology, Director, Parkinson's Disease Center and Movement Disorders Clinic, Baylor College of Medicine, Houston, Texas, USA*

Mandar S. Jog*, M.D., Ph. D.   *London Health Sciences Center, London, Ontario, Canada*

Vern C. Juel, M.D.   *Associate Professor, Department of Neurology, University of Virginia, Charlottesville, Virginia, USA*

Ryuji Kaji, M.D., Ph.D.   *Professor and Chairman, Department of Neurology, Tokushima University, Tokushima, Japan*

Christopher G. Kalhorn, M.D.   *Department of Neurosurgery, Baylor College of Medicine, Houston, Texas, USA*

Un Jung Kang*, M.D.   *University of Chicago, Chicago, Illinois, USA*

Barbara Illowsky Karp*, M.D.   *National Institute of Neurological Disorders and Stroke, Bethesda, Maryland, USA*

Serdar Kesken, M.D.   *Neurologist, Department of Neurology, SSK Teperik Hospital, Izmir, Turkey*

Marina Konakova, Ph.D.   *Postdoctoral Researcher, Department of Neurology, Cedars Sinai Medical Center, Los Angeles, California, USA*

Paul Krack, M.D.   *Department of Neurology, University Hospital; Department of Biological and Clinical Neurosciences, Joseph Fourier University, Grenoble, France*

Cristina Lampuri, B.A.   *Medical Student, State University of New York at Buffalo School of Medicine and Biomedical Sciences, Buffalo, New York, USA*

Richard J. Lederman, M.D., Ph.D.   *Neurologist, Department of Neurology, The Cleveland Clinic Foundation, Cleveland; Associate Professor, Department of Neurology, Ohio State University College of Medicine, Columbus, Ohio, USA*

Joanne C. Leung   *Molecular Neurogenetics Unit, Department of Neurology, Massachusetts General Hospital, Boston, Massachusetts, USA*

Sue E. Leurgans*   *Rush Presbyterian St. Luke's Medical Center, Chicago, Illinois, USA*

Mark F. Lew*, M.D.   *Associate Professor, Department of Neurology, University of Southern California, Keck School of Medicine, University of Southern California, Los Angeles, California, USA*

Vanessa K. Lim, Ph.D.   *Philip Wrightson Post-doctoral Fellow, Department of Sport and Exercise Science, The University of Auckland, Auckland, New Zealand*

Andres M. Lozano, M.D. *Division of Neurosurgery, Toronto Western Hospital, Toronto, Ontario, Canada*

Jonathan W. Mink, M.D., Ph.D. *Associate Professor, Departments of Neurology, Neurobiology, and Pediatrics, University of Rochester School of Medicine; Chief, Department of Child Neurology, Golisano Children's Hospital at Strong Hospital, Rochester, New York, USA*

Anjum Misbahuddin, M.R.C.P. *Clinical Research Fellow, Department of Clinical Neuroscience, Royal Free and University College Medical School, London, United Kingdom*

Nagako Murase, M.D. *Research Fellow, Human Cortical Physiology Section, National Institutes of Health, Bethesda, Maryland, USA*

Michael E. R. Nicholls, Ph.D. *Department of Psychology, School of Behavioural Sciences, University of Melbourne, Melbourne, Australia*

Nobuyoshi Nishiyama, Ph.D. *Associate Professor, Graduate School of Pharmaceutical Sciences, The University of Tokyo, Tokyo, Japan*

Yoshiko Nomura, M.D. *Assistant Director, Segawa Neurological Clinic for Children, Tokyo, Japan*

Shelley R. Oberlin, M.S. *Research Assistant, Department of Neurology, David Geffen School of Medicine at the University of California at Los Angeles, Los Angeles, California, USA*

Casey A. O'Farrell, MSc. *Neurogenetics Laboratory, Mayo Clinic Jacksonville, Jacksonville, Florida, USA*

William G. Ondo, M.D. *Associate Professor, Department of Neurology, Baylor College of Medicine, Houston, Texas, USA*

Laurie J. Ozelius, Ph.D. *Assistant Professor, Department of Molecular Genetics, Albert Einstein College of Medicine, Bronx, New York, USA*

Rosa Patiño-Picirrillo, M.D., C.C.R.C. *Clinical Research Coordinator, Department of Neurology–Research, The Cleveland Clinic Florida, Weston, Florida, USA*

Joel S. Perlmutter, M.D. *Professor, Departments of Neurology, Radiology and Neurobiology, Washington University School of Medicine; Head, Movement Disorders Center, Barnes-Jewish Hospital St. Louis, Missouri, USA*

Alessandra Pesenti, M.D. *Ph.D. Student, Department of Clinical Neurology, University of Milan; Clinical Resident Fellow, Department of Clinical Neurology, IRCCS—Ospedale Maggiore Milano, Milan, Italy*

Giselle M. Petzinger*, M.D. *University of Southern California, Los Angeles, California, USA*

Mark R. Placzek, B.Sc. *Research Assistant, Department of Clinical Neuroscience, Royal Free and University College Medical School, London, United Kingdom*

Pierre Pollak, M.D., Ph.D. *Department of Neurology, University Hospital; Department of Biological and Clinical Neurosciences, Joseph Fourier University, Grenoble, France*

Alberto Priori, M.D., Ph.D. *Consultant Neurologist, Department of Clinical Neurology, IRCCS—Ospedale Maggiore Milano; Associate Professor, Department of Clinical Neurology, University of Milan, Milan, Italy*

Stefan Pulst *Director, Division of Neurology, Carmen and Louis Warschaw Chair in Neurology; Cedars-Sinai Medical Center; Professor of Medicine and Neurobiology, David Geffen School of Medicine at the University of California at Los Angeles, Los Angeles, California, USA*

David Riley*, M.D. *University Hospitals of Cleveland, Cleveland, Ohio, USA*

Chester Robson, D.O. *Chief Resident, Department of Family Medicine, La Grange Memorial Hospital, La Grange, Illinois, USA*

Daniel Rogers, M.D., F.R.C.Psych. *Department of Neuropsychiatry, Frenchay Hospital, Bristol, United Kingdom*

John C. Rothwell, M.A., Ph.D. *Head, Sobell Department of Neuroscience and Movement Disorders, Institute of Neurology, Queen Square, London, United Kingdom*

James B. Rowe *National Hospital for Neurology, London, United Kingdom; Wellcome Department of Imaging Neuroscience, Institute of Neurology, London, United Kingdom*

John Rowe *Department of Clinical Psychology, East London and The City Mental Health Trust, Homerton Hospital, London, United Kingdom*

Manjit K. Sanghera, Ph.D. *Assistant Professor, Department of Neurosurgery, Baylor College of Medicine, Houston, Texas, USA*

Rachel Saunders-Pullman, M.D., M.P.H. *Assistant Professor of Neurology, Department of Neurology, Beth Israel Medical Center, New York, New York, USA*

Gottfried Schlaug, M.D. *Department of Neurology, Harvard Medical School, Beth Israel Deaconess Medical Center, Boston, Massachusetts, USA*

Stephan U. Schuele, M.D. *Assistant Professor, Senior Resident, Department of Neurology and Medical Center for Performing Artists, The Cleveland Clinic Foundation, Cleveland, Ohio, USA*

Lauren Seeberger*, M.D. *Colorado Neurological Institute, Englewood, Colorado, USA*

Masaya Segawa, M.D. *Director, Segawa Neurological Clinic for Children, Tokyo, Japan*

Elaina G. Sexton, M.S. *Graduate Program, Department of Biological Sciences, The University of Alabama, Tuscaloosa, Alabama, USA*

Vicki Shanker, M.D. *Department of Neurology, Albert Einstein College of Medicine, Bronx, New York, USA*

Janet Shriberg, M.S., M.P.H. *Department of Neurology, Beth Israel Medical Center, New York, New York, USA*

Hartwig R. Siebner *Sobell Department of Motor Neuroscience and Movement Disorders, Institute of Neurology, London, United Kingdom; Department of Neurology, Christian-Albrechts-University, Kiel, Germany*

Andrew Singleton, Ph.D. *Molecular Genetics Section, Laboratory of Neurogenetics, National Institute on Aging, National Institutes of Health, Bethesda, Maryland, USA*

Damien J. Slater *Molecular Neurogenetics Unit, Department of Neurology, Massachusetts General Hospital; Program in Neuroscience, Harvard Medical School, Boston, Massachusetts, USA*

Mark Stacy*, M.D. *Barrow Neurological Institute, Phoenix, Arizona, USA*

David G. Standaert *Assistant Professor, Department of Neurology, Harvard Medical School; Department of Neurology, Massachusetts General Hospital, Charlestown, Massachusetts USA*

Glenn T. Stebbins*, M.D. *Rush Presbyterian St. Luke's Medical Center, Chicago, Illinois, USA*

Oksana Suchowersky*, M.D. *University of Calgary, Calgery, Alberta, Canada*

Michael R. Swenson*, M.D. *University of Louisville, Louisville, Kentucky, USA*

Russell H. Swerdlow M.D. *Assistant Professor, Department of Neurology, University of Virginia, Charlottesville, Virginia, USA*

Daniel Tarsy*, M.D. *Beth Israel Deaconess Medical Center, Boston, Massachusetts, USA*

Maja Trošt, M.D. *Center for Neurosciences, North Shore-Long Island Jewish Research Institute, Manhasset, New York; Department of Neurology, Division of Neurology, University Medical Centre Ljubljana, Zaloska, Ljubljana, Slovenia*

Joel M. Trugman*, M.D. *University of Virginia Health System, Charlottesville, Virginia, USA*

Daniel Truong*, M.D. *The Parkinson's and Movement Disorder Institute, Fountain Valley, California, USA*

Joseph Tsui*, M.B.B.S. *University Hospital, Vancouver, Brittish Columbia, Canada*

Paul Tuite*, M.D. *University of Minnesota, Minneapolis, Minnesota, USA*

Ryo Urushihara, B.S. *Post-graduate Fellow, Department of Integrative Physiology, The University of Tokushima School of Medicine, Tokushima, Japan*

Fatma Uzunel, R.N. *Registered Nurse, Department of Neurology, Dokuz Eylül University, Izmir, Turkey*

Enza Maria Valente, M.D., Ph.D. *Research Assistant, Department of Neurogenetics, C.S.S. Mendel Institute, Rome, Italy*

Laurent Vercueil, M.D. *Neurologist, Department of Neurology, Grenoble University Hospital, Grenoble, France*

Kendall J. Vermilion, B.S. *Wayne State University College of Medicine, Detroit, Michigan*

Ramachandran Viswanathan, M.D. *Institute of Neurology, National Hospital for Neurology and Neurosurgery, Queen Square, London, United Kingdom*

Thomas T. Warner, Ph.D., F.R.C.P. *Reader, Department of Clinical Neuroscience, Royal Free and University College Medical School; Consultant Neurologist, Royal Free Hospital, London, United Kingdom*

G. Frederick Wooten, M.D. *Professor, Department of Neurology, University of Virginia, Charlottesville, Virginia, USA*

Joanne Wuu*, Sc.M. *Rush Presbyterian St. Luke's Medial Center, Chicago, Illinois, USA*

Lichuan Yang, M.D. *Department of Neurology and neuroscience, Weill Medical College of Cornell University, Ithaca, New York, USA*

Masayuki Yokochi, M.D., Ph.D. *Director, Department of Neurology, Tokyo Metropolitan Ebara Hospital, Tokyo, Japan*

Shoko Yukishita *Medical Technician, Molecular Laboratory Section, Segawa Neurological Clinic for Children, Tokyo, Japan*

*A member of the Dystonia Study Group

Preface

The Fourth International Dystonia Symposium, sponsored by the Dystonia Medical Research Foundation and the National Institutes of Health, was held in Atlanta, Georgia, on June 13–15, 2002. This monograph represents the proceedings of that symposium. This is the fourth volume on dystonia published in *Advances in Neurology*; each volume represents the proceedings of an international symposium. Whereas the first three volumes were published approximately ten years apart, the rapid advances in recent years had led the fourth volume to come out only five years after the third volume. Since the third symposium was held, there have been new genetic discoveries, including the cloning of the gene for Oppenheim (DYT1) dystonia, the development of an animal model with this gene, and more investigations as to the biology of this gene and its protein, TorsinA. This protein utilizes ATP and is thought to be a chaperone protein in the endoplasmic reticulum, with a function in repairing damaged proteins. In addition, genes have been mapped for families with other types of dystonia.

The symposium and this volume cover six major themes: pathophysiology, the clinical features and biology of Oppenheim dystonia, reviews of other genetic forms of dystonia, positron emission tomography (PET), focal dystonias including musicians' cramps, and therapeutics, including new developments in the surgical therapy of dystonia.

New concepts in pathophysiology are the loss of surround inhibition leading to the development of the abnormal movements, deficits in the sensory system whereby distortion of sensory feedback may play a pathophysiologic role, and experimental work on primates that develop focal dystonia apparently due to aberrant neuroplasticity as a result of repetitive motor performance. TorsinA synthesis is greatest in the dopamine neurons of the substantia nigra. In rodents, TorsinA synthesis is greatest in young animals, and in the cholinergic neurons of the striatum, then the protein is reduced with age. Both knock-in and knock-out TorsinA mice have been developed, and are being studied for clues to the development and treatment of dystonia.

At least 14 dystonia genes have been mapped at the present time, and some of them have now been identified. For the benefit of the readers of this monograph, these gene loci are listed here, where AD represents autosomal dominant, and AR, autosomal recessive.

DYT1 = 9q34, TorsinA, AD, young-onset, limb-onset (Oppenheim dystonia)

DYT2 = AR in Spanish gypsies, unconfirmed

DYT3 = Xq13.1, Lubag in Filipino males (X-linked dystonia-parkinsonism)

DYT4 = a whispering dysphonia family

DYT5 = 14q22.1, GTP Cyclohydrolase-1, AD (known as Dopa-Responsive Dystonia) (also Tyrosine hydroxylase deficiency = 11p11.5, AR, can respond to levodopa)

DYT6 = 8p21-q22, AD, mixed type, in the Mennonite/Amish population

DYT7 = 18p, AD, Familial torticollis, but localization is now in doubt

DYT8 = 2q33-q35, AD, Paroxysmal nonkinesigenic dyskinesia (PNKD) (FDP1) (Mount-Rebak syndrome)

DYT9 = 1p21, AD, Paroxysmal dyskinesia with spasticity (CSE)

DYT10 = 16p11.2-q12.1, AD, Paroxysmal kinesigenic dyskinesia (PKD)
(another PKD on 16q13-q22.1)
(also Paroxysmal exertional dyskinesia with infantile convulsions on 16p12-q11.2

DYT11 = 7q21-q23, epsilon-sarcoglycan, AD, Myoclonus-dystonia; Also 18p11 AD

DYT12 = 19q, AD, Rapid-Onset Dystonia-Parkinsonism
DYT13 = 1p36.13-p36.32, AD, cranial-cervical-brachial
DYT14 = 14q13, AD, DRD

There are a number of other genetic forms of dystonia that have not yet been labeled as "DYT," and we list these to be more complete.

Deafness-dystonia (Mohr-Tranebjaerg syndrome), X-linked recessive; faulty assembly of the DDP1/TIMM8a-TIMM13 complex

Aromatic amino acid decarboxylase deficiency; AR

6-Pyruvoyltetrahydropterin synthase deficiency, AR

Pterin-4a-carbinolamine dehydratase deficiency, AR

Dihydropteridine reductase deficiency; AR

Sepiapterin reductase deficiency; AR

Neurodegenerative disorder with iron accumulation Type 1 (formerly called Hallervorden-Spatz syndrome), pantothenate kinase deficiency, AR, 20p12.3-p13

Neuroferritinopathy, 19q13.3, ferritin light polypeptide, AD

Cervical dystonia, polymorphism in the dopamine (D5) receptor gene

Blepharospasm, polymorphism in the dopamine (D5) receptor gene

Utilizing PET scans with motor sequence learning tasks, non-manifesting carriers of the mutated *DYT1* gene were found to have altered activation of brain regions, from frontal to posterior parietal cortical areas. Other PET studies have found that the D2 receptor pathway in the basal ganglia is impaired.

Dystonia that occurs in professional musicians often leads to the end of their careers. Musicians with task-specific focal dystonia show abnormalities in sensory processing and sensorimotor integration. Embouchure dystonia in horn and woodwind players have involvement of the perioral muscles, used to control the force and direction of airflow into the mouthpiece. Keyboard instrumentalists with dystonia are affected predominantly in the right hand, as are those utilizing plucking instruments, while string players display predominantly left hand dystonia. Immobilization of the affected limb is to be tested in a clinical trial.

A consensus was reached that patients with primary dystonia have a better outcome with surgery (usually deep brain stimulation today) than those with secondary dystonia. There is no good explanation as to why patients might have a delay of benefit after surgery, and why the benefit may be lost after several years. Physiological recordings during surgery reveal altered firing patterns in the pallidum, but why surgery at this target can alleviate dystonia remains unclear. There is still uncertainty as to the ideal patient for surgery, the best target, the degree of benefit, the duration of benefit, and the adverse effects for the various surgical procedures. More work and careful observations are required.

Stanley Fahn, M.D.
Mahlon DeLong M.D.
Mark Hallett, M.D.

Acknowledgments

We are grateful for the support by the National Institutes of Health, the Dystonia Medical Research Foundation (DMRF), and numerous individual donors. Our special thanks goes to Ms. Kim Kuman of the DMRF who tirelessly stayed on top of organizing the symposium and bringing in the chapters for this volume, which will be the latest update on what's happening in torsion dystonia.

Dystonia 4: Advances in Neurology, Vol. 94. Edited by Stanley Fahn, Mark Hallett, and Mahlon R. DeLong. Lippincott Williams & Wilkins, Philadelphia © 2004.

1

Dystonia: Abnormal Movements Result from Loss of Inhibition

Mark Hallett

Human Motor Control Section, National Institute of Neurological Disorders and Stroke, National Institutes of Health, Bethesda, Maryland

Dystonia is characterized by excessive movement. The excessive movement leads to involuntary movements, distorted voluntary movements and abnormal postures. While it can be present at rest, it is brought out more by attempted voluntary movement. Electromyogram (EMG) studies have revealed that there is excessive co-contraction of antagonist muscles and there is overflow activation of extraneous muscles (1). With phasic movements, there are prolonged EMG bursts. Given that the central nervous system operates as a balance between excitation and inhibition, excessive movement could arise from increased excitability or reduced inhibition. Evidence has been accumulating that dystonia is generated by a loss of inhibition.

The central nervous system is complex, and there are multiple types of central nervous system inhibition. The concept is now emerging that the defective inhibition in dystonia is "surround inhibition." Surround inhibition is a concept well accepted in sensory physiology. For example, receptive fields in the visual cortex are organized such that light in the center of the field activates a cell, while light in the periphery inhibits it. Such a pattern helps to sharpen borders and is an important step in the formation of patterns and objects. Surround inhibition is not so well known in the motor system, but it is a logical concept. When making a movement, the brain must ac-

tivate the motor system. It is possible that the brain just activates the specific movement. On the other hand, it is more likely that the one specific movement is generated, and, simultaneously, other possible movements are suppressed. The suppression of unwanted movements would be surround inhibition. This should produce a more precise movement, just as surround inhibition in sensory systems produces more precise perceptions. If such surround inhibition in the motor system is lacking, it would not be surprising that a disorder like dystonia would emerge.

This chapter makes three arguments. First, that inhibition is decreased in dystonia. Second, that surround inhibition is a mechanism of function of the motor system, and, in particular, that the basal ganglia mechanisms can contribute to surround inhibition. Third, that there is some evidence that surround inhibition is lacking in dystonia.

DECREASED INHIBITION IN DYSTONIA

Rothwell and colleagues (2) first demonstrated that there was deficient reciprocal inhibition in dystonia. Reciprocal inhibition is represented at multiple levels in the central nervous system and can be studied as a spinal reflex. Reciprocal inhibition is reduced in patients with dystonia, including those with

generalized dystonia, writer's cramp, spasmodic torticollis, and blepharospasm (2–7).
Valls-Solé and Hallett (8) have evaluated the
effects of radial nerve stimulation on the
EMG activity of the wrist flexor muscles during a sustained contraction, demonstrating reduced reciprocal inhibition during movement.

Other spinal and brainstem reflexes have
been studied, and a common result is that inhibitory processes are reduced. Another example that has been extensively studied is the
blink reflex. Abnormalities of blink reflex recovery were first identified for blepharospasm (9), and have also been demonstrated
in generalized dystonia, spasmodic torticollis,
and spasmodic dysphonia (10). In the last two
conditions, abnormalities can be found even
without clinical involvement of the eyelids.
Similarly, abnormalities are seen with perioral

reflexes (11) and exteroceptive silent periods
(12).

Several studies have shown hyperexcitability of the motor cortex in dystonia. Transcranial magnetic stimulation (TMS) shows increased excitability of the motor cortex (13).
The likely explanation of the hyperexcitability is loss of inhibition. Ridding et al. (14)
studied intracortical inhibition with the "double pulse paradigm." Motor evoked potentials
(MEPs) are inhibited when conditioned by a
prior subthreshold TMS stimulus to the same
position at intervals of 1 to 5 ms. Inhibition
was less in both hemispheres of patients with
focal hand dystonia (Fig. 1-1). Inhibition can
also be evaluated with double pulses at longer
intervals with the muscle under study either at
rest or contracted. Chen et al. (15) investigated this type of inhibition in patients with

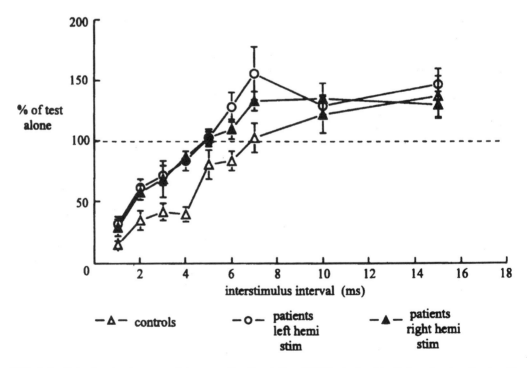

FIG. 1-1. Paired-pulse transcranial magnetic stimulation (TMS) study of both hands of patients with hand dystonia and normal controls. The percentage amplitude change of the conditioned motor evoked potentials (MEPs) is plotted against the paired pulse interval. Note the loss of inhibition in both hands of the patients compared with normal. (From Ridding MC, Sheean G, Rothwell JC, et al. Changes in the balance between motor cortical excitation and inhibition in focal, task specific dystonia. *J Neurol Neurosurg Psychiatry* 1995;59:493–498, with permission.)

writer's cramp and found a deficiency only in the symptomatic hand and only with background contraction. This abnormality is particularly interesting since it is restricted to the symptomatic setting, as opposed to many other physiologic abnormalities in dystonia that are more generalized.

Chen et al. (15) also found that the silent period following an MEP was slightly shorter for the symptomatic hemisphere in patients with focal hand dystonia. A nonsignificant trend was also seen by Ikoma et al. (13) earlier. Moreover, the silent period is shorter during a dystonic contraction than during a voluntary movement with the same intensity (16). These results also indicate a deficiency of inhibition.

There is also loss of inhibition produced by cutaneous stimulation. Stimulation of the median nerve or index finger leads to inhibition of MEPs in hand and forearm muscles at various intervals becoming maximal at 200 ms. Patients with focal hand dystonia show facilitation instead (17).

Movement-related cortical potentials (MRCPs) associated with self-paced finger movement in patients with hand dystonia show a diminished NS' (negative slope) component (thought to be generated in the motor cortex) (18,19). A focal abnormality of the contralateral central region was confirmed with an analysis of event-related desynchronization of the EEG prior to movement which showed a localized deficiency in desynchronization of beta frequency activity (20). Feve et al. (21) studied MRCPs in patients with symptomatic dystonia including those with lesions in the striatum, pallidum, and thalamus. With bilateral lesions, patients showed deficient gradients for the Bereitschaftspotential and NS' bilaterally and lack of vertex predominance for the Bereitschaftspotential and contralateral predominance for NS'. With unilateral lesions, the problem was worse for the symptomatic hand. The contingent negative variation (CNV) is the EEG potential that appears between a warning and a go stimulus in a reaction-time task. The CNV shows deficient late negativity with head turning in pa-

tients with torticollis (22) and hand movement in patients with writer's cramp (23). The late negativity represents motor function similar to the MRCP. Such defective negativity in the MRCP and CNV are consistent with loss of inhibition in cortical processing.

An MRCP is seen prior to muscle relaxation as well as contraction, and this phenomenon has been investigated in dystonia (24). Studies of normal subjects making wrist extension movements and initiating relaxation from a tonic wrist extension showed a prominent negativity over the contralateral central area, similar for the two types of movement. In patients with focal hand dystonia, the negativity was maximal in the contralateral central region for the contraction task, but for the relaxation task the negativity was maximal at the midline and symmetrically distributed. At the contralateral central area, the negativity in the dystonia group was diminished significantly in the relaxation task compared with the contraction task. Thus, cortical activity is abnormal for voluntary inhibition as well as activation.

Another failure of cortical inhibition was found when patients with dystonia observed, but did not respond to, a series of stimuli that ordinarily triggered a learned motor sequence (25). In normal subjects, during inhibition, there was reduced MEP amplitude in muscles that would have been involved in the task and an increase in alpha power in the EEG, suggesting cortical inactivity. These findings were not present in patients with focal hand dystonia.

It should be noted that loss of cortical inhibition in motor cortex can give rise to dystonic-like movements in primates. Matsumura et al. (26) showed that local application of bicuculline, a γ-aminobutyric acid (GABA) antagonist, onto the motor cortex led to disordered movement and changed the movement pattern from reciprocal inhibition of antagonist muscles to co-contraction (26). In a second study, they showed that bicuculline caused cells to lose their crisp directionality, converted unidirectional cells to bidirectional cells, and increased firing rates of most cells, including making silent cells into active ones (27). There is preliminary evidence from magnetic resonance spectroscopy that GABA is diminished in the motor cortex region in patients with hand dystonia (28).

SURROUND INHIBITION IS A FUNCTION OF THE NORMAL MOTOR SYSTEM AND AIDED BY THE BASAL GANGLIA

The concepts that the motor system makes a movement by activating one pattern and inhibiting others, and that the basal ganglia play a role in this process have been discussed for many years. The idea might have been original to Denny-Brown, but was emphasized in my own work as well (29). There is now explicit evidence that inhibition of unselected tasks actually occurs.

Leocani et al. (30) evaluated corticospinal excitability of both hemispheres during the auditory reaction-time (RT) tasks using TMS (30). Nine right-handed subjects performed right and left thumb extensions in simple

(SRT), choice (CRT), and go/no-go auditory RT paradigms. TMS, which induced MEPs simultaneously in the extensor pollicis brevis muscles bilaterally, was applied at different latencies from the tone. For all paradigms, MEP amplitudes on the side of movement increased progressively in the 80 to 120 ms before EMG onset, while the resting side showed inhibition (Fig. 1-2). The inhibition was significantly more pronounced for right than for left thumb movements. After no-go tones, bilateral inhibition occurred at a time corresponding to the mean RT to go tones. Corticospinal inhibition on the side not to be moved suggests that suppression of movement is an active process. Proof that this is active rather than passive comes from studies of no-go trials by Waldvogel et al. (31) and Sohn et al. (32). During the period of MEP suppression, intracortical inhibition was determined to be increased using the paired-pulse TMS method. Further evidence supporting this effect as cortical comes from the observation of Liepert et al. (33), who showed that the inhibition of the contralateral hand, while

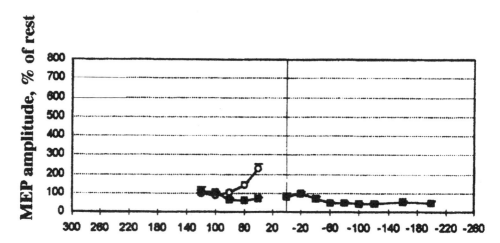

FIG. 1-2. Percentage amplitude change of motor evoked potentials (MEPs) during a reaction time task. *Open circles* are from one abductor pollicis brevis (APB) muscle that is the agonist of the movement, and the *closed squares* are from the APB muscle on the other hand, which is not involved in the movement. Zero time is the electromyogram (EMG) onset of the agonist muscle. Note the inhibition of the APB on the nonmoving side both before and during the movement. (From Leocani L, Cohen LG, Wassermann EM, et al. Human corticospinal excitability evaluated with transcranial magnetic stimulation during different reaction time paradigms. *Brain* 2000;123:1161–1173, with permission.)

demonstrable with TMS, could not be demonstrated with transcranial electrical stimulation. Preliminary results from Sohn et al. show that with movement of one finger there is widespread inhibition of muscles in the contralateral limb (34) and some inhibition of muscles in the ipsilateral limb when those muscles are not involved in any way in the movement (unpublished results).

In another experiment, Liepert et al. (35) studied changes in intracortical inhibition associated with two motor tasks requiring a different selectivity in fine motor control of small hand muscles [abductor pollicis brevis (APB) muscle, and fourth dorsal interosseous (4DIO) muscle]. In experiment 1, subjects completed four sets (5-minute duration each) of repetitive thumb movements at 1 Hz. In experiment 2, the subjects produced the same number of thumb movements, but complete relaxation of 4DIO was demanded. Following free thumb movements, amplitudes of MEPs in response to both single and paired TMS showed a trend to increase with the number of exercise sets in both APB and 4DIO. By contrast, more focal, selective thumb movements involving APB with relaxation of 4DIO caused an increase in MEP amplitudes after single and paired pulses only in APB, while there was a marked decrease in MEPs after paired pulses, but not after single TMS, in the actively relaxed 4DIO. Intracortical inhibition within the hand representation appears to vary according to the selective requirements of the motor program. Performance of more focal tasks may be associated with a decrease in intracortical inhibition in muscles engaged in the repetitive action, while at the same time intracortical inhibition may be increased in an actively relaxed muscle.

Can the basal ganglia influence inhibition? The full effect of the basal ganglia upon the cortex is unknown, but there is some evidence that the basal ganglia do affect cortical inhibition. The first line of evidence of this influence is the effect of basal ganglia disorders on the silent period following TMS. In Parkinson's disease, the silent period is shorter than normal and can be improved with dopaminergic treatment (36,37). In Huntington's disease, the silent period is longer than normal (38). Moreover, the clinical assessment of degree of chorea correlates with silent period length. The second line of evidence is the dopaminergic control of short interval: intracortical inhibition. Bromocriptine given to normal subjects will increase the amount of inhibition (39). Third, thalamocortical influences on the cortex can be both excitatory and inhibitory, and, in some circumstances, the inhibitory influence is more profound (40). It is not unreasonable to think, therefore, that if cortical inhibition is diminished in dystonia the basal ganglia could be responsible.

The basal ganglia are anatomically organized to work in a center-surround mechanism. This idea of center-surround organization was one of the possible functions of the basal ganglia circuitry suggested by Alexander and Crutcher (41). This was followed up nicely by Mink (42), who detailed the possible anatomy. The direct pathway has a focused inhibition in the globus pallidus, while the subthalamic nucleus has divergent excitation. The direct pathway (with two inhibitory synapses) is a net excitatory pathway and the indirect pathway (with three inhibitory synapses) is a net inhibitory pathway. Hence the direct pathway can be the center and the indirect pathway the surround of a center-surround mechanism (Fig. 1-3).

Tremblay and Filion (43) studied the reactions of single cells in the globus pallidus to stimulation in the striatum. The great majority of responses consisted of an initial inhibition, at a mean latency of 14 ms, followed by excitation, at a mean latency of 35 ms. The early inhibition was always displayed by neurons located in the center of the pallidal zone of influence of each striatal stimulation site, and was ended and often curtailed by excitation. At the periphery of the zone, excitation occurred alone or as the initial component of responses. The authors state, "This topological arrangement suggests that excitation is used, temporally, to control the magnitude of the central striatopallidal inhibitory signal and, spatially,

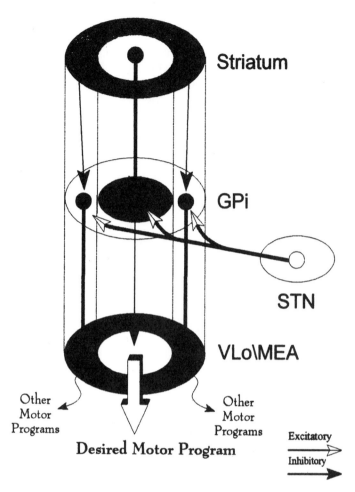

FIG. 1-3. Model diagram of the basal ganglia to show how it might function for surround inhibition. The center is the direct pathway and produces the desired movement. The outside is the indirect pathway and functions to suppress unwanted movements. GPi, internal division of the globus pallidus; STN, subthalamic nucleus; VLo/MEA, oralis portion of the ventrolateral nucleus of the thalamus and the midbrain extrapyramidal area. (From Mink JW. The basal ganglia: focused selection and inhibition of competing motor programs. *Prog Neurobiol* 1996;50:381–425, with permission.)

to focus and contrast it onto a restricted number of pallidal neurons." In interpreting these data, it is important to remember that the output of the globus pallidus is inhibitory, so that inhibition would be the "center" signal and excitation the "surround" signal.

The cortex also has anatomic and functional connections that allow for surround inhibition. Activation of a region gives rise to activity in short inhibitory interneurons that inhibit nearby neurons. This pattern has been well characterized in models of focal epilepsy where neurons surrounding a focus are inhibited (44).

SURROUND INHIBITION IS LACKING IN DYSTONIA

Using imaging to assess dopamine and dopamine receptors, several studies concur that there is a loss of D2 receptors in the putamen (45–48). The meaning of this is not clear, but it could indicate that there is a reduction in the influence of the indirect pathway.

Bütefisch et al. (49) have tested whether task-dependent modulation of inhibition within the motor cortex is impaired in dystonia using an experimental design similar to that of Liepert et al. (35) described above. Paired-pulse TMS at short interstimulus time intervals was used to measure cortical inhibition in muscles that acted as agonist (APB) and synergist (4DIO) in a selective and nonselective task. The synergistic muscle was activated in the nonselective task but not in the selective task. Following the selective task, the conditioned MEP of the synergist decreased in normal subjects, while the conditioned MEPs of the agonist increased. In contrast, conditioned MEP of both synergistic and agonist muscles increased in the dystonic subjects. In the nonselective task, the conditioned amplitudes of both muscles increased in normal and dystonic subjects. These results suggest that task-dependent cortical inhibition is disturbed in patients with dystonia.

As noted earlier, preliminary data from Sohn et al. (unpublished) show that there is inhibition of the ADM (abductor digiti minimi) (an uninvolved muscle in the "surround") when the flexor digitorum superficialis (FDS) of finger two is activated. Additional preliminary data from Sohn et al. (unpublished) show that this effect is less in patients with focal hand dystonia.

There are also data from sensory function that are compatible with loss of inhibition. Tinazzi et al. (50) studied median and ulnar nerve somatosensory evoked potentials (SEPs) in patients who had dystonia involving at least one upper limb. They compared the amplitude of spinal N13, brainstem P14, parietal N20 and P27, and frontal N30 SEPs obtained by stimulating the median and ulnar nerves simultaneously (MU), the amplitude value being obtained from the arithmetic sum of the SEPs elicited by stimulating the same nerves separately (M + U). The MU:(M + U) ratio indicates the interaction between afferent inputs from the two peripheral nerves. No significant difference was found between SEP amplitudes and latencies for individually stimulated median and ulnar nerves in dystonic patients and normal subjects, but recordings in patients yielded a significantly higher percentage ratio for spinal N13, brainstem P14, and cortical N20, P27, and N30 components. The SEP ratio of central components obtained in response to stimulation of the digital nerves of the third and fifth fingers was also higher in patients than in controls, but the difference did not reach a significant level. The authors state, "These findings suggest that the inhibitory integration of afferent inputs, mainly proprioceptive inputs, coming from adjacent body parts is abnormal in dystonia. This inefficient integration, which is probably due to altered surrounding inhibition, could give rise to an abnormal motor output and might therefore contribute to the motor impairment present in dystonia."

CONCLUSION

While further evidence is needed, it appears that surround inhibition is an important mechanism in motor control and that it may be a principal function of the basal ganglia. Its dysfunction may be the central problem in dystonia. Learning how to influence surround inhibition may be helpful in symptomatic treatment.

REFERENCES

1. Cohen LG, Hallett M. Hand cramps: clinical features and electromyographic patterns in a focal dystonia. *Neurology* 1988;38:1005–1012.
2. Rothwell JC, Obeso JA, Day BL, et al. Pathophysiology of dystonias. *Adv Neurol* 1983;39:851–863.
3. Nakashima K, Rothwell JC, Day BL, et al. Reciprocal inhibition in writer's and other occupational cramps and hemiparesis due to stroke. *Brain* 1989;112:681–697.
4. Panizza ME, Hallett M, Nilsson J. Reciprocal inhibition in patients with hand cramps. *Neurology* 1989;39:85–89.
5. Panizza M, Lelli S, Nilsson J, et al. H-reflex recovery curve and reciprocal inhibition of H-reflex in different kinds of dystonia. *Neurology* 1990;40:824–828.
6. Chen RS, Tsai CH, Lu CS. Reciprocal inhibition in writer's cramp. *Mov Disord* 1995;10:556–561.
7. Deuschl G, Seifert G, Heinen F, et al. Reciprocal inhibition of forearm flexor muscles in spasmodic torticollis. *J Neurol Sci* 1992;113:85–90.
8. Valls-Solé J, Hallett M. Modulation of electromyographic activity of wrist flexor and extensor muscles in patients with writer's cramp. *Mov Disord* 1995;10:741–748.
9. Berardelli A, Rothwell JC, Day BL, et al. Pathophysiol-

ogy of blepharospasm and oromandibular dystonia. *Brain* 1985;108:593–608.

10. Cohen LG, Ludlow CL, Warden M, et al. Blink reflex excitability recovery curves in patients with spasmodic dysphonia. *Neurology* 1989;39:572–577.

11. Topka H, Hallett M. Perioral reflexes in orofacial dyskinesia and spasmodic dysphonia. *Muscle Nerve* 1992; 15:1016–1022.

12. Nakashima K, Thompson PD, Rothwell JC, et al. An exteroceptive reflex in the sternocleidomastoid muscle produced by electrical stimulation of the supraorbital nerve in normal subjects and patients with spasmodic torticollis. *Neurology* 1989;39:1354–1358.

13. Ikoma K, Samii A, Mercuri B, et al. Abnormal cortical motor excitability in dystonia. *Neurology* 1996;46: 1371–1376.

14. Ridding MC, Sheean G, Rothwell JC, et al. Changes in the balance between motor cortical excitation and inhibition in focal, task specific dystonia. *J Neurol Neurosurg Psychiatry* 1995;59:493–498.

15. Chen R, Wassermann E, Caños M, et al. Impaired inhibition in writer's cramp during voluntary muscle activation. *Neurology* 1997;49:1054–1059.

16. Filipovic SR, Ljubisavljevic M, Svetel M, et al. Impairment of cortical inhibition in writer's cramp as revealed by changes in electromyographic silent period after transcranial magnetic stimulation. *Neurosci Lett* 1997; 222:167–170.

17. Abbruzzese G, Marchese R, Buccolieri A, et al. Abnormalities of sensorimotor integration in focal dystonia: a transcranial magnetic stimulation study. *Brain* 2001; 124:537–545.

18. Deuschl G, Toro C, Matsumoto J, et al. Movement-related cortical potentials in writer's cramp. *Ann Neurol* 1995;38:862–868.

19. van der Kamp W, Rothwell JC, Thompson PD, et al. The movement related cortical potential is abnormal in patients with idiopathic torsion dystonia. *Mov Disord* 1995;5:630–633.

20. Toro C, Deuschl G, Hallett M. Movement-related electroencephalographic desynchronization in patients with hand cramps: evidence for motor cortical involvement in focal dystonia. *Ann Neurol* 2000;47:456–461.

21. Feve A, Bathien N, Rondot P. Abnormal movement related potentials in patients with lesions of basal ganglia and anterior thalamus. *J Neurol Neurosurg Psychiatry* 1994;57:100–104.

22. Kaji R, Ikeda A, Ikeda T, et al. Physiological study of cervical dystonia. Task-specific abnormality in contingent negative variation. *Brain* 1995;118:511–522.

23. Ikeda A, Shibasaki H, Kaji R, et al. Abnormal sensorimotor integration in writer's cramp: study of contingent negative variation. *Mov Disord* 1996;11:638–690.

24. Yazawa S, Ikeda A, Kaji R, et al. Abnormal cortical processing of voluntary muscle relaxation in patients with focal hand dystonia studied by movement-related potentials. *Brain* 1999;122:1357–1366.

25. Hummel F, Andres F, Altenmuller E, et al. Inhibitory control of acquired motor programmes in the human brain. *Brain* 2002;125:404–420.

26. Matsumura M, Sawaguchi T, Oishi T, et al. Behavioral deficits induced by local injection of bicuculline and muscimol into the primate motor and premotor cortex. *J Neurophysiol* 1991;65:1542–1553.

27. Matsumura M, Sawaguchi T, Kubota K. GABAergic inhibition of neuronal activity in the primate motor and premotor cortex during voluntary movement. *J Neurophysiol* 1992;68:692–702.

28. Levy LM, Hallett M. Impaired brain GABA in focal dystonia. *Ann Neurol* 2002;51:93–101.

29. Hallett M, Khoshbin S. A physiological mechanism of bradykinesia. *Brain* 1980;103:301–314.

30. Leocani L, Cohen LG, Wassermann EM, et al. Human corticospinal excitability evaluated with transcranial magnetic stimulation during different reaction time paradigms. *Brain* 2000;123:1161–1173.

31. Waldvogel D, van Gelderen P, Muellbacher W, et al. The relative metabolic demand of inhibition and excitation. *Nature* 2000;406:995–998.

32. Sohn YH, Wiltz K, Hallett M. Effect of volitional inhibition on cortical inhibitory mechanisms. *J Neurophysiol* 2002;88:333–338.

33. Liepert J, Dettmers C, Terborg C, et al. Inhibition of ipsilateral motor cortex during phasic generation of low force. *Clin Neurophysiol* 2001;112:114–121.

34. Sohn YH, Jung HY, Kaelin-Lang A, et al. Excitability of ipsilateral motor cortex during phasic voluntary hand movement. *Neurology* 2002;58(suppl 3):A447.

35. Liepert J, Classen J, Cohen LG, et al. Task-dependent changes of intracortical inhibition. *Exp Brain Res* 1998;118:421–426.

36. Cantello R, Gianelli M, Bettucci D, et al. Parkinson's disease rigidity: magnetic motor evoked potentials in small hand muscles. *Neurology* 1991;41:1449–1456.

37. Priori A, Berardelli A, Inghilleri M, et al. Motor cortical inhibition and the dopaminergic system. Pharmacological changes in the silent period after transcranial brain stimulation in normal subjects, patients with Parkinson's disease and drug-induced parkinsonism. *Brain* 1994;117:317–323.

38. Roick H, Giesen HJ, Lange HW, et al. Postexcitatory inhibition in Huntington's disease. *Mov Disord* 1992;7: 27.

39. Ziemann U, Tergau F, Bruns D, et al. Changes in human motor cortex excitability induced by dopaminergic and anti-dopaminergic drugs. *Electroencephalogr Clin Neurophysiol* 1997;105:430–437.

40. Ashby P, Lang AE, Lozano AM, et al. Motor effects of stimulating the human cerebellar thalamus. *J Physiol (Lond)* 1995;489:287–298.

41. Alexander GE, Crutcher MD. Functional architecture of basal ganglia circuits: neural substrates of parallel processing. *Trends Neurosci* 1990;13:266–271.

42. Mink JW. The basal ganglia: focused selection and inhibition of competing motor programs. *Prog Neurobiol* 1996;50:381–425.

43. Tremblay L, Filion M. Responses of pallidal neurons to striatal stimulation in intact waking monkeys. *Brain Res* 1989;498:1–16.

44. Collins RC. Use of cortical circuits during focal penicillin seizures: an autoradiographic study with [14C]deoxyglucose. *Brain Res* 1978;150:487–501.

45. Horstink CA, Booij J, Berger HJC, et al. Striatal D2 receptor loss in writer's cramp. *Mov Disord* 1996;11 (suppl 1):209.

46. Perlmutter JS, Stambuk MK, Markham J, et al. Decreased [18F]spiperone binding in putamen in idiopathic focal dystonia. *J Neurosci* 1997;17:843–850.

47. Perlmutter JS, Stambuk MK, Markham J, et al. Decreased [18F]spiperone binding in putamen in dystonia. *Adv Neurol* 1998;78:161–168.

48. Naumann M, Pirker W, Reiners K, et al. Imaging the pre- and postsynaptic side of striatal dopaminergic synapses in idiopathic cervical dystonia: a SPECT study using [123I] epidepride and [123I] beta-CIT. *Mov Disord* 1998;13:319–323.

49. Bütefisch CM, Boroojerdi B, Battaglia F, et al. Task dependent intracortical inhibition is impaired in patients with task specific dystonia. *Mov Disord* 2000;15(suppl 3):153.

50. Tinazzi M, Priori A, Bertolasi L, et al. Abnormal central integration of a dual somatosensory input in dystonia. Evidence for sensory overflow. *Brain* 2000;123:42–50.

Dystonia 4: Advances in Neurology, Vol. 94. Edited by Stanley Fahn, Mark Hallett, and Mahlon R. DeLong. Lippincott Williams & Wilkins, Philadelphia © 2004.

2

Sensory Deficits in Dystonia and Their Significance

Ryuji Kaji, Nagako Murase, Ryo Urushihara, and Kotaro Asanuma

Department of Neurology, Tokushima University Hospital, Tokushima, Japan

Dystonia is defined as a syndrome of sustained muscle contractions frequently causing twisting or repetitive movements or abnormal postures. The most prevalent are focal dystonias, which include cervical dystonia (spasmodic torticollis), blepharospasm, and writer's cramp. In the earliest full description of spasmodic torticollis made by Destarac (1), a peculiar benefit of tactile sensory stimulation to the nearby skin in correcting abnormal posture was already noted as *geste antagonistique,* which is presently known as a *sensory trick.* Another example of sensory phenomena in dystonia is that bright light aggravates the symptoms of blepharospasm. Conversely, avoiding brightness by wearing dark sunglasses usually ameliorates them.

Botulinum toxin injection became the treatment of choice for these focal dystonias. During the course of botulinum treatment, patients with cervical dystonia often show changes in the pattern of muscles involved: previously silent agonist muscles (e.g., anterior part of the trapezius muscle) come into action after weakening hyperactive muscles (e.g., sternocleidomastoid muscle on the same side) (Fig. 2-1). The net result is therapeutic resistance to the injection, as if the patient were destined to maintain a fixed abnormal posture. This phenomenon indicates that abnormal muscle contraction in dystonia is not programmed for individual muscles but as an abnormal body image in which any muscle can be recruited to attain the abnormal posture. In other words the abnormal program is written in proprioceptive sensory rather than motor language. This also highlights the sensory aspect in dystonia.

Based on these clinical observations, we reasoned that it might be possible to alter the abnormal motor output in dystonia by stimulating or blocking muscle afferents; in writer's cramp, dystonic muscle contractions were reproduced by stimulating group Ia afferents by high-frequency vibration (tonic vibration reflex, TVR) and were abolished by blocking the afferents with diluted lidocaine (muscle afferent block) (2). These findings indicated an abnormal link between sensory input and motor output in dystonia, and prompted a hypothesis that dystonia is a sensory disorder (3).

Another line of evidence for sensory abnormalities came from an animal model of dystonia produced by imposing a precision-required repetitive handgrip task on monkeys, whose primary somatosensory cortex showed markedly disorganized sensory representation of the digits (4). Similar abnormalities were inferred in patients with hand dystonia using source localization of somatosensory evoked potentials (SEPs) after digit stimulation (5). Indeed, abnormal hand representation in the somatosensory cortex should disturb normal motor-sensory integration in writing; if extraneous

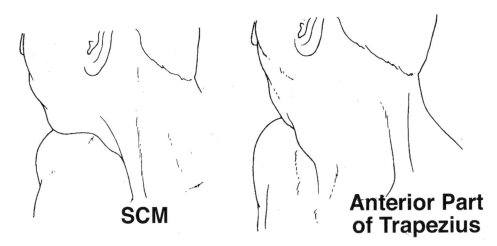

FIG. 2-1. Change in the pattern of muscle activation in a patient with cervical dystonia. *Left:* Before botulinum toxin injection, left sternocleidomastoid (SCM) and right posterior neck muscles were hyperactive. *Right:* Two weeks after injecting the toxin into these muscles, a previously silent muscle (anterior part of trapezius) was activated to maintain the abnormal posture.

sensory input is fed back for subsequent movement, this would set up a vicious cycle, causing further dilapidation of motor control.

Further studies showed abnormal kinesthesia (6) and spatial or temporospatial sensory discrimination (7,8) in writer's cramp or hand dystonia. SEP studies in hand dystonia also demonstrated abnormal summation of dual SEP input, which indicates insufficient central surround inhibition at sensory relay nuclei (9). These studies point to deficits in sensory processing or sensorimotor integration in dystonia.

In this review, we will focus on writer's cramp or hand dystonia, in which both sensory input and motor output are easily controlled.

PREMOVEMENT GATING OF SOMATO-SENSORY EVOKED POTENTIALS

To explore this sensorimotor link, we have developed a method to evaluate processing sensory input for motor control using SEPs (10). It was known that SEPs are attenuated or *gated* during movement of the stimulated limb. This gating was ascribed to the central process of actively modulating sensory input for motor control (central gating) and interference by pe-

ripheral feedback afferents activated by the movement (peripheral gating). To sort out the central gating, we took advantage of a reaction time paradigm; the warning signal (S1) was a sound and the imperative signal (S2) was electric stimulation to the median nerve of the hand to be moved (Fig. 2-2A). The latter electric stimuli triggered median SEPs at the same time. Because the reaction time always exceeded 70 ms, gating of SEP components up to this latency was never contaminated by peripheral feedback afferents, and all SEP gating in this paradigm was central. In normal subjects, the gated component was the frontal N30 component in median SEPs, whereas the P40 component was gated in tibial SEPs (Fig. 2–2B) (11). Interestingly, N30 in the median SEP was not gated for foot movement, nor was P40 in tibial SEPs for hand movement. This signifies that these SEP components were specifically attenuated before the movement of the stimulated limb; this central gating occurs selectively for the input from the body part to be moved.

Using this method, Murase et al. (12) studied gating of median SEPs before hand movements in patients with writer's cramp, and found the lack of normal gating of frontal

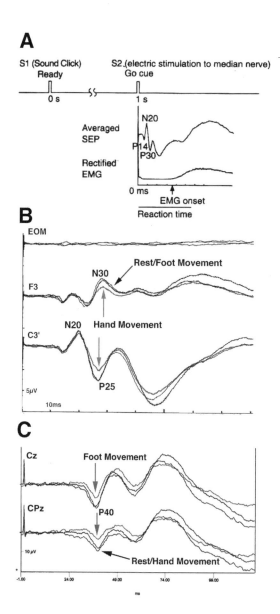

FIG. 2-2. Premovement gating of somatosensory evoked potentials (SEPs). **A:** Paradigm. **B:** Median SEPs. Only hand movement gated N30/P25 component. No gating was seen for foot movement (rest/foot movement). **C:** Tibial SEPs. Only foot movement gated P40 component. No gating was seen for hand movement (rest/hand movement).

N30 in hand dystonia (Fig. 2-3A). We subsequently found the lack of normal gating of P40 of tibial SEPs in patients with leg dystonia (Fig. 2-3B) (13). These findings point to a specific abnormality in utilizing sensory input from the affected body part for motor control in dystonia.

In normal subjects, these SEP components were *gated*, possibly because part of the SEP generators had been busy processing information and not synchronized by the external stimuli. This may be interpreted as the input channels being opened for the limb prior to its movement. Dystonia patients lack this process for the affected limb, thus interfering with the sensory feedback control for the execution of the motor program.

Dystonia has been regarded as a disorder of basal ganglia or their connections to the thalamus and the motor cortices. Animal and human studies suggest that basal ganglia play an important role in gating sensory inputs for guiding

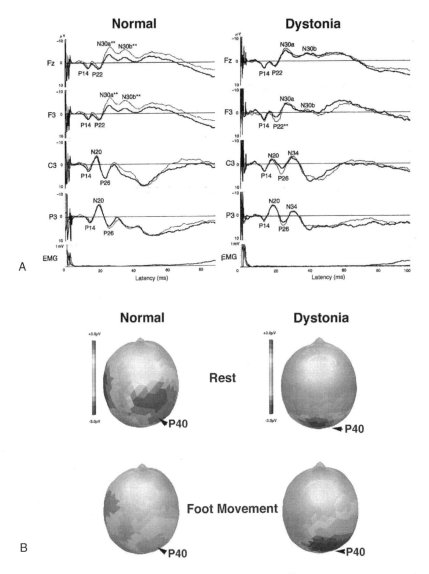

FIG. 2-3. A: Premovement gating of N30 component in median somatosensory evoked potentials (SEPs) (grand averages). Gating was lost in hand dystonia patients *(right)*. (Adapted from Murase N, Kaji R, Shimaz H, et al. Abnormal premovement gating of somatosensory input in writer's cramp. *Brain* 2000;123 (pt. 9):1813–1829.) **B:** Premovement gating of P40 component in tibial SEPs (grand averages). Mapping of the cortical potentials at the peak latency of P40 recorded from 64 channels over the scalp. Gating was lost in leg dystonia *(right)*.

movements (14,15). One of the main hypotheses for the function of the basal ganglia is to control or select automatic movements after learning. In fact, a human study showed activation of the pallidum after learning a motor task, and it was argued that the basal ganglia act as a flexible system for learning the association of

sensory cues and movements (16). If this flexibility in associating sensory input and motor output is lost by, for instance, repetitious execution of a learned motor act such as writing, a fixed input-output mismatch may be the consequence. Thus, dystonia may be viewed as a disorder of *motor subroutine* in which sensory input and motor output are defined for controlling frequently used movement (17).

MANIPULATING CORTICAL EXCITABILITY IN DYSTONIA

Neuroimaging studies in writer's cramp or hand dystonia using positron emission tomography (PET) invariably showed hyperactive premotor cortex (18,19). In normal subjects, Penhune and Doyon (20) investigated PET activation during early and late phases of motor learning. It was demonstrated that during early learning, cerebellar mechanisms are involved in adjusting sensory input to produce accurate motor output. During late learning, the basal ganglia were activated for automatization of the task, when premotor and parietal cortices became involved. Therefore, abnormal gating of N30 or P40 components in dystonia is likely through hypermetabolism of the premotor cortex interfering with the modulation of parietal SEP generators.

Recent studies using transcranial magnetic stimulation (TMS) showed deficient paired-pulse inhibition and shortened cortical silent period in hand dystonia, both indicating deficient intracortical inhibition or increased excitability in the primary motor area (M1). De-

velopment of repetitive transcranial magnetic stimulation (rTMS) made it possible to manipulate the cortical excitability for an extended period after stimulation. Munchau et al. (21) have succeeded in affecting the excitability of M1 through low-frequency subthreshold rTMS over the premotor area. Enomoto et al. (22) showed that median SEP amplitudes can be altered by low-frequency rTMS over M1. Low-frequency (<1 Hz) rTMS generally exerts inhibitory rather than excitatory influence over the cortex being stimulated.

MODULATING N30 BY REPETITIVE TRANSCRANIAL MAGNETIC STIMULATION OVER THE PREMOTOR AREA

Based on the above findings, we have attempted to modulate frontal N30 component in median SEPs by rTMS (23). In 11 normal subjects, we applied low-frequency (0.2 Hz) subthreshold rTMS (250 stimuli) over primary motor, supplementary motor, and premotor cortices. Stimulation (or inhibition in effect) of premotor cortices, but not other cortices, significantly increased the amplitude of frontal N30-parietal P25 components in median SEPs (Fig. 2-4). The decreased ampli-

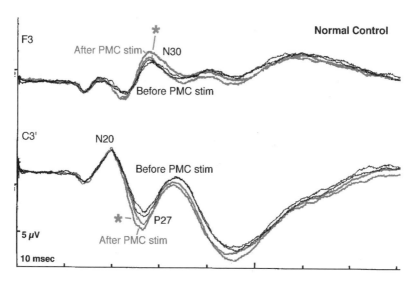

FIG. 2-4. Median somatosensory evoked potentials (SEPs) before and after repetitive transcranial magnetic stimulation (rTMS) over premotor cortex (PMC). "After PMC stim" indicates the recording immediately after rTMS, and asterisk denotes 1 hour after rTMS. Note the lasting effect of rTMS.

tude of N30 preceding the movement, or premovement gating, in normal subjects may therefore be interpreted as excitation of the premotor cortex in preparation for a movement. Given the hypermetabolism of the premotor area and the lack of normal premovement gating of N30, it is reasonable to speculate that the premotor cortex in dystonia is so hyperactive that it is no longer possible to modulate the excitability of the sensorimotor cortex for controlling movement. In support of this view, our preliminary findings indicate that rTMS over the premotor area does not alter N30 amplitude in dystonics (24).

THERAPEUTIC IMPLICATIONS

In seven patients with hand dystonia, we tried to apply low-frequency (0.2 Hz) subthreshold (85% of resting motor threshold) rTMS (250 stimuli) over primary motor, supplementary motor, and premotor areas in a single-blind study (25). The handwritings of these subjects were evaluated with a computer-aided program to register the error and the pen pressure of pen tracking. There was an improvement in tracking error after stimulation (or inhibition in effect) of premotor area with significant prolongation of the cortical silent period. This underscores the pivotal role of the premotor area in sensorimotor disintegration in hand dystonia. In this study, the stimulation over premotor cortex was then repeated every 2 weeks for 10 months in one subject, resulting in a lasting clinical benefit (Fig. 2-5). The latter finding needs more observations to conclude that rTMS has efficacy as a therapy, but it may become a useful adjunct to the standard therapy.

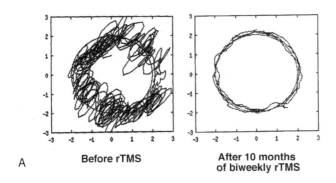

A   Before rTMS   After 10 months
                               of biweekly rTMS

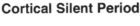

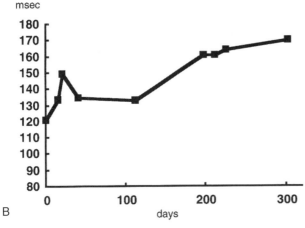

B

FIG. 2–5. **A:** Handwriting of a patient with hand dystonia in a task of tracking a target that circles three times at a fixed speed. *Left:* Before rTMS sessions. *Right:* After 10 months of biweekly sessions of rTMS over premotor area. **B:** Cortical silent periods recorded from the same subject.

CONCLUSION

Dystonic symptoms are influenced by sensory input applied near the affected body part. Hand dystonia patients may show overt abnormalities in temporal and/or spatial discrimination in the hand. In focal dystonia, opening the input channel from the affected body part is impaired prior to its movement, and the link between sensory input and motor output seems deranged. This sensorimotor mismatch seems mediated in part by hyperactive premotor areas, which may be suppressed by low-frequency subthreshold rTMS.

ACKNOWLEDGMENTS

This work was supported by Grant-in-Aids for Scientific Researches from the Japanese Ministry of Science, Sports, and Culture, and those for Health Science Researches from the Japanese Ministry of Health, Labor, and Welfare and Health Science Research Foundation of Japan.

REFERENCES

1. Destarac. Torticolis spasmodique et spasmes functionels. *Rev Neurol* 1901;9:591–597.
2. Kaji R, Rothwell JC, Katayama M, et al. Tonic vibration reflex and muscle afferent block in writer's cramp. *Ann Neurol* 1995;38(2):155–162.
3. Hallett M. Is dystonia a sensory disorder? *Ann Neurol* 1995;38(2):139–140.
4. Byl NN, Merzenich MM, Jenkins WM. A primate genesis model of focal dystonia and repetitive strain injury: I. Learning-induced dedifferentiation of the representation of the hand in the primary somatosensory cortex in adult monkeys. *Neurology* 1996;47(2):508–520.
5. Bara-Jimenez W, Catalan MJ, Hallett M, et al. Abnormal somatosensory homunculus in dystonia of the hand. *Ann Neurol* 1998;44(5):828–831.
6. Grunewald RA, Yoneda Y, Shipman JM, et al. Idiopathic focal dystonia: a disorder of muscle spindle afferent processing? *Brain* 1997;120(pt 12):2179–2185.
7. Bara-Jimenez W, Shelton P, Hallett M. Spatial discrimination is abnormal in focal hand dystonia. *Neurology* 2000;55(12):1869–1873.
8. Sanger TD, Tarsy D, Pascual-Leone A. Abnormalities of spatial and temporal sensory discrimination in writer's cramp. *Mov Disord* 2001;16(1):94–99.
9. Tinazzi M, Priori A, Bertolasi L, et al. Abnormal central integration of a dual somatosensory input in dystonia. Evidence for sensory overflow. *Brain* 2000;123(pt 1):42–50.
10. Shimazu H, Kaji R, Murase N, et al. Pre-movement gating of short-latency somatosensory evoked potentials. *NeuroReport* 1999;10(12):2457–2460.
11. Asanuma K, Urushihara R, Nakamura K, et al. Pre-movement gating of somatosensory evoked potentials after tibial nerve stimulation. *NeuroReport* 2003;14(pt. 3):375–379.
12. Murase N, Kaji R, Shimazu H, et al. Abnormal pre-movement gating of somatosensory input in writer's cramp. *Brain* 2000;123(pt 9):1813–1829.
13. Asanuma K, Urushihara R, Nakamura K, et al. Abnormal premovement sensory processing in leg dystonia. *(Submitted)*.
14. Lidsky TI, Manetto C, Schneider JS. A consideration of sensory factors involved in motor functions of the basal ganglia. *Brain Res* 1985;356(2):133–146.
15. Romo R, Ruiz S, Crespo P, et al. Representation of tactile signals in primate supplementary motor area. *J Neurophysiol* 1993;70(6):2690–2694.
16. Passingham RE, Toni I, Schluter N, et al. How do visual instructions influence the motor system? *Novartis Found Symp* 1998;218:129–141.
17. Kaji R, Shibasaki H, Kimura J. Writer's cramp: a disorder of motor subroutine? [editorial; comment]. *Ann Neurol* 1995;38(6):837–838.
18. Ceballos-Baumann AO, Brooks DJ. Basal ganglia function and dysfunction revealed by PET activation studies. *Adv Neurol* 1997;74:127–139.
19. Eidelberg D, Moeller JR, Ishikawa T, et al. The metabolic topography of idiopathic torsion dystonia. *Brain* 1995;118(pt 6):1473–1484.
20. Penhune VB, Doyon J. Dynamic cortical and subcortical networks in learning and delayed recall of timed motor sequences. *J Neurosci* 2002;22(4):1397–1406.
21. Munchau A, Bloem BR, Irlbacher K, et al. Functional connectivity of human premotor and motor cortex explored with repetitive transcranial magnetic stimulation. *J Neurosci* 2002;22(2):554–561.
22. Enomoto H, Ugawa Y, Hanajima R, et al. Decreased sensory cortical excitability after 1 Hz rTMS over the ipsilateral primary motor cortex. *Clin Neurophysiol* 2001;112(11):2154–2158.
23. Urushihara R, Murase N, Asanuma K, et al. Modulation of frontal N30 by repetitive transcranial magnetic stimulation over premotor cortex. *(Submitted)*.
24. Murase N, Urushihara R, Asanuma K, et al. Lack of modulation of frontal N30 by rTMS over premotor cortex in hand dystonia. *(In preparation)*.
25. Murase N, Kaji R, Ikeda A, et al. Short-term effect of low-frequency repetitive transcranial magnetic stimulation in upper limb dystonia. *Neurology* 2002;58(suppl 3):A394.

Dystonia 4: Advances in Neurology, Vol. 94. Edited by Stanley Fahn, Mark Hallett, and Mahlon R. DeLong. Lippincott Williams & Wilkins, Philadelphia © 2004.

3

Focal Hand Dystonia May Result from Aberrant Neuroplasticity

Nancy N. Byl

Department of Physical Therapy and Rehabilitation Science, School of Medicine, University of California, San Francisco, California

Individuals who perform jobs demanding high levels of stressful repetitive movements can develop acute pain in the upper limb (1). Some of these individuals may proceed to develop persistent, chronic pain or unusual, disabling symptoms of fatigue and incoordination referred to as "occupational hand cramps" or "focal hand dystonia" (2–5). Dystonia is a syndrome of sustained, uncontrollable, muscle co-contractions, causing abnormal twisting, intermittent, and/or static posturing (6–8). A dystonia that involves a particular body part (e.g., hand, neck, foot) is called a "focal limb dystonia." If the limb dystonia occurs only during the performance of a target task, it may be called a task specific or action dystonia (9). Limb dystonias are rated for severity (10,11) and categorized by the extent of dysfunction: (a) *simple cramp*, movements are abnormal in relation to a single task; (b) *dystonic cramps,* movements are abnormal from the outset, in relation to more than one task; or (c) *progressive cramps*, abnormal movements begin in relation to a single task and later become abnormal while performing other tasks. Limb and action dystonias may also be classified by occupation (e.g., musician's cramps, writer's cramp, drummer's cramp, golfer's yip, keyboarder's cramp). Focal hand dystonias (FHDs) are most common (12).

The etiology of FHD is still considered idiopathic, with successful treatment approaches still considered controversial among movement awareness trainers, neurologists, physical therapists, neurosurgeons, and neuroscientists (13). Proposed theories for the origin of FHD include abnormalities associated with genetics (14), basal ganglia-thalamic-cortical circuits (15,16), inhibition (17—21), cortical potentials/asynchronization (22–25), neuroenzyme availability [e.g., adrenocorticotropic hormone (ACTH) and dopamine] (26), sensorimotor integration (18,27–31), somatosensory differentiation (30,32–38), musculoskeletal mobility (39–41), peripheral nerve mobility (42–44), or peripheral trauma (45). The etiology may also result from negative neural adaptation associated with overuse (2–4,46).

Simple, target-specific hand dystonias are difficult to explain based on general neurophysiologic dysfunction. However, a nervous system that maintains a tenuous adaptation due to genetic or structural deficits may be tipped out of balance by stressful overuse, trauma, or degeneration (4,32,40). Aberrant learning is consistent with direct observations and self-reported patient histories highlighting behaviors that involve (a) rapid, near simultaneous, stereotypical movements of adjacent digits; (b) extended periods of co-contractions of agonists and antagonists; (c) precise motor control; (d) sophisticated "feedback-related" modulation; (e) spaced, intense practice behaviors carried out over long periods of time; (f) goal orientation and attention; or (g) modification in instrumentation or strategies of performance (2–5,14,46–48).

NEUROPLASTICITY AND THE SENSORIMOTOR LEARNING HYPOTHESIS: ONE ETIOLOGY OF FOCAL HAND DYSTONIA

Selective spatial and spectral cell assemblies with sharp segregation must be present to permit efficient, coordinated voluntary movements. Interestingly, these event-by-event, complex signal representations are highly plastic (49,50). Positive learning can be measured clinically by improved efficiency and quality of movement and structurally as increased size of somatotopic and functional representations, decreased size of the somatosensory receptive fields, increased processing efficiency, modified amplitude and density of somatosensory evoked responses, improvement in distinct, orderly representations of the digits, and increased accuracy in the sensorimotor feedback loop (34,51–64). Negative learning has the opposite effect on these neural parameters (2,3,32,46–48) (see Figure 3-1).

Rewarded practice and spaced repetition over time classically lead to improved performance (21,39,64–66). Interestingly, patients with FHD report that increased practice leads to deterioration in performance efficiency, performance quality, and unusual fatigue (5,11,12). Excessive fatigue can produce negative, compensatory postural adaptations and muscle tension. As performance deteriorates, practice is intensified, particularly as reported by musicians (12). Ultimately, the fingers seem to develop a life of their own, uncontrollably curling or extending when performing the target task (13). The *sensorimotor learning*

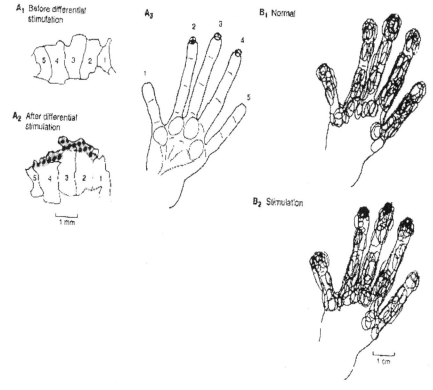

FIG. 3-1. Positive learning: Normal representation. The digits are normally organized from D1 to D5 and from proximal to distal (Z1) with each neuron associated with a small receptive field (A3). Attended, rewarded, repetitive sensory stimulation increases the area of cortical representation, (A2) the density of receptive fields (B2), while decreasing the size and specificity of the location of receptive fields on the stimulated surface (B2).

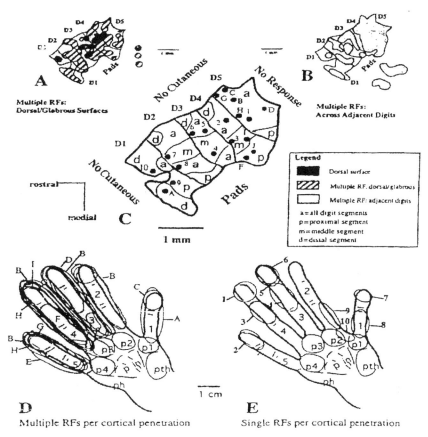

FIG. 3-1. *(Cont.)* Negative learning: Dedifferentiation. Dedifferentiation of the hand in primates with focal hand dystonia following repetitive, rapid, rewarded, opening and closing of the hand: reduced area of cortical representation (C); large receptive fields (D and E), receptive fields and overlapping adjacent digits (B) and overlapping dorsal and glabrous.

hypothesis proposes that the nervous system has a finite capacity for neural adaptation (2,3, 46–48). As operative movements become more efficient and stereotypic, the temporal inputs can become nearly simultaneous, losing their individual differentiation. Then, the stereotypic repetition leads to degradation in the somatotopic representations in the sensory, motor, and related pathways (2,3,46–48).

Cortical networks appear to engage both excitatory and inhibitory neurons by strong input perturbation. Within given cortical areas, pyramidal cells cannot be effectively reexcited by another perturbation for tens to hundreds of milliseconds (54,56,65). These "integration times" are primarily dictated by the time for recovery from inhibition, which dominates

poststimulus excitability. The cortex continues to define its representation of the temporal aspects of behaviorally important inputs by generating more synchronous representations of sequenced input perturbations or events. The time constants both govern and limit the ability of the cortex to "chunk," that is, to separately represent by distributed, coordinated discharge successive events within its processing channels (2,3,46–48,62).

Although the typical manifestation of FHD is characterized by temporary and fixed extreme positions of the limb, there is increasing evidence that the underlying dysfunction has an important sensory component (36). Clinically, patients with FHD demonstrate poor sensory discrimination in response to active

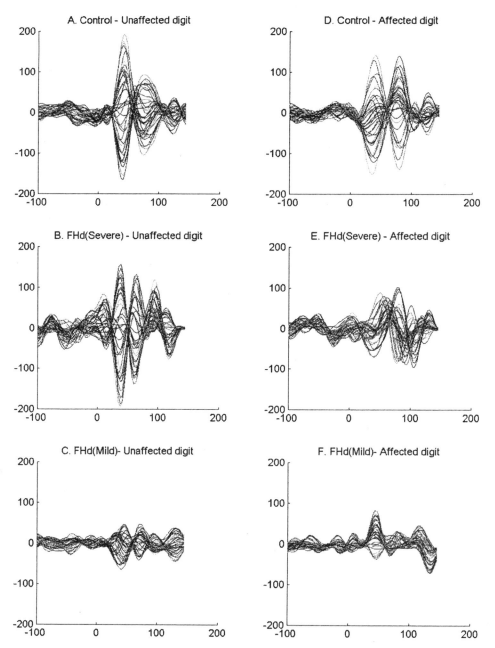

FIG. 3-2. Examples of Somatosensory Evcoked Field Responses Following Sensory Stimulation: Controls and Subjects with FHd.

and passive stimuli (31,38,67–69) (e.g., abnormal graphesthesia, stereognosis, kinesthesia, spatial-temporal discrimination). These findings are also consistent with reports that patients with idiopathic FHD demonstrate abnormal perception and increased abnormal dystonic posturing following vibration of the tendon or muscle belly (18), reduction in dystonic posturing with anesthesia of the muscle spindle (28), or specific cutaneous stimulation (sensory trick) (36). Structurally, using electrophysiologic mapping techniques, Byl et al. (2,3), Blake et al. (46), and Wang et al. (47,48) have reported significant dedifferentiation of the sensory representation of the hand in non-human primates where motor dysfunction resulted from highly repetitive, stereotypical, digital opening and closing movements or specific target movements of the hand. In these naive primates, the area of representation was either diminished or enlarged, and the receptive fields increased more than 10 times normal size, with the evoked neural response engaging a broad neuronal network not only across adjacent digits but also across dorsal and glabrous surfaces (2,3,46,47). Using magnetoencephalography, similar degradation has been reported in human subjects [e.g., altered amplitude, location, oscillation frequency, pattern, and duration of the somatosensory evoked potential (SEP) field response with decreased finger spread and poor sequential finger order] (22,32,35) (see Figure 3-2). Sanger et al. (38) reported that simultaneous sensory stimulation of adjacent digits was associated with a neural firing intensity less than the expected serial sum of each digit observed in normal subjects (D2 plus D3 alone).

The *sensorimotor learning hypothesis* may represent an "abnormal gain in the sensorimotor feedback loop." Sanger and Merzenich (37) proposed the computational model of focal dystonia that not only is consistent with our learning hypothesis, but also can explain several features of focal dystonia. For example, gain can be imbalanced by expansion or shrinkage of the sensory cortical representation of a limb; specific increased, simultaneous neuronal network of firing; coupling of multiple sensory signals; or voluntary coactivation of muscles. The loop through the deep nuclei of the cortex, basal ganglia, and thalamus, combined with the sensorimotor loop gain, contributes to a stable or unstable state. If only certain mechanical pathways are unstable, then a focal dystonia rather than a generalized dystonia can develop.

TREATMENT OF FOCAL HAND DYSTONIA BASED ON THE PRINCIPLES OF NEUROPLASTICITY

All patients need a complete neurologic examination. In most cases, this examination is interpreted as normal, except when the patient is observed performing the target task (13,70). Some patients demonstrate subtle abnormalities such as reduced arm swing, loss of smooth controlled grasping, or a physiologic tremor. Both hands should be carefully evaluated. It is important to carefully define the abnormal movements and which fingers are most involved. Even though one or more digits may be observed going into flexor spasm, the extensors of the fingers are usually contracting simultaneously with other digits uncontrollably extending. In other cases, the wrist flexes and ulnarly deviates with excessive pronation or supination at the elbow. It is important to determine whether a contraction of the flexors drives the co-contraction of the extensors or vice versa. All patients should be videotaped while performing the target task to provide a basis for scoring, noting the time of onset for the dystonia and measuring change over time. It is important to analyze which normal movements have been preserved. It is also important to provide some type of rating scale to score the severity of the movement dysfunction (10,11). Other measurements from the neurologic and physical examination should be recorded as objectively as possible (e.g., range of motion, strength, vascular restriction, peripheral nerve entrapment, sensory performance, fine motor skills, sympathetic signs like sweating). Sensibility testing should include psychomotor tests such as localization, graphesthesia, stereognosis, spatial orientation, and/or kinesthesia (31,67,68,70–73).

Dynamic electromyography (EMG) can be included as part of the diagnostic workup to confirm the presence of classic co-contraction of antagonists and agonists, excessive or reduced firing amplitude, and inability to release contractions (74). Nerve conduction studies usually are normal, but reduced conduction in the ulnar nerve is sometimes reported (42). Brain imaging, scanning, and tomography are sometimes used to help rule out other diagnoses (e.g., tumors, malformations, etc.), but are not necessarily considered standard tests for FHD. Positive emission tomography (PET), functional magnetic resonance imaging (fMRI), SEP, and magnetic source imaging

(MSI) are reserved more for research than diagnosis (22–24). High-speed three-dimensional (3D) video images and force and acceleration data have also been used to characterize the dystonia (13). In addition, technology is gaining acceptance in motor research laboratories to help document computer assisted digital timing and force information (75).

The treatment for occupational hand cramps should include an ergonomic evaluation of the workstation, tool redesign, and evaluation of the unique demands imposed by the instrument interface with avoidance of excessive forces and unnecessary overuse. Treatment must allow normal cortical segregation to be reestablished, which necessitates stopping the abnormal movements and reducing the risk factors (e.g., limitations in motion, weakness, postural imbalance, peripheral nerve entrapment, neurovascular compression at the thoracic outlet, hydration, nutrition). The whole person is affected by the problem, both physically and mentally (13,65). A positive environment must be created for learning, for addressing self-image, motivation, and commitment to recover, along with attention to neurophysiologic, sensory, and biomechanical parameters of fine motor control (13,65). While increasing reports of success have been reported for constraint-induced therapy (76,77), sensitization (70), conditioning (78), limb immobilization (79), electrical muscle stimulation (13), and biofeedback and training with assistive devices (80) rationalized on the basis of neuroplasticity, sensorimotor training based on the principles of learning-based neural adaptation is the recommended treatment strategy.

If the somatosensory cortex is plastic and goal-attended behaviors can enhance cortical representation, then it is critical that highly attended, nonstereotypical, spaced rewarded repetitive sensorimotor activities, progressed in difficulty, be aimed at restoring the normal sensory and motor representations of the hand as well as the recovery of normal fine motor control. If aberrant large receptive fields and excessive receptive fields overlap across the cortex with clumping of the orderly representation of the digits, and imbalance in the sensorimotor feedback loop gain are the consequence

of excessive, repetitive overuse of the hands in focal dystonia, then sensory training must stimulate normal cortical segregation with heavy recruitment of neurons on the contralateral hemisphere (21,49,58–61,64,66,72,81–83).

Heavily attended sensory signals presented to a limited skin surface should be the signal that leads to redifferentiating the hand representation in the primary sensory cortex (21,39,60,61,64,82–92). Retraining can be difficult in the context of severe cramping. Techniques to reduce the spasms and enable individuals to participate more productively in retraining must be carefully evaluated (e.g., finding a position to train with minimal abnormal movements, using an assistive device to inhibit the abnormal movements, implementing limb immobilization techniques or injecting botulinum toxin to reduce the severity of spasms) (13). However, taking or injecting medications without retraining allows the person to continue to perform the job using the abnormal movements that strengthen the negative learning.

Tasks that depend on slowly adaptive sensory afferents (SAI afferents) include roughness estimation, reading Braille or embossed letters, or performing grating orientation discrimination (72,81,85,86,88,89). Tasks that involve primarily rapidly adaptive (RA) afferents include flutter discrimination and recognition of small surface asperities. Two mechanoreceptor systems have small receptive fields and low mechanical thresholds that can be stimulated to force discriminative decisions to redifferentiate the sensory map (72,81, 85,86). These psychophysical tasks must be presented in a way that is heavily attended in order to drive coincident delivery of neuromodulators with a neural signal about which the cortex can reorganize (49,54–56,60,61,64). Tasks should involve a defined skin surface within a training session so that segregation demands have cues only from a limited portion of the skin surface at one time. The tasks should include active exploration as well as passive stimulation (a sensory stimulus is delivered to the skin) (69).

Cross-modality effects have been measured with training with different modalities and can be incorporated into training programs (e.g., somatosensory sensory training improves auditory discrimination) (57). All sensory tasks should be heavily practiced prior to reengaging the patient in fine motor tasks. Sensory exploration and sensitivity should be integrated concurrently as fine motor task training begins (both on the nontarget and then the target task). There must be variability in the practiced movements to integrate uncorrelated movement components, each with only a few relevant sensory neurons (54,65, 66). This is comparable to behaviors uncoupling the pathologically coupled modes. Experience-based reshaping of cortical representation can be mediated by dynamic plastic operations of the brain, with subject–environment interactions affecting organizational features of the somatosensory cortex.

Sensory discrimination tasks must be done without increasing muscle tension. If muscle co-contractions are triggered on the affected side, then the sensory task should be initiated with the unaffected side until there is familiarity and comfort with the task. All of the sensory tasks should be carried out with the patient blindfolded or with the eyes closed to minimize visual guiding. The sensory training should be done with a variety of stimuli with the patient positioned in supine, prone, or even inverted positions to access all possible sensory maps and possibly enable normal task performance (e.g., a drummer may be able to drum normally while supine, but unable while sitting or standing). Ultimately, the sensory retraining needs to progress to the target instrument, the performance position, and the target task (11,77).

The most dystonic fingers are identified, and sensory retraining may begin with the adjacent dystonic digits and not the most involved digit. When multiple adjacent digits are involved, the sensory retraining should target the pads of the fingers and then the lateral and medial surfaces between the adjacent digits. Patients should carry games, objects, coins, puzzles, and shapes in their pockets in order to constantly challenge meaningful sensory exploration and decision making. Patients need to work on sensory retraining for an hour to 1.5 hours a day (can be spread throughout the day) (2,3).

As patients improve in somatosensory processing, mental rehearsal of the target and similar target task can facilitate physical performance (93). Neurons involved in functional tasks can be engaged by using alternate limbs (e.g., when writing with the toes, the somatotopic map for the foot-toes is activated along with the functional map for writing) (94). Normal movement and task performance must be reinforced. When the target task is broken down into small, simple components, the patient may be able to execute the tasks normally. Further, mirrors can be used to reinforce normal, controlled fine-motor movement. For example, when the unaffected hand is placed in front of the mirror, the mirror image looks like the affected hand. With the affected hand placed behind the mirror, the individual concentrates on making the affected side look like the mirror image (68,95–97).

To assist in the recovery of isolated agonist and antagonist movements, it is important to determine whether the agonist drives the firing of the antagonist or vice versa. Often the antagonist is the muscle that is firing first, even though the agonist motion is observed. The patient must learn to inhibit this. Biofeedback can be used to reinforce training in all activities of daily living (ADLs) including the target task. Biofeedback can be electrical, auditory, or cutaneous (e.g., temporary taping of the digit can increase sensory feedback and control). Attention will be needed to keep all other fingers quiet when practicing an isolated movement of an individual digit. The restoration of normal fine motor control must include specific well-controlled practice at variable speeds. A metronome may be used to change speeds.

Byl et al. reported the effectiveness of sensorimotor training in two case studies (68,95), three case reports (98), and one quasi-experimental, repeated measures design study ($n =$ 12) (95,96). These pilot studies supplemented with other plasticity studies reinforce the evidence that somatosensory reeducation can facilitate restoration of normal somatosensory representation of the hand as well as normal fine motor control (58,59,63,64,66). The training was associated with 70% to 90% improvement in sensory discrimination, fine motor control, target-specific motor control, and return to work (95,96). A significant constraint in this learning-based paradigm was the contingency that patients had to be motivated to work on training activities at home. This required high levels of compliance. Keeping each individual challenged and committed to goal-directed, specific, repetitive, retraining activities is critical in rehabilitation. Unfortunately, limitations in health care reimbursement for the treatment of chronic problems such as FHD can interfere with the opportunity for mentored treatment.

CONCLUSION

At this time, there is no consensus regarding the etiology of FHD or the most effective intervention strategy. However, evidence is accumulating in support of the *sensorimotor learning hypothesis* based on the theory of aberrant neuroplasticity. This could explain the origin of one type of FHD, specifically, the type that occurs in occupations with excessive, repetitive hand use. The sensorimotor learning hypothesis provides a logical foundation on which to create effective treatment strategies. To confirm structural and functional changes, randomized clinical trials across multiple sites are needed to compare the effectiveness of sensorimotor retraining, botulinum toxin injections, and other traditional and nontraditional intervention strategies for patients with FHD.

REFERENCES

1. Barr AE, Barbe MF. Pathophysiological tissue changes associated with repetitive movement: a review of the evidence. *Phys Ther* 2002;82:173–187.
2. Byl N, Merzenich M, Jenkins W. A primate genesis model of focal dystonia and repetitive strain injury: I. Learning-induced de-differentiation of the representation of the hand in the primary somatosensory cortex in adult monkeys. *Ann Neurol* 1996;47:508–520.
3. Byl N, Merzenich M, Cheung S, et al. A primate model for studying focal dystonia and repetitive strain injury: effects on the primary somatosensory cortex. *Phys Ther* 1997;77:727–739.
4. Chen R, Hallett M. Focal dystonia and repetitive motion disorders. *Clin Orthop Rel Res* 1998;351:102–106.
5. Fry H, Hallett M, Mastroianni T, et al. Incoordination in pianists with overuse syndrome. *Neurology* 1998;51:512–519.
6. Crossman AR, Brotchie JM. Pathophysiology of dystonia. *Adv Neurol* 1998;78:19–26.
7. Hallett M. Physiology of dystonia. *Adv Neurol* 1998;78:11–18.
8. Lim VK, Altenmuller E, Bradshaw JL. Focal dystonia; current theories. *Hum Move Sci* 2001;20;875–914.
9. Utti R, Vengernoetz FJG, Tsui JKC. Limb dystonia. In: Tsui JKC, Calne DB, eds. *Handbook of dystonia.* New York: Marcel Dekker, 1995:143–148.
10. Fahn S, Marsden CD, Calne D. Classification and investigation of dystonia. In: Marsden CD, Fahn S, eds. *Movement disorders,* vol 2. London: Butterworth, 1987:332–353.
11. Tubiana R. Incidence: classification of severity and results of therapy. In: Winspur I, Parry CBW, eds. *The musician's hand.* London: Martin Dunitz, 1998:164–l67.
12. Hochberg F, Harris S, Blartert T. Occupational hand cramps: professional disorders of motor control. *Hand Injury Sports Perform Arts* 1990;6:427–428.
13. Altenmueller E. Causes and cures of focal limb dystonia in musicians. In: Scott R, Black J, eds. *Health and the musician: proceedings of the 1997 York Conference.* London: BAPAM, 1997:G.1–12.
14. Gasser T, Bove C, Ozelius L, et al. Haplotype analysis at the DYT1 locus in Ashkenazi Jewish patients with occupational hand dystonia. *Mov Disord* 1996;11:163–166.
15. DeLong MR. Primate models of movement disorders of basal ganglia origin. *Trends Neurosci* 1990;13:281–285.
16. Karbe H, Holfhof V, Rudolf J. Positron emission tomography demonstrates frontal cortex and basal ganglia hypometabolism in dystonia. *Neurology* 1992;42:1540–1544.
17. Hughes M, McLellan DL. Increased co-activation of the upper limb muscles in writer's cramp. *J Neurol Neurosurg Psychiatry* 1985;48:782–787.
18. Kaji R, Rothwell J, Katayama M, et al. Tonic vibration reflex and muscle afferent block in writer's cramp. *Ann Neurol* 1995;38:155–162.
19. Panizza M, Hallett M, Nilsson J. Reciprocal inhibition in patients with hand cramps. *Neurology* 1989;39:85–89.
20. Ridding M, Sheean G, Rothwell J, et al. Changes in the balance between motor cortical excitation and inhibition in focal, task specific dystonia. *J Neurol Neurosurg Psychiatry* 1995;59:493–498.
21. Yazawa S, Ikeda A, Kaji R, et al. Abnormal cortical processing of voluntary muscle relaxation in patients with focal hand dystonia studied by movement-related potentials. *Brain* 1999;122:1357–1366.
22. Mavroudais N, Caroyer J, Brunko E, et al. Abnormal motor evoked responses to transcranial magnetic stimulation in focal dystonia. *Neurology* 1995;45:1671–1677.
23. Oga T, Honda M, Toma K, et al. Abnormal cortical mechanisms of voluntary muscle relaxation in patients with writer's cramp: an fMRI study. *Brain* 2002;124:895–914.
24. Tempel L, Perlmutter J. Abnormal cortical responses in patients with writer's cramp. *Neurology* 1993;43:2252–2257.
25. Toro C, Deuschl G, Hallett M. Movement-related electroencephalographic desynchronization in patients with hand cramps. Evidence for motor cortical involvement. *Ann Neurol* 2000;47:456–461.
26. Juliano SL, Ma W, Eslin D. Cholinergic depletion prevents expansion of topographic maps in somatosensory cortex. *Proc Natl Acad Sci USA* 1991;88:780–784.

27. Abruzzese G, Marchese R, Buccolieri A, et al. Abnormalities of sensorimotor integration in focal dystonia: a transcranial magnetic stimulation study. *Brain* 2001; 124:537–545.

28. Grunewald F, Rayoneda Y, Shipman JM, et al. Idiopathic focal dystonia is a disorder of muscle afferent processing. *Brain* 1997;120(pt 12):2179–2185.

29. Ikeda A, Shibasaki H, Kaji R, et al. Abnormal sensorimotor integration in writer's cramp: study of contingent negative variation. *Mov Disord* 1999;17(6):683–690.

30. Odergren T, Iwasaki N, Borg J, et al. Impaired sensory motor integration during grasping in writer's cramp. *Brain* 1996;119(pt 2):569–583.

31. Tinassi M, Frasson E, Bertolasi L, et al. Temporal discrimination of somesthetic stimuli is impaired in dystonic patients. *NeuroReport* 1999;10:1547–1550.

32. Bara-Jiminez W, Catalan M, Hallett M. Abnormal somatosensory homunculus in dystonia of the hand. *Ann Neurol* 1998;44(5):828–831.

33. Byl NN, McKenzie A, Nagarajan SS. Differences in somatosensory hand organization in a healthy flutist and flutist with focal hand dystonia: a case report. *J Hand Ther* 2000;301–309.

34. Elbert T, Pantev C, Wienbruch C, et al. Increased cortical representation of the fingers of the left hand in string players. *Science* 1995;270:305–307.

35. Elbert T, Candia V, Altenmuller F, et al. Alternation of digital representation in somatosensory cortex in focal hand dystonia. *NeuroReport* 1998;9:3571–3575.

36. Hallett M. Is dystonia a sensory disorder? *Ann Neurol* 1995;38:139–140.

37. Sanger TD, Merzenich MM. Computational model of the role of sensory disorganization in focal task-specific dystonia. *J Neurophysiol* 2000;84:2458–2464.

38. Sanger TD, Pascual-Leone A, Tarsay D, et al. Nonlinear sensory cortex response to simultaneous tactile stimuli in writer's cramp. *Mov Disord* 2002;27:105–108.

39. Lederman SJ. Tactile roughness of grooved surfaces: The touching process and effects of macro-microsurface structure. *Percept Psychophys* 1974;16:385–395.

40. Topp K, Byl N. Repetitive strain injury-focal hand dystonia: anatomical analysis in owl monkeys. *Mov Disord* 2000;14(2):295–306.

41. Wilson F, Wagner C, Homberg V, et al. Interaction of biomechanical and training factors in musicians with occupational cramps/focal dystonia. *Neurology* 1991;4(3 suppl 1):292–296.

42. Charness M. The relationship between peripheral nerve injury and focal dystonia in musicians. *Am Acad Neurol* 1993;162:21–27.

43. Katz R, Williams C. Focal dystonia following soft tissue injury: three case reports with long term outcomes. *Arch Phys Med Rehabil* 1990;71:345–349.

44. Quartarone A, Girlanda P, Risitano G. Focal hand dystonia in a patient with thoracic outlet syndrome. *J Neurol Neurosurg Psychiatry* 1998;65:272–274.

45. Jancovic J. Can peripheral trauma induce dystonia and other movement disorders? Yes. *Mov Disord* 2001; 16:7–11.

46. Blake D, Byl N, Cheung S, et al. Sensory representation abnormalities that parallel the genesis of focal dystonia in a primate model. *Somatosens Mot Res* 2002;19: 347–357.

47. Wang X, Merzenich MM, Sameshima K, et al. Remodeling of hand representation in adult cortex determined by timing of tactile stimulation. *Nature* 1995;378:71–75.

48. Wang X, Merzenich MM, Sameshima K, et al. Afferent input integration and segregation in learning are input timing dependent. *Neurosci Abst* 1994;20:1427.

49. Jenkins W, Merzenich M, Ochs M, et al. Functional reorganization of primary somatosensory cortex in adult owl monkeys after behaviorally controlled tactile stimulation. *J Neurophysiol* 1990;53:82–104.

50. Kaas JH, Merzenich MM, Killackey HP. The reorganization of somatosensory cortex following peripheral nerve damage in adult and developing mammals. *Annu Rev Neurosci* 1983;6:325–356.

51. Merzenich MM, Kaas JH, Wall J, et al. Topographic reorganization of somatosensory cortical areas 3b and 1 in adult monkeys following restricted deafferentiation. *Neuroscience* 1983;8(1):33–55.

52. Merzenich MM, Kaas JH, Wall J, et al. Progression of change following median nerve section in the cortical representation of the hand in areas 3b and 2 in adult owl and squirrel monkeys. *Neuroscience* 1983;10(3): 639–665.

53. Merzenich M, Nelson R, Stryker M, et al. Somatosensory cortical map changes following digit amputation in adult monkeys. *J Comp Neurol* 1984;224:591–605.

54. Merzenich MM. Development and maintenance of cortical somatosensory representations: functional "maps" and neuroanatomic repertoires. In: Barnard KE, Brazelton TB, eds. *Touch: the foundation of experience.* Madison: International University Press, 1999:47–71.

55. Merzenich MM, Jenkins WM. Cortical plasticity, learning and learning dysfunction. In: Jules B, Kovacs I, eds. *Maturational windows and adult cortical plasticity.* New York: Addison-Wesley, 1995:247–272.

56. Merzenich MM, Wright B, Jenkins WM, et al. Cortical plasticity underlying perceptual, motor and cognitive skill development: implications for neurorehabilitation. *Cold Springs Harb Symp Quant Biol* 1996;61:1–8.

57. Nagarajan SS, Blake DT, Wright BA, et al. Practice-related improvements in somatosensory, integration discrimination is temporarily specific but generalizes across skin location, hemisphere and modality. *J Neurosci* 1999;18(4):1559–1663.

58. Nudo R, Wise BS, Fuentes F, et al. Neural substrates for the effects of rehabilitative training on motor recovery after ischemic infarct. *Science* 1996;272:1791–1795.

59. Nudo RJ, Millikin GW. Reorganization of movement representations in primary motor cortex following focal ischemic infarcts in adult squirrel monkeys. *J Neurosci* 1996;75:2144–2149.

60. Recanzone G, Jenkins W, Hradek G, et al. Progressive improvement in discriminative abilities in adult owl monkeys performing a tactile frequency discrimination task. *J Neurophysiol* 1992;67:1015–1030.

61. Recanzone GH, Merzenich MM, Jenkins WM. Frequency discrimination training engaging a restricted skin surface results in an emergence of a cutaneous response zone in cortical area 3a. *J Neurophysiol* 1992; 67:1057–1070.

62. Sur M, Merzenich MM, Kaas JH. Magnification, receptive-field area and "hypercolumn" size in areas 3b somatosensory cortex in owl monkey. *J Comp Neurol* 1980;44:295–311.

63. Xerri C, Coq JO, Merzenich MM, et al. Experience-induced plasticity of cutaneous maps in the primary somatosensory cortex of adult monkeys and rats. *J Physiol (Paris)* 1996;90:277–287.

64. Xerri C, Merzenich MM, Jenkins W, et al. Representa-

tional plasticity in cortical area 3b paralleling tactual-motor skill acquisition in adult monkeys. *Cerebral Cortex* 1999;9:264–276.

65. Byl N, Merzenich MM. Principles of neuroplasticity: implications for neurorehabilitation and learning. In: *Downey and Darling's physiological basis of rehabilitation medicine.* Butterworth-Heineman, Woburn, MA Silver Chair, 2001.

66. Classen J, Liepert J, Wise SP, et al. Rapid plasticity of human cortical movement representation induced by practice. *J Neurophysiol* 1997;79:1117–1123.

67. Byl N, Hamati D, Melnick M, et al. The sensory consequences of repetitive strain injury in musicians: focal dystonia of the hand. *J Back Musculoskel Rehabil* 1996; 7:27–39.

68. Byl NN, Topp KS. Focal hand dystonia. *Phys Ther Case Rep* 1998;1:39–52.

69. Vega-Bermudez F, Johnson KO, Hsiao SS. Human tactile pattern recognition: active versus passive touch, velocity effects, and patterns of confusion. *J Neurophysiol* 1996;65:531–546.

70. Champagne P. Functional assessment and rehabilitation of musician's focal dystonia. In: Tubiana R, Amadio PC, eds. *Medical problems of the instrumentalist musician.* Martin Dunitz, Paris, Fr 2000:343–362.

71. Ayres J. *Sensory integration praxis test.* Los Angeles: Western Psychological Association, 1989.

72. Blake DT, Hsiao SS, Johnson KO. Neural coding mechanisms in tactile pattern recognition: the relative contributions of slowly and rapidly adapting mechanoreceptors to perceived roughness. *J Neurosci* 1997;17: 7680–7689.

73. Dellon AI. *Somatosensory testing and rehabilitation.* American Occupational Therapy Association, Bethesda MD 1997.

74. Cohen L, Hallett M. Hand cramps: clinical features and electromyographic patterns in focal dystonia. *Neurology* 1988;38:1005–1012.

75. Wilson F. Digitizing digital dexterity: a novel application for MIDI recordings of keyboard performance. *Psychomusicology* 1992;11:79.

76. Candia V, Elbert T, Altenmuller E, et al. A constraint-induced movement therapy for focal hand dystonia in musicians. *Lancet* 1999;353:42–43.

77. Taub E, Crago JE, Uswatte G. Constraint-induced movement therapy: a new approach to treatment in physical medicine. *Rehabil Psychol* 1988;43:152–170.

78. Liversedge LA, Sylvester JD. Conditioning techniques in the treatment of writer's cramp. *Lancet* 1994;6(4): 1147–1149.

79. Priori A, Pesenti A, Scarlato G, et al. Limb immobilization for the treatment of focal occupational dystonia. *Neurology* 2001;56:405–409.

80. Mai N, Marguardt C. Treatment of writer's cramp: Kinematic measures as assessment tools for planning and evaluating handwriting training procedures. In: Fause C, Keuss P, Vinler G, eds. *Advances in handwriting and drawing.* Europia Paris: 1994:445–461.

81. Burton H, Sinclair RJ. Representation of tactile roughness in thalamus and somatosensory cortex. *Can J Physiol Pharmacol* 1994;72:546–557.

82. Druschky K, Kaltenhauser M, Hummel C, et al. Somatotopic organization of the ventral and dorsal finger surface representations in human primary sensory cortex evaluated by magnetoencephalography. *NeuroImage* 2002;15:182–189.

83. Evans PM, Craig JC, Rinker MA. Perceptual processing of adjacent and nonadjacent tactile nontargets. *Percept Psychophys* 1992;52:571–581.

84. Craig JC. Anomalous sensations following prolonged tactile stimulation. *Neuropsychologia* 1993;31:277–291.

85. Johnson KO, Hsiao SS. Evaluation of the relative roles of slowly and rapidly adapting afferent fibers in roughness perception. *Can J Physiol Pharmcol* 1994;72: 488–497.

86. Johnson KO. Reconstruction of population response to a vibratory stimulus in quickly adapting mechanoreceptive afferent fiber populations innervating glabrous skin of the monkey. *J Neurophysiol* 1974;37:67–72.

87. Kalaska JF. Central neural mechanisms of touch and proprioception. *Can J Physiol Pharmacol* 1994;72: 542–545.

88. LaMotte RH and Whitehouse J. Tactile detection of a dot on a smooth surface: peripheral neural events. *J Neurophysiology* 1986;56:1109–1128.

89. LaMotte RH, Srinivasan MA. Neural encoding of shape: responses of cutaneous mechanoreceptors to a wavy surface stroked across the monkey fingerpad. *J Neurophysiol* 1996;76:377–379.

90. Phillips J, Johnson K, Hsiao S. Spatial pattern representation and transformation in monkey somatosensory cortex. *Proc Natl Acad Sci USA* 1988;85:1317–1321.

91. Schubotz R, Friederici AD. Electrophysiological correlates of temporal and spatial information processing. *NeuroReport* 1997;8:1981–1986.

92. Van Boven RW, Johnson KO. The limit of tactile spatial resolution in humans: grating orientation. *Neurology* 1994;44(12):2361–2366.

93. Porro CA, Francescato MP, Cettolo V, et al. Primary motor and sensory cortex activation during motor performance and motor imagery: a functional magnetic resonance imaging study. *J Neurosci* 1996;16: 7688–7698.

94. Rijintjes M, Dettmers C, Buchel C, et al. A blueprint for movement: functional and anatomical representation in the human motor system. *J Neurosci* 1999;19(18): 8043–8048.

95. Byl NN, Nagarajan SS, Newton N, et al. Effect of sensory discrimination training on structure and function in a musician with focal hand dystonia. *Phys Ther Case Rep* 2000;3:94–113.

96. Byl NN, McKenzie A. Treatment effectiveness of patients with a history of repetitive hand use and focal hand dystonia: a planned prospective follow up study. *J Hand Ther* 2000;13:289–301.

97. Yang TT, Gallen C, Schwartz B, et al. Sensory maps in the human brain. *Nature* 1994;368:592–593.

98. Byl N, Nagarajan SS, McKenzie A. Effectiveness of sensory retraining: three case studies of patients with focal hand dystonia. Abstract and poster. Society of Neuroscience annual meeting, New Orleans, LA November 6, 2000.

Dystonia 4: Advances in Neurology, Vol. 94. Edited by Stanley Fahn, Mark Hallett, and Mahlon R. DeLong. Lippincott Williams & Wilkins, Philadelphia © 2004.

4

Basal Ganglia Neuronal Discharge in Primary and Secondary Dystonia

*Manjit K. Sanghera, *Robert G. Grossman, *Christopher G. Kalhorn, *Winifred J. Hamilton, †William G. Ondo, and †Joseph Jankovic

*Department of Neurosurgery, Baylor College of Medicine, Houston, Texas. †Department of Neurology, Baylor College of Medicine, Houston, Texas

The dystonias are a heterogeneous group of movement disorders characterized by repetitive, writhing movement of the limbs involving the simultaneous contraction of agonist and antagonist muscle groups. Classification of the dystonias can be made on the basis of anatomic distribution as focal, segmental, hemi-, or generalized. The dystonias can also be classified by etiology (1,2) as primary genetic dystonia (1° DYS), in which there is generally early onset, a typical pattern of progression, and a family history of the disease (1° DYS is often associated with mutation of the *DYT1* gene); secondary dystonia (2° DYS), which is associated with brain injury and may involve lesions of the basal ganglia (BG) or thalamus (3,4); and primary idiopathic dystonia (idiopathic DYS), in which no cause can be identified and which does not resemble 1° DYS clinically.

The presence of a lesion in the BG in some cases of 2° DYS (3–5) and the amelioration of 1° DYS and some cases of 2° DYS following posteroventral pallidotomy (PVP) (6–9) suggests that the BG may play an important role in the genesis of DYS. The mechanisms by which a BG lesion induces DYS and PVP ameliorates DYS, however, are poorly understood, in part due to the lack of substantial published data on the behavior of neurons in the BG in DYS.

We analyzed the discharge rates and patterns of neurons in the putamen (Put), globus pallidus externa (GPe), and globus pallidus interna (GPi) in patients who underwent PVP for the treatment of DYS. Neuronal activity in the DYS patients was compared with that in patients with Parkinson's disease (PD) who also underwent PVP. The effect of anesthesia on neuronal activity was also investigated, as were differences in neuronal activity among DYS patients who benefited from PVP and those who did not. These data have been reported in detail elsewhere (10).

PATIENTS AND METHODS

Sixteen DYS patients, seven male and nine female (mean age 19.6 ± 12.6 years; range 8 to 57 years) with severe generalized or hemidystonia who were refractory to medical treatment, underwent PVP (Table 4-1). Seven patients were classified as having 1° DYS based on either the presence of the mutated form of the *DYT1* gene (four patients) or on clinical presentation (three patients). Five patients were classified as having 2° DYS secondary to brain injury that was visualized on

TABLE 4-1. *Characteristics of dystonia patients and their outcome after posteroventral pallidotomy*

Patient ID	Symptom type	Awake or anes	DYT1	Age (yrs)	Onset (yrs)	Surgery	UDRS pre-surg	UDRS post-surg	% Improve	BFM pre-	BFM post-	% Improve
Primary genetic dystonia												
1	Gen	Awake	NT	19	9.5	R PVP	30	NT	—	22	NT	—
2	Gen	Anes	Yes	15	7	Bi simul PVP	68	12	82%	50	12	76%
3	Gen	Anes	Yes	10	8	Bi staged PVP	36	21	42%	26	19	27%
4	Gen	Anes	NT	51	9	Bi staged PVP	83	26	69%	57	15	74%
5	Gen	Anes	Yes	13	8	Bi simul PVP	81	20	75%	48	17	65%
6	Gen	Anes	Yes	16	12	Bi simul PVP	41	2	71%	27	10	63%
7	Gen	Anes	No	17	7	Bi simul PVP	101	27	73%	59	17	71%
Secondary dystonia												
8	Gen	Awake	NT	57	40	R PVP	NT	NT	—	NT	NT	—
9	Gen	Awake	NT	15	6	Bi simul PVP	82	74	10%	56	45	19%
10	Hemi	Awake	NT	18	9	L PVP	37	15	59%	25	13	48%
11	Hemi	Anes	NT	21	10	L PVP	38	11	71%	23	6	73%
12	Gen	Anes	NT	19	9	Bi simul PVP	86	63	27%	56	43	23%
Idiopathic dystonia												
13	Gen	Awake	NT	48	42	R PVP	28	20	29%	18	18	0%
14	Gen	Anes	No	15	5	Bi simul PVP	78	66	15%	49	46	6%
15	Gen	Anes	No	11	2	Bi simul PVP	88	54	38%	58	36	38%
16	Gen	Anes	NT	8	0.4	Bi staged PVP	51	34	33%	31	25	19%

Anes, anesthetized; Bi, bilateral; BFM, Burke-Fahn-Marsden scale (higher = more impairment); *DYT1,* mutated form of *DYT1* gene; Gen, generalized dystonia; Hemi, hemidystonia; improve, improvement; NT, not tested; PVP, posteroventral pallidotomy; simul, simultaneous; surg, surgery; UDRS, United Dystonia Rating Scale (higher = more impairment).

magnetic resonance imaging (MRI) scans, and four patients were classified as having idiopathic DYS.

We compared BG neuronal activity in these 16 DYS patients with that in 78 patients with PD (43 males and 35 females; mean age 62.1 ± 9.2 years; range 39 to 78 years) who were levodopa-responsive and who exhibited severe "off" rigidity and dopa-induced dyskinesias. The demographic features, the MRI characteristics of the PVP lesions, and the motor and neuropsychological outcomes of subgroups of these patients have been previously published (7,11–15).

General inhalation anesthesia [1.5–4.6% desflurane (Suprane, Baxter, Dearfield, IL)] was used during PVP for 11 DYS and six PD patients. When necessary, patients also received low doses of intravenous midazolam (<1.5 mg; Versed, Roche, Nutley, NJ) and/or fentanyl (75–100 μg; Sublimaze, Taylor, Decatur, IL) 2 to 3 hours prior to intraoperative microelectrode recording. All antiparkinsonian and antidystonia medications were withdrawn on the night prior to surgery.

Clinical Assessment

Patients with DYS were assessed before surgery, and at approximately 3 weeks, 6 months, 9 months and 12 months after surgery using the Unified Dystonia Rating Scale (UDRS) (16,17) and the Burke-Fahn-Marsden (BFM) dystonia scale (18). Standardized videotape assessments were utilized. The accuracy of lesion placement was evaluated by MRI within 3 weeks of PVP. Postoperative outcome was expressed as the percentage change from the preoperative UDRS and BFM rating scale scores (Table 4-1). The postsurgical outcome of a subgroup of these DYS patients has been previously reported in a comparison of the efficacy of PVP and thalamotomy (9).

Operative Procedures

The surgical technique for stereotactic PVP has been described in detail elsewhere (10). Basically, the patient's head was placed in a Leksell G frame and the anterior-posterior commissure (AC-PC) line was identified on computed tomographic (CT) scans (19). The target point in the posteroventral region of the GPi was chosen at 20 mm lateral to the midline, 4 mm below the AC-PC line and 3 mm anterior to the midcommissural point. Neuronal signals were recorded with a tungsten or Pt/Ir electrode (impedance of 0.5–1.0 M) and displayed and stored on a Axon Guideline (GS 3000) system for off-line analysis using DATAPAC 2K2 software (Run Technologies, Mission Viejo, CA).

Macrostimulation was performed at the target site in all awake patients to locate the proximity of the optic nerve and the internal capsule. If no optic or capsular responses were evoked, two radiofrequency lesions were made, one above the other, 2 mm apart, by withdrawing the electrode along the electrode tract. The lesions were made with the electrode tip temperature at 75°C for 60 seconds. The verification of the lesion site and the lesion dimensions were visualized in postoperative MRI scans and have been described previously (12).

Off-line analysis of the neurophysiologic properties of recorded neurons was performed on well-isolated neurons. For each neuron, the mean discharge rate, mean interspike interval (ISI), and auto- and cross-correlation histograms were analyzed. The dispersion of the ISI was used to calculate the degree of variance of the neuronal discharge pattern from the variance of ISI/mean ISI (8). Statistical analysis was performed using SigmaStat, v. 2.03 (SPSS Science; Chicago, IL). An alpha of 0.05 was used to determine statistical significance.

RESULTS

There were readily observable differences in the discharge rates and patterns of Put, GPe, and GPi neurons in PD and DYS patients. In PD patients, for example, spontaneously discharging GPe and GPi neurons were abundant, and their action potentials were stable, of large amplitude (0.5–0.8 mV) and could be recorded over a distance of 50 to 100 μm. The "pausing" and "bursting" discharge patterns of GPe neurons, and the rapid, regular discharge of GPi neurons were apparent (19,20).

In DYS patients, spontaneously discharging neurons were less frequently encountered. In general, pallidal neurons were fragile and difficult to isolate, and their action potentials were often of small amplitude. There were also "silent" neurons whose presence was indicated by the occurrence of a brief injury potential followed by electrical silence.

Characteristics of Putamen Neurons

Recordings were obtained from 34 Put neurons in 16 DYS patients and from 19 neurons in 78 PD patients. The great majority of Put neurons discharged slowly and had, in general, irregular discharge patterns. However, in one patient with idiopathic DYS (patient 15), the Put neurons recorded had discharge rates up to 33 Hz, which we have not observed in PD.

The effect of anesthesia on Put neurons was minimal both in DYS and in PD. However, there was a tendency for Put neurons to discharge at a slightly higher rate in awake PD patients (Table 4-2).

Characteristics of GPe Neurons

In DYS patients, GPe neurons generally had a poor signal-to-noise ratio and a large variation in their discharge rates. There were no significant differences in the discharge rates among the three DYS groups (Table 4–2). Individual neurons in the GPe were classified as having one of four types of discharge pattern: irregular, regular, bursting, or

TABLE 4-2. *Mean ± standard deviation (SD) discharge rate (Hz) and mean ± SD dispersion (ms) of putamen (Put), globus pallidus externa (GPe), and globus pallidus interna (GPi) neurons in awake and anesthetized dystonia and Parkinson's disease patients*

Patient ID	Awake or anes	Put discharge rate; dispersion	GPe discharge rate; dispersion	GPi discharge rate; dispersion
Primary genetic dystonia (*n* = 7)				
1	Awake	—	38; 29 (1)	33.4 ± 8.4; 54.0 ± 8.2 (5)
2	Anes	2.2 ± 0.9; 38.5 ± 4.9 (2)	33.6 ± 26.3; 78.4 ± 99.0 (4)	30.3 ± 23.3; 60.8 ± 35.6 (8)
3	Anes	2.2 ± 1.5; 36.3 ± 4.5 (3)	21.9 ± 10.4; 50.8 ± 27.8 (9)	30.6 ± 15.6; 49.1 ± 30.1 (7)
4	Anes	2.9 ± 0.7; 49.1 ± 18.4 (2)	19.2 ± 13.8; 75.4 ± 8.7 (5)	19.1 ± 9.1; 72.3 ± 28.6 (9)
5	Anes	1.3 ± 1.1; 28.5 ± 9.2 (2)	8.0 ± 2.8; 68.0 ± 2.8 (2)	28.8 ± 12.7; 82.1 ± 23.4 (15)
6	Anes	3.1 ± 2.4; 97.3 ± 11.9 (8)	18.4 ± 12.1; 104.0 ± 37.1 (7)	29.4 ± 2.6; 43.1 ± 22.8 (5)
7	Anes	2.8 ± 1.7; 35.0 ± 10.0 (2)	15.3 ± 4.0; 90.7 ± 63.3 (3)	5.0 ± 9.2; 134.5 ± 53.7 (6)
Secondary dystonia (*n* = 5)				
8	Awake	5.2 ± 0.9; 81.2 ± 29.4 (2)	21; 39 (1)	70.8 ± 21.8; 14.1 ± 5.7 (11)
9	Awake	3.2 ± 0.4; 31.0 ± 7.1 (2)	13; 35 (1)	23.7 ± 9.3; 86.0 ± 15.1 (3)
10	Awake	2.0 ± 1.8; 22.5 ± 6.3 (2)	—	24.3 ± 12.0; 52.5 ± 26.8 (8)
11	Anes	—	45.7 ± 17.6; 13.3 ± 9.2 (3)	20.5 ± 9.2; 72.0 ± 74.9 (2)
12	Anes	1.3 ± 0.7; 76.5 ± 12.0 (2)	13; 61 (1)	10.7 ± 4.2; 59.0 ± 43.5 (3)
Idiopathic dystonia (*n* = 4)				
13	Awake	—	21.5 ± 17.6; 86.5 ± 84.2 (2)	38.7 ± 13.0; 35.0 ± 35.3 (6)
14	Anes	1.9 ± 0.4; 33.0 (2;1)	12.3 ± 1.2; 115.0 ± 77.7 (3)	19.8 ± 9.0; 117.2 ± 144.7 (9)
15	Anes	22.2 ± 11.4; 42.0 ± 35.9 (4)	2.5; 82 (1)	15.6 ± 10.0; 90.6 ± 62.1 (11)
16	Anes	3.2; 41 (1)	—	12.6 ± 3.8; 62.8 ± 31.0 (5)
Parkinson's disease (*n* = 78)				
n = 72	Awake	3.8 ± 1.6; 37.8 ± 20.6 (11)	50.1 ± 20.8; 14.5 ± 10.6 (118)	86.2 ± 24.3; 21.7 ± 25.8 (147)
n = 6	Anes	2.6 ± 1.7; 25.3 ± 19.3 (8)	33.9 ± 16.4; 75.9 ± 66.0 (29)	35.6 ± 18.0; 39.8 ± 222.1 (25)

Number of recorded neurons in parentheses.

clustering (Fig. 4-1; Table 4-3). The discharge pattern of the majority of GPe neurons was highly irregular, and their ISI histograms tended to be either positively or negatively skewed. Greater irregularity of the discharge pattern was correlated with greater separation of the modal and mean discharge frequencies.

Regularly discharging neurons displayed higher discharge rates and lower dispersion of the ISI as indicated by the symmetrical, near normal distribution of their ISI histograms (Fig. 4-1). The greater the regularity of the discharge pattern, the closer were the modal and mean discharge frequencies.

A third group of GPe neurons discharged in a "bursting" pattern (Fig. 4-1). The spikes within the burst often exhibited decremental amplitude. The ISI histogram of bursting neurons could be either unimodal, with positively skewed longer intervals, or bimodal, consisting of a large primary peak that was either positively skewed or near normally distributed, followed by a smaller secondary peak that was normally distributed. The discharge rate within the bursts ranged from 104 to 183 Hz. The number of spikes within the bursts ranged from 5 to 10 spikes. The duration of the bursts ranged from 19 to 191 ms, with the interburst interval ranging from 190 to 2,422 ms. Bursting neurons were found in all three DYS groups. However, no significant differences were found in the discharge rate, num-

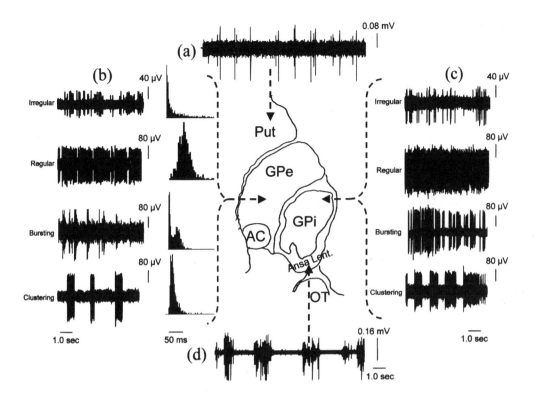

FIG. 4-1. Firing patterns of basal ganglia (BG) neurons encountered in an electrode trajectory to the posteroventral globus pallidus interna (GPi) in dystonia (DYS) patients. Neuronal discharges are displayed on a 1.0-second time scale. **A:** Slow firing, irregularly discharging neurons were characteristic of the putamen (Put) neurons. **B:** Discharge patterns of globus pallidus externa (GPe) neurons. GPe neurons discharged in one of four patterns: irregular, regular, bursting, or clustering. The histogram of the interspike interval (ISI) corresponding to each discharge pattern is displayed on the right panel. Bin width = 2 ms. **C:** Discharge patterns of GPi neurons. GPi neurons also displayed one of four patterns: irregular, regular, bursting, or clustering. The dispersion of the ISI and the distribution of the ISI histogram corresponding to each of the discharge patterns in the GPi were similar to those seen in the GPe. **D:** At a depth corresponding to the base of the GPi, where no spontaneous discharges typical of GPi neurons were observed, discharges that were largely negative in polarity were often evoked with each advance of the microelectrode. These discharges most likely correspond to the microelectrode passing through the ansa lenticularis. AC, anterior commissure; Ansa Lent., ansa lenticularis; OT, optic tract.

ber of spikes within the burst, duration of the burst, or the interburst interval among the three DYS groups.

The fourth neuronal discharge pattern observed in GPe neurons was a "clustering" of discharges (Fig. 4–1). There was little variation in spike amplitude within the clusters. The discharging neurons often displayed a very regular ISI within the cluster, and the clusters themselves tended to occur at regular intervals. The ISI histogram of these neurons resembled that of regular, tonically discharging GPe neurons.

There was no significant difference in the GPe neuronal discharge rate between awake ($n = 5$) and anesthetized ($n = 11$) DYS patients (Table 4-2). The irregularity of GPe neuronal discharge increased under anesthesia, but this

TABLE 4-3. *Mean discharge rate ± SD and mean dispersion ± SD of the interspike interval of pallidal neurons in regular, irregular, bursting, and clustering patterns in all dystonia patients (n = 16)*

	GPe				GPi			
	Irregular	Regular	Bursting	Clustering	Irregular	Regular	Bursting	Clustering
Primary genetic dystonia (31 GPe and 55 GPi neurons recorded)								
Discharge rate (Hz)	15.1 ± 6.5	36.2 ± 24.6	22.8 ± 9.1	17.8 ± 10.2	25.9 ± 10.9	39.9 ± 21.3	25.0 ± 11.7	16.6 ± 9.9
Dispersion (ms)	74.1 ± 41.2	32.4 ± 27.3	109.6 ± 2.4	115.0 ± 69.8	81.6 ± 40.0	18.4 ± 8.4	68.0 ± 20.1	89.6 ± 27.1
No. neurons recorded (%)	19 (63%)	5 (16%)	5 (16%)	2 (6%)	37 (67%)	7 (13%)	4 (7%)	7 (13%)
Secondary dystonia (6 GPe and 27 GPi neurons recorded)								
Discharge rate (Hz)	30.5 ± 24.7	44.5 ± 24.8	17 ± 5.7	0	54.7 ± 21.5	30.7 ± 18.8	27	18.3 ± 0.5
Dispersion (ms)	29.5 ± 7.8	9.5 ± 2.1	50 ± 15.6	0	24.2 ± 16.2	6.3 ± 5.5	49	84.0 ± 0.5
No. neurons recorded (%)	2 (33%)	2 (33%)	2 (33%)	0	13 (48%)	6 (22%)	1 (4%)	7 (26%)
Idiopathic dystonia (6 GPe and 31 GPi neurons recorded)								
Discharge rate (Hz)	2.5	23.5 ± 14.9	13.0 ± 4.8	0	24.8 ± 15.0	27.3 ± 7.5	29.0 ± 14.0	15.0 ± 10.3
Dispersion (ms)	82.0	29.5 ± 3.5	127.0 ± 32.1	0	60.8 ± 41.3	11.4 ± 5.0	12.5 ± 147.8	125.5 ± 110.6
No. neurons recorded (%)	1 (17%)	3 (50%)	2 (34%)	0	18 (58%)	5 (16%)	2 (6%)	6 (19%)

difference was not statistically significant. In anesthetized PD patients, there was a significant decrease in the discharge rate of GPe neurons and a significant increase in the irregularity of their discharge when compared with awake PD patients ($p < .05$; Table 4-2).

Characteristics of GPi Neurons

The number of discharging GPi neurons, their signal-to-noise ratio, and their stability were greater than in GPe neurons in all DYS patients. The discharge rate of GPi neurons varied considerably among the DYS groups: 5 to 80 Hz in 1° DYS; 6 to 112 Hz in 2° DYS; and 5 to 53 Hz in idiopathic DYS (Table 4–2). In one 2° DYS patient (patient 8), the mean discharge rate was high, similar to that seen in PD patients. Neither the discharge rate nor the dispersion of the ISI was significantly different among the three DYS groups.

As observed for GPe neurons, four different patterns of discharge were noted among the GPi neurons: irregular, regular, bursting,

and clustering (Fig. 4–1). The ISI characteristics were similar to those of GPe neurons. Irregularly discharging neurons comprised the majority of neurons in the GPi, and the discharge rates and dispersion of their ISI were similar in all three DYS groups.

The regularly discharging GPi neurons had higher discharge rates (range 12–112 Hz) and lower dispersion values (range 9–31 ms) than did the irregularly discharging GPe neurons.

Neurons discharging in a "bursting" pattern in the GPi were present in all three DYS patient groups. The mean discharge rate within the bursts, the number of spikes in a burst, the duration of the bursts, and the interburst interval were not significantly different from those observed in bursting neurons in the GPe.

"Clustering" GPi neurons exhibited the lowest mean discharge rate and the highest ISI dispersion of all neurons (Table 4-3). Clustering neurons were observed in all three DYS groups. Within the clusters, the mean discharge rate, the number of spikes within the cluster, the cluster duration, and the interval between clusters were not significantly different from those observed in clustering neurons in the GPe.

The discharge rate of GPi neurons in DYS patients was not significantly affected by anesthesia (Table 4-2). However, there was a tendency for the discharge pattern in anesthetized patients to be more irregular when compared with the pattern observed in awake patients. In anesthetized PD patients, however, there was a significant decrease in the GPi discharge rate and a significant increase in the dispersion of the ISI (Table 4-2) ($p < .05$).

Outcome Following Posteroventral Pallidotomy in Patients with Dystonia and Parkinson's Disease

Pre- and postoperative outcomes, using the UDRS and BFM rating scales, generally demonstrated a robust benefit of PVP in 1° genetic DYS patients (mean improvement: 69% UDRS and 63% BFM; Table 4-1). One 1° DYS patient (patient 1) was unable to return for postoperative examination but was reported to be doing "very well" by his neurologist. As noted in Table 4-1, one 1° DYS patient (patient 3) benefited by only 42% and 27% (UDRS and BFM, respectively).

Two 2° DYS patients with hemidystonia (patients 9 and 10) significantly benefited from PVP (mean improvement: 59% and 71% with UDRS, respectively, and 48% and 73% with BFM, respectively). Two 2° DYS patients with generalized dystonia who had bilateral simultaneous PVP had minimal improvement (mean improvement: 10% and 27% with UDRS, and 19% and 23% with BFM), and one 2° DYS (patient 8) with hemidystonia experienced only a transient beneficial effect. Idiopathic DYS patients did not greatly benefit from PVP.

Overall, the data suggest that, for DYS patients, PVP is most beneficial for patients with 1° genetic DYS ($p < .05$). No correlation between outcome and pallidal discharge rate, discharge pattern, the age of onset, or the duration of DYS before PVP was found.

Pallidotomy had beneficial effects on the motor symptoms of patients with PD, and relieved levodopa-induced dyskinesias, as has been previously reported (10,11).

DISCUSSION

In this study we have recorded from pallidal neurons in DYS and PD patients under sufficiently similar physiologic conditions to suggest the following: (a) the discharge rates of Put neurons are very low in both DYS and in PD; (b) the discharge rates of both GPe and GPi neurons are much lower and more variable in DYS than in PD in both awake and anesthetized patients; (c) in DYS, the discharge rates and discharge patterns of GPe and GPi neurons are similar, whereas in PD patients the GPe discharge rate is lower than that recorded in the GPi; (d) there are no statistically significant differences in the discharge rates and patterns of GPe and GPi neurons in patients whose DYS is ameliorated by PVP and those who do not benefit; and (e) there are noticeable differences in the quality of neuronal recordings between patients with DYS and PD, suggesting a physical difference in the state of the globus pallidus.

Our finding of similar discharge rates and patterns in primary genetic, secondary, and idiopathic DYS does not explain why PVP is more efficacious in relieving dystonic symptoms associated with mutation of the *DYT1* gene compared with DYS of other origins. However, given the sources of variability encountered in making intraoperative recordings, an analysis of recordings made in a larger number of patients might reveal differences in the relative proportions of neurons exhibiting different discharge properties in DYS of different etiologies.

REFERENCES

1. Bressman SB. Dystonia. *Curr Opin Neurol* 1998;11: 363–372.
2. Fahn S, Bressman SB, Marsden CD. Classification of dystonia. In: Fahn S, Marsden CD, DeLong MR, eds. *Advances in Neurology: Dystonia 3.* Philadelphia: Lippincott-Raven, 1998:1–10.

3. Chuang C, Fahn S, Frucht SJ. The natural history and treatment of acquired hemidystonia: Report of 33 cases and review of the literature. *J Neurol Neurosurg Psychiatry* 2002;72:59–67.

4. Marsden CD, Obeso JA, Zarranz JJ, et al. The anatomical basis of symptomatic hemidystonia. *Brain* 1985; 108:463–483.

5. Pettigrew LC, Jankovic J. Hemidystonia: a report of 22 patients and a review of the literature. *J Neurol Neurosurg Psychiatry* 1985;48:650–657.

6. Lozano AM, Kumar R, Gross RE, et al. Globus pallidus internus pallidotomy for generalized dystonia. *Mov Disord* 1997;12:865–870.

7. Ondo WG, Desaloms JM, Jankovic J, et al. Pallidotomy for generalized dystonia. *Mov Disord* 1998;13:693–698.

8. Vitek JL, Chockkan V, Zhang JY, et al. Neuronal activity in the basal ganglia in patients with generalized dystonia and hemiballismus. *Ann Neurol* 1999;46:22–35.

9. Yoshor D, Hamilton WJ, Ondo W, et al. Comparison of thalamotomy and pallidotomy for the treatment of dystonia. *Neurosurgery* 2001;48:818–826.

10. Sanghera MK, Grossman RG, Kalhorn CG, et al. Basal ganglia neuronal discharge in primary and secondary dystonia in patients undergoing pallidotomy. *Neurosurgery* 2003;52:1358–1373.

11. Desaloms JM, Krauss JK, Lai EC, et al. Posteroventral medial pallidotomy for treatment of Parkinson's disease: preoperative magnetic resonance imaging features and clinical outcome. *J Neurosurg* 1998;89:194–199.

12. Krauss JK, Desaloms JM, Lai EC, et al. Microelectrode-guided posteroventral pallidotomy for treatment of Parkinson's disease: postoperative magnetic resonance imaging analysis. *J Neurosurg* 1997;87:358–367.

13. Lai EC, Jankovic J, Krauss JK, et al. Long-term efficacy of posteroventral pallidotomy in the treatment of Parkinson's disease. *Neurology* 2000;55:1218–1222.

14. Rettig GM, York MK, Lai EC, et al. Neuropsychological outcome after unilateral pallidotomy for the treatment of Parkinson's disease. *J Neurol Neurosurg Psychiatry* 2000;69:326–336.

15. York MK, Levin HS, Grossman RG, et al. Neuropsychological outcome following unilateral pallidotomy. *Brain* 1999;122:2209–2220.

16. Comella CL, Leurgans S, Chmura TA, et al. The United Dystonia Rating Scale: initial concurrent validity testing with other dystonia scales. *Neurology* 1999;52 (suppl 2):A292(abst).

17. Comella CL, Dystonia Study Group. Rating scales for dystonia: a multicenter assessment of three dystonia rating scales: the Unified Dystonia Rating Scale (UDRS), the Burke-Fahn-Marsden (BFM) and the Global Dystonia Rating Scale (GDS). *Neurology* 2001;56(suppl 3):A387(abst).

18. Burke RE, Fahn S, Marsden CD, et al. Validity and reliability of a rating scale for the primary torsion dystonias. *Neurology* 1985;35:73–77.

19. Lozano A, Hutchison W, Kiss Z, et al. Methods for microelectrode-guided posteroventral pallidotomy. *J Neurosurg* 1996;84:194–202.

20. Sterio D, Beric A, Dogali M, et al. Neurophysiological properties of pallidal neurons in Parkinson's disease. *Ann Neurol* 1994;35:586–591.

Dystonia 4: Advances in Neurology, Vol. 94. Edited by Stanley Fahn, Mark Hallett, and Mahlon R. DeLong. Lippincott Williams & Wilkins, Philadelphia © 2004.

5

Evidence of Widespread Impairment of Motor Cortical Inhibition in Focal Dystonia: A Transcranial Magnetic Stimulation Study in Patients with Blepharospasm and Cervical Dystonia

*Raif Cakmur, *Berril Donmez, *Fatma Uzunel, *Huriye Aydin, and †Serdar Kesken

*Department of Neurology, Dokuz Eylül University, Medical School, Izmir, Turkey.
†Tepecik Hospital, Izmir, Turkey

The genetic basis for various forms of primary dystonia has been well recognized, but little is known about the cause of focal dystonias. Genetic studies strongly support the concept that most cases of focal dystonia are entities distinct from generalized dystonia (1). In focal dystonia, only a single area of the body is involved, but there is also evidence of more generalized disturbances (2–10). Therefore, the question as to whether focal and segmental dystonias are separate and distinct or are *forme frustes* of generalized dystonia has not been entirely resolved (1).

Transcranial magnetic stimulation (TMS) has proved to be a useful tool to study the pathophysiology of a number of disorders including dystonia, because it produces both excitatory and inhibitory effects (11,12). The cortical silent period (SP, or postexcitatory inhibition), as assessed by single pulse TMS, is thought to originate largely from the inhibitory function of cortical or subcortical structures, with spinal mechanisms participating only in the early part (13–15). Activation of intracortical inhibitory circuits, most likely by the activation of γ-aminobutyric acid (GABA)ergic in-

terneurons, may play an essential part in its generation (16,17). The duration of SP, therefore, may provide information about the excitability of intracortical inhibitory neurons or axons. Significant changes of SP have been reported in different basal ganglia disorders, indicating an important influence of basal ganglia function over intracortical inhibitory interneuron excitability (2–5,18–22).

Although the exact pathophysiology of focal dystonia is not yet fully understood, neurophysiologic studies have provided new insights. First, hyperexcitability of brainstem and spinal motoneuronal pools has been demonstrated in many reflex studies (cranial reflexes and reciprocal inhibition) (6–8,23–28). More recently, impairment of the cortical mechanisms of motor control, as assessed by single- and double-pulse TMS, has been demonstrated in different types of focal dystonia (2–5,29–33). All the evidence suggests that focal dystonia results from abnormal commands descending from the cortex, presumably secondary to distorted basal ganglia control, leading to abnormal regulation of inhibitory interneuronal mechanisms at the brainstem and spinal cord level.

In idiopathic focal dystonia, there are observations of more generalized disturbances at the segmental level and in the brainstem, which do not seem to be limited to the affected region. Evidence for this comes from findings of reduced reciprocal inhibition of forearm muscles and enhanced blink reflex excitability (6–10,24,25). Shortening of SP evoked by single-pulse TMS in the affected muscles of different types of focal dystonia has been reported (2–4,29,32). However, there have been conflicting results indicating the existence and lack of widespread changes in cortical inhibitory control responsible for the generation of postexcitatory inhibition in focal dystonia (2–5,29,34).

The aim of this study is to determine whether a generalized disturbance of intracortical inhibitory mechanisms reflected by SP evoked by TMS can be observed in the two most common forms of focal dystonia—cervical dystonia and blepharospasm—supporting the hypothesis of focal dystonia as a more generalized disorder. We therefore studied SP in cranial, cervical, and hand muscles in 40 patients with focal dystonia (20 essential blepharospasm and 20 cervical dystonia) and 20 normal controls.

PATIENTS AND METHODS

Subjects

We studied 60 subjects, including 20 patients with essential blepharospasm, 20 patients with idiopathic cervical dystonia, and 20 healthy controls. The demographic features of the patients and controls are shown in Table 5-1. The patients who were diagnosed as focal dystonia with adult onset were included in the study. All patients had a normal neurologic examination except for dystonia, and had normal neuroimaging (computed tomography and magnetic resonance imaging). The patients who were taking central acting drugs (e.g., benzodiazepines, anticholinergics) or who had contraindications for TMS were excluded. All patients and controls gave their informed consent to participate in the study. For ten patients (nine patients in the cervical dystonia group and one patient in the blepharospasm group) who had received botulinum toxin type A (BTX-A) injections, TMS was performed when symptoms demanded treatment, but not before 4 months from the last injection. The severity of neurologic disability was evaluated on a scale between 0 and 5 for patients with blepharospasm (0, normal; 1, inconvenienced; 2, independent, with moderate function; 3, independent, with poor function; 4, dependent outside the home; 5, blind) and on the Toronto Western Spasmodic Torticollis Rating Scale (TWSTRS) for patients with cervical dystonia (35,36).

Stimulation Technique

TMS was performed with a Magstim 200 stimulator connected to a 90-mm circular coil placed over the vertex (Magstim Company Ltd., Spring Gardens, UK). The maximal transient magnetic field produced around the coil was 2.0 tesla. The coil was placed tangentially to the scalp and centered over the

TABLE 5-1. *Demographic features of the patients and controls*

	Blepharospasm group ($n = 20$)	Cervical dystonia group ($n = 20$)	Control group ($n = 20$)
Sex (F/M)	12/8	14/6	12/8
Age (years)[a]	65.1 ± 7.6 (51–76)	50.3 ± 13.0 (27–73)	57.8 ± 9.8 (35–69)
Duration of symptoms (years)[a]	10.9 ± 7.8 (4–36)	11.4 ± 8.1 (1–25)	—
BTX-A treatments per patient[a]	9.4 ± 4.9 (0–17)	3.21 ± 4.9 (0–17)	—

[a]Mean ± SD (range).
BTX-A, botulinum toxin type A.

vertex with its edge overlying the arm area of the motor cortex. The direction of the current in the coil seen from above was clockwise. The orientation of the coil was in the anterior-posterior direction with the handle posterior. Electromyographic (EMG) recordings were made from the left side of the body from the orbicularis oculi, orbicularis oris, sternocleidomastoid, and abductor pollicis brevis muscles in all subjects. Ag-AgCl surface electrodes were used for all recordings. For cranial recordings, electrodes were placed over the orbicularis oculi and orbicularis oris muscles, and a common reference was used over the tip of the nose. For cervical recordings, an active recording electrode was located over the sternocleidomastoid muscle between the upper two thirds and the lower third of the muscle belly and the reference electrode over sternoclavicular joint 1. For upper extremity recordings, electrodes were placed over the belly and tendon of the abductor pollicis brevis muscle, about 3 cm apart from each other. The EMG was recorded using the Neuropack MEB 2200 EMG/EP device (Nihon Kohden Corp., Tokyo, Japan). Signals were filtered (200 Hz to 5 kHz) and full-wave rectified. EMG activity was recorded for 200 ms before and 800 ms after delivering the magnetic stimuli.

The patients and controls were comfortably positioned on a bed in a quiet room with their eyes closed. Threshold and latency values were obtained from the abductor pollicis brevis muscle at rest while monitoring background EMG activity throughout the recording to avoid facilitation of motor evoked potentials (MEPs) by slight contraction. The resting motor threshold (RMT) for the abductor pollicis brevis was determined according to the criteria outlined by the IFCN committee (12). The RMT was defined as the lowest intensity able to produce an EMG response over $100\mu V$ in at least 50% of ten successive trials. The shortest latencies of MEPs were measured on both sides from three consecutive responses obtained with a stimulus intensity of $2\times$ RMT. The SP was evaluated at the maximum output of the stimulator, while the

subject sustained the maximum voluntary contraction of the target muscle (2,3). The TMS for every single muscle was performed each time. The interference pattern of EMG activity was monitored throughout SP recording. For measurements of SP, at least five artifact-free traces were obtained and superimposed to demonstrate the constancy of the EMG suppression. The SP was taken from the end of the excitatory response to the shortest latency at which the tonic EMG activity returned to its prestimulus level. SP measurements were taken manually with cursors by the same investigator (B.D.), who was blinded to the diagnosis.

Statistical Analysis

We found that all the variables followed normal distribution with the Kolmogorov-Smirnov goodness-of-fit test. The one-way analysis of variance (ANOVA) test was used to investigate differences between groups, and when a significant difference ($p < .05$) was found, Student's unpaired t-test was used to determine in which of the two groups significant differences occurred. Correlations between disability scores and SP durations for each group were evaluated by Pearson's correlation coefficient. Statistical analyses were performed by using the SPSS program.

RESULTS

The procedure was well tolerated by all subjects and no adverse reactions were reported. For RMT, latency, and amplitude values of MEPs in the abductor pollicis brevis muscle, no significant differences were found between groups (Table 5-2). In all subjects, high-intensity TMS elicited SP in target muscles. Results of the duration of SP in controls and in patients with blepharospasm and cervical dystonia are shown in the Fig. 5-1 and Table 5-3. The duration of the silent period in the abductor pollicis brevis muscle did not differ between groups ($p > .05$). Statistically significant differences for the duration of the SP in the orbicularis oculi, orbic-

TABLE 5-2. *Results of motor evoked potentials (MEPs) in abductor pollicis brevis muscle in blepharospasm, cervical dystonia, and control groups*

	Blepharospasm group ($n = 20$)	Cervical dystonia group ($n = 20$)	Control group ($n = 20$)	p
Resting motor threshold (RMT) (%)[a]	44.9 ± 11.2	45.2 ± 11.8	42.0 ± 7.4	ns
MEP latency (ms)[a]	21.6 ± 1.0	20.6 ± 1.5	21.5 ± 1.4	ns
MEP amplitude (mV)[a]	3.1 ± 2.1	2.4 ± 1.5	2.0 ± 1.7	ns

[a]Mean ± SD; ns: $p > .05$.

ularis oris, and sternocleidomastoid muscles were found between groups (Fig. 5-2). When compared to controls, the mean cortical SP was significantly shorter in upper and lower facial muscles (orbicularis oculi and orbicularis oris muscles) in both the blepharospasm and cervical dystonia groups. Only the patients with cervical dystonia showed shorter SP in the sternocleidomastoid muscle compared to controls. The mean value for the SP for the sternocleidomastoid muscle in the blepharospasm group was shorter than that of the control group, but the difference did not reach statistical significance. Mean TWSTRS score for patients with cervical dystonia was 13.7 [standard deviation (SD): 3.1, range: 8–20]. Mean disability score for blepharospasm patients was 3.2 (SD: 0.71, range: 2.5–5). There was an inverse correlation between the severity of neurologic disability and the duration of SP in the orbicularis oculi ($p < .01$) and the orbicularis oris ($p < .05$) muscles in patients with blepharospasm.

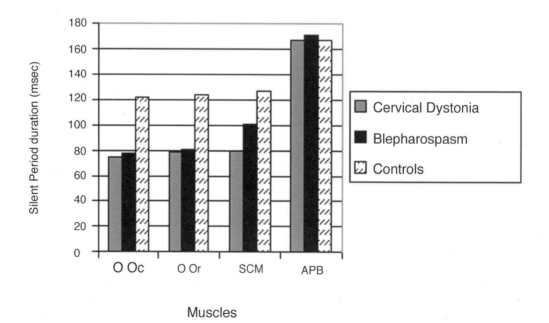

FIG. 5-1. Mean duration of the silent period in orbicularis oculi (O Oc), orbicularis oris (O Or), sternocleidomastoid (SCM), and abductor pollicis brevis (APB) muscles in cervical dystonia, blepharospasm, and control groups.

TABLE 5-3. *Duration of the silent period (SP) in orbicularis oculi (O. Oculi), orbicularis oris (O. Oris), sternocleidomastoid (SCM), and abductor pollicis brevis (APB) muscles in blepharospasm, cervical dystonia, and control groups*

	Blepharospasm group ($n = 20$)	Cervical dystonia group ($n = 20$)	Control group ($n = 20$)
O. Oculi SP (ms)[a]	78.7 ± 37.4*	75.8 ± 32.2*	122.3 ± 31.7
O. Oris SP (ms)[a]	81.6 ± 35.6*	79.7 ± 24.0*	124.4 ± 31.8
SCM SP (ms)[a]	101.8 ± 27.3	80.9 ± 36.3[†]	127.1 ± 42.8
APB SP (ms)[a]	171.5 ± 45.3	167.1 ± 44.0	167.8 ± 36.1

[a]Mean ± SD.
*Significant difference between control and patient groups ($p \leq .001$).
[†]Significant difference between blepharospasm and cervical dystonia groups ($p \leq .05$).

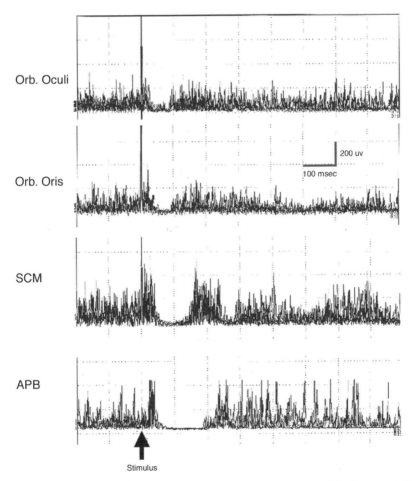

FIG. 5-2. Raw data from a patient with cervical dystonia demonstrating the silent period (SP) in orbicularis oculi (O Oculi), orbicularis oris (O Oris), sternocleidomastoid (SCM), and abductor pollicis brevis (APB) muscles.

DISCUSSION

The purpose of this study was to investigate the cortical excitability in patients with blepharospasm and cervical dystonia. To do this we used the technique of TMS over the motor cortex. The RMT, latency, and amplitude of MEPs, and the duration of the SP can be used to measure the excitability of the motor system with single-pulse TMS. In focal dystonia, the RMT, latency, and amplitude of MEPs at rest did not differ from controls in previous studies (2,4,5,29–32,34). These findings may suggest a normal corticomotoneuron connection and normal excitability of cortical motor areas in focal dystonia. We also found that these parameters in abductor pollicis brevis muscle were normal in both the blepharospasm and cervical dystonia groups. By contrast, major changes in excitability became evident when the SP was recorded with high-intensity TMS in our study. These findings support the results of previous studies (2,3).

The pathophysiology leading to the clinical manifestations of focal dystonia remains obscure. Our finding of the shortening of SP in patients with focal dystonia may indicate an impairment of the mechanisms of inhibitory motor control, as previously reported (2–4,29,31,32). Although the mechanisms of SP are not precisely known, cortical SP is currently attributed to the activation of intracortical inhibitory circuits, with spinal mechanisms participating only in the early part (13–15,37). Moreover, an exclusive cortical origin of the SP, especially for the facial muscle SP, was also suggested (3,38,39). Therefore, abnormalities of SP in our focal dystonia patients occur at cortical level. In general, a short SP could be the result of reduced excitability of cortical inhibitory interneurons as a consequence of dysfunction in the motor cortex or of reduced facilitation of inhibitory interneurons from subcortical or other cortical structures (3). The shortening of the SP was also reported in patients with brain damage involving the primary motor cortex (39,40) and in patients with Parkinson's disease (19,41). Since motor cortex lesions are unlikely in focal dystonia, the shortening of the SP in our patients is probably due to an altered basal ganglia output influencing the activity of intracortical inhibitory interneurons, as in patients with Parkinson's disease. A decrease of intracortical inhibition with paired stimuli TMS has also been reported in patients with task-specific dystonia (2,3,5,29, 30). However there have been conflicting results on this subject (4,32).

Although impairment of the cortical mechanisms of motor control assessed by single- and double-pulse TMS has been demonstrated in the affected muscles of different types of focal dystonia (2–5,29–33), our findings suggest that disturbance of the cortical inhibitory control may be more widespread than clinical symptoms of the disease. Other groups have also provided some evidence for the existence of a generalized disturbance of the inhibitory system in focal dystonia (2–4,32,33). Bilateral impairment of the inhibitory mechanisms occurring after the period of postexcitatory inhibition revealed by paired TMS in patients with unilateral task-specific dystonia has been reported (4,5). The shortening of the SP in bilateral cervical muscles in patients with spasmodic torticollis has been elicited with high-intensity TMS (2). The delay of SP onset was found in the sternocleidomastoid muscle of both the affected and unaffected side of patients with torticollis (32). Curra et al. (3) found a shortened SP in cranial districts not involved in cranial dystonia and suggested more widespread impairment of the cortical inhibitory mechanisms. In addition to affected muscles, we found the shortening of the SP in cranial muscles of patients with cervical dystonia and in perioral muscles of patients with blepharospasm. If the abnormality of the central mechanisms is more generalized than is apparent in focal dystonias, the question that arises is how far these changes extend beyond the clinically affected site. In the present study, the duration of the SP in the hand muscle in patients with blepharospasm and cervical dystonia did not differ significantly from that of the control group.

Schwenkreis et al. (34) have also reported the lack of any difference between cervical dystonia patients and controls in SP duration by TMS from the hand muscle. Therefore, these findings may indicate that there may be a somatotopy of impairment of the inhibitory mechanisms related to the site of maximal dystonic symptoms, so that the motor control of the body parts relatively distant from the clinically affected site would be less influenced than those that are closer.

In previous studies, a positive correlation between SP duration and the degree of neurologic disability has been reported (2). Curra et al. (3) suggested that the greater SP shortening observed in patients with blepharospasm plus oromandibular dystonia than in patients with blepharospasm alone is likely to be related to the greater severity of dystonia. Although we could not find any correlation with the TWSTRS scores in patients with cervical dystonia, there was an inverse correlation between SP duration and the degree of neurologic disability in patients with blepharospasm.

Reduced spinal cord and brainstem inhibition is a common finding in dystonia (42). In blink reflex recovery curve studies, inhibition of the brainstem circuits mediating the R2 response was found to be reduced in patients with blepharospasm (6–10). Moreover, the same abnormality was also found in patients with cranial and cervical dystonia whose dystonia spares the orbicularis oculi muscle (6–10,24,25). In patients with focal arm dystonia, however, excitability of the blink reflex R2 response was found to be normal in these studies. Therefore, the results of the present study parallel the results of blink reflex recovery curve studies in focal dystonia. In a recent study, Sommer et al. (43) found that the intracortical inhibition is inversely and significantly correlated with R2 inhibition. They concluded that the correlation of intracortical inhibitory interneurons and ipsilateral blink reflex interneurons may indicate a common influence, possibly from basal ganglia, on either circuit, or a direct influence of cortical circuits on brainstem circuits via corticopontine pathways. Our results may support the idea that abnormality of motoneuronal inhibition in the brainstem, which has been demonstrated by blink reflex studies, is most likely the consequence of abnormal commands descending from cortical areas.

In conclusion, the present study provides further evidence for widespread changes in the activity of cortical inhibitory interneurons responsible for the generation of postexcitatory inhibition in focal dystonia. Abnormalities outside the clinically involved territory may represent an underlying predisposition to dystonia or subclinical alterations in focal dystonia. Because of parallelism with the results of blink reflex recovery curve studies, our results indicate a possible correlation of intracortical inhibition and brainstem interneuronal activity. Recently, existence of an inverse correlation between intracortical and brainstem inhibition has been reported in healthy subjects (43). Therefore, our findings may also support the idea that focal dystonia is a consequence of an abnormal supraspinal command signal rather than a primary disorder of spinal and brainstem circuitry.

REFERENCES

1. Fahn S. Generalized dystonia. In: Tsui JKC, Calne DB, eds. *Handbook of dystonia.* New York: Marcel Dekker, 1995:193–211.
2. Amadio S, Panizza M, Pisana F, et al. Transcranial magnetic stimulation and silent period in spasmodic torticollis. *Am J Phys Med Rehabil* 2000;79:361–368.
3. Curra A, Romaniello A, Berardelli A, et al. Shortened cortical silent period in facial muscles of patients with cranial dystonia. *Neurology* 2000;54:130–135.
4. Rona S, Berardelli A, Inghilleri M, et al. Alterations of motor cortical inhibition in patients with dystonia. *Mov Disord* 1998;13:118–124.
5. Ridding MC, Sheean G, Rothwell JC, et al. Changes in the balance between motor cortical excitation and inhibition in focal, task specific dystonia. *J Neurol Neurosurg Psychiatry* 1995;59:493–498.
6. Eekhof JL, Aramideh M, Bour LJ, et al. Blink reflex recovery curves in blepharospasm, torticollis spasmodica, and hemifacial spasm. *Muscle Nerve* 1996;19:10–15.
7. Nakashima K, Rothwell JC, Thompson PD, et al. The blink reflex in patients with idiopathic torsion dystonia. *Arch Neurol* 1990;47:413–416.
8. Tolosa E, Montserrat L, Bayes OA. Blink reflex studies in focal dystonias: enhanced excitability of brainstem interneurons in cranial dystonia and spasmodic torticollis. *Mov Disord* 1988;3:61–69.

9. Pauletti G, Berardelli A, Cruccu G, et al. Blink reflex and the masseter inhibitory reflex in patients with dystonia. *Mov Disord* 1993;8:495–500.

10. Panizza M, Lelli S, Nilsson J, et al. H reflex recovery curve and reciprocal inhibition of H reflex in different kinds of dystonia. *Neurology* 1990;40:824–828.

11. Hallet M. Transcranial magnetic stimulation: negative effects. *Adv Neurol* 1995;67:107–113.

12. Rossini PM, Barker AT, Berardelli A, et al. Non-invasive electrical and magnetic stimulation of the brain, spinal cord and roots: basic principles and procedures for routine clinical application. Report of an IFCN committee. *Electroencephalogr Clin Neurophysiol* 1994;91: 79–92.

13. Brasil-Neto JP, Cammarota J, Valls-Sole J, et al. Role of intracortical mechanisms in the late part of the silent period to transcranial stimulation of the human motor cortex. *Acta Neurol Scand* 1995;92:383–386.

14. Roick H, Von Giesen HJ, Benecke R. On the origin of the postexcitatory inhibition seen after transcranial magnetic brain stimulation in awake human subjects. *Exp Brain Res* 1993;94:489–498.

15. Inghilleri M, Berardelli A, Cruccu G, et al. Silent period evoked by transcranial magnetic stimulation of the human motor cortex and cervicomedullary junction. *J Physiol* 1993;466:521–534.

16. Siebner HR, Dressnandt J, Auer C, et al. Continuous intrathecal baclofen infusions induced a marked increase of the transcranially evoked silent period in a patient with generalized dystonia. *Muscle Nerve* 1998;21: 1209–1212.

17. Werhahn KJ, Kunesch E, Noachtar S, et al. Differential effects on motorcortical inhibition induced by blockade of GABA uptake in humans. *J Physiol* 1999;517: 591–597.

18. Nakashima K, Wang Y, Shimoda M, et al. Shortened silent period produced by magnetic cortical stimulation in patients with Parkinson's disease. *J Neurol Sci* 1995; 130(2):209–214.

19. Priori A, Berardelli A, Inghilleri M, et al. Motor cortical inhibition and the dopaminergic system. *Brain* 1994; 117:317–323.

20. Priori A, Berardelli A, Inghilleri M, et al. Electromyographic silent period after transcranial brain stimulation in Huntington's disease. *Mov Disord* 1994;9:178–182.

21. Ridding MC, Inzelberg R, Rothwell JC. Changes in excitability of motor cortical circuitry in patients with Parkinson's disease. *Ann Neurol* 1995;37:181–188.

22. Modugno N, Curra A, Giovannelli M, et al. The prolonged cortical silent period in patients with Huntington's disease. *Clin Neurophysiol* 2001;112:1470–1474.

23. Aramideh M, Eekhof JLA, Bour LJ, et al. Electromyography and recovery of the blink reflex in involuntary eyelid closure: a comparative study. *J Neurol Neurosurg Psychiatry* 1995;58:692–698.

24. Berardelli A, Rothwell JC, Day BL, et al. Pathophysiology of cranial dystonia. *Adv Neurol* 1988;50:525–535.

25. Cohen LG, Ludlow CL, Warsden M, et al. Blink reflex excitability recovery curves in patients with spasmodic dysphonia. *Neurology* 1989;39:572–577.

26. Valls-Sole J, Hallett M. Modulation of electromyographic activity of wrist flexor and extensor muscles in patients with writer's cramp. *Mov Disord* 1995;10: 741–748.

27. Cruccu G, Pauletti G, Agostino R, et al. Masseter inhibitory reflex in movement disorders. Huntington's chorea, Parkinson's disease, dystonia and unilateral masticatory spasm. *Electroencephalogr Clin Neurophysiol* 1991;81:24–30.

28. Nakashima K, Thompson PD, Rothwell JC, et al. An exteroceptive reflex in the sternocleidomastoid muscle produced by electrical stimulation of the supraorbital nerve in normal subjects and patients with spasmodic torticollis. *Neurology* 1989;39:1354–1358.

29. Chen R, Wassermann EM, Canos M, et al. Impaired inhibition in writer's cramp during voluntary muscle activation. *Neurology* 1997;49:1054–1059.

30. Ikoma K, Samii A, Mercuri B, et al. Abnormal cortical motor excitability in dystonia. *Neurology* 1996;46: 1371–1376.

31. Mavroudakis N, Caroyer JM, Brunko E, et al. Abnormal motor evoked responses to transcranial magnetic stimulation in focal dystonia. *Neurology* 1995;45:1671–1677.

32. Curra A, Berardelli A, Rona S, et al. Excitability of motor cortex in patients with dystonia. *Adv Neurol* 1998:78:33–40.

33. Odergren T, Rimpilainen I, Borg J. Sternocleidomastoid muscle responses to transcranial magnetic stimulation in patients with cervical dystonia. *Electroencephalogr Clin Neurophysiol* 1997;105:44–52.

34. Schwenkreis P, Vorgerd M, Malin JP, et al. Assessment of postexcitatory inhibition in patients with focal dystonia. *Acta Neurol Scand* 1999;100:260–264.

35. Elston JS. The management of blepharospasm and hemifacial spasm. *J Neurol* 1992;239:5–8.

36. Consky ES, Basinski A, Belle L, et al. The Toronto Western Spasmodic Torticollis Rating Scale (TW-STRS): assessment of validity and inter-rater reliability. *Neurology* 1990;40(suppl):445.

37. Fuhr P, Agostino R, Hallett M. Spinal motor neuron excitability during the silent period after cortical stimulation. *Electroencephalogr Clin Neurophysiol* 1991;81: 257–262.

38. Cruccu G, Inghilleri M, Berardelli A, et al. Cortical mechanisms mediating the inhibitory period after magnetic stimulation of the facial motor area. *Muscle Nerve* 1997;20:418–424.

39. Schnitzler A, Benecke R. The silent period after transcranial magnetic stimulation is of exclusive cortical origin: evidence from isolated cortical ischemic lesions in man. *Neurosci Lett* 1994;180:41–45.

40. von Giesen HJ, Roick H, Benecke R. Inhibitory actions of motor cortex following unilateral brain lesions as studied by magnetic brain stimulation. *Exp Brain Res* 1994;99:84–96.

41. Cantello R, Gianelli M, Bettucci D, et al. Parkinson's disease rigidity: magnetic motor evoked potentials in a small hand muscle. *Neurology* 1991;41:1449–1456.

42. Berardelli A, Rothwell JC, Hallett M, et al. The pathophysiology of primary dystonia. *Brain* 1998;121: 1195–1212.

43. Sommer M, Heise A, Tergau F, et al. Inverse correlation of intracortical inhibition and brain-stem inhibition in humans. *Clin Neurophysiol* 2002;113:120–123.

Dystonia 4: Advances in Neurology, Vol. 94. Edited by Stanley Fahn, Mark Hallett, and Mahlon R. DeLong. Lippincott Williams & Wilkins, Philadelphia © 2004.

6

Modulation of Cortical Activity by Repetitive Transcranial Magnetic Stimulation (rTMS): A Review of Functional Imaging Studies and the Potential Use in Dystonia

*Saša R. Filipović, †Hartwig R. Siebner, ‡James B. Rowe, §Carla Cordivari, ‖Willibald Gerschlager, ¶John C. Rothwell, **Richard S. J. Frackowiak, and ¶Kailash P. Bhatia

*Sobell Department of Motor Neuroscience and Movement Disorders, London, and Burden Neurological Institute, Bristol, United Kingdom. †Sobell Department of Motor Neuroscience and Movement Disorders, London, United Kingdom and Department of Neurology, Christian-Albrechts-University, Kiel, Germany. ‡National Hospital for Neurology, London and Wellcome Department of Imaging Neuroscience, London, United Kingdom. §Division of Neurophysiology, Institute of Neurology, University College London, United Kingdom. ‖Sobell Department of Motor Neuroscience and Movement Disorders, London, United Kingdom and Department of Neurology, University of Vienna, Vienna, Austria. ¶Sobell Department of Motor Neuroscience and Movement Disorders, London, United Kingdom. **Wellcome Department of Imaging Neuroscience, London, United Kingdom*

FUNCTIONAL IMAGING STUDIES IN DYSTONIA

During the last decade, functional imaging studies have provided important new insights into the pathophysiology of primary (idiopathic) dystonia. Basically, there were two types of studies that examined two different aspects of dystonia pathophysiology. A first group of studies focused on underlying dysfunctions that were independent of the manifestation of dystonia. Initial positron emission tomography (PET) studies using 18-fluorodeoxyglucose (FDG), which have looked at regional glucose utilization at rest, did not find any consistent difference in regional metabolism between patients with primary dystonia and normal subjects (1–3). Similarly, using FDG PET, Eidelberg et al. (4) were also not able to detect any significant difference in metabolism at rest between patients with idiopathic dystonia (although the majority of them being with the action-induced type) and a control group of healthy subjects. However, by applying a statistical model of regional metabolic covariation on FDG-PET data at rest, they were able to demonstrate what they called "a significant topographic profile characterized by relative bilateral increases in the metabolic activity" in the premotor cortex (PMC) and supplementary motor area (SMA), "associated with relative covariate hypermetabolism" of the lentiform nucleus, pons, and midbrain, contralaterally. In addition, subject scores for this covariance profile correlated significantly with ratings on a dystonia severity scale. Interestingly, a pattern of increased metabolism in basal ganglia, thalamus, and premotor-motor cortex at rest has been independently found by FDG-PET in patients with isolated cervical dystonia (5).

Other studies explored the neuronal substrate of motor dysfunction in dystonia. Instead of looking at neuronal activity at rest, activation PET studies with ^{15}O-labeled water (H$_2$^{15}O PET), which measure cerebral blood flow as an index of neuronal metabolic activity, have been looking at whether there is an abnormal activation pattern related to the execution of various movements and tasks. Compared with healthy controls, the movement-related activation during freely selected joystick movements in patients with both generalized and focal arm primary dystonia has been found to be increased in the striatum and its frontal lobe association projection areas [including PMC and dorsolateral prefrontal cortex (DLPFC)] (6,7). This was accompanied by a decrease in activation in executive motor areas, such as the primary sensorimotor cortex (6,7). However, some other studies, using different motor tasks, were not able to confirm movement-related overactivation in frontal premotor areas (8,9). The inconsistency has opened a debate as to whether frontal overactivity exists in dystonia, and if so, whether it is the cause of dystonic contraction or is a mere reflection of compensatory mechanisms to overcome difficulties in task performance due to motor impairment imposed by dystonia.[1]

---

[1]The results of activation functional imaging studies of movement disorders are generally vulnerable to the ambiguities in interpretation due to methodologic problems caused by the very nature of these diseases. Patients with movement disorders are often unable to accomplish satisfactory muscle relaxation at rest. Also, regarding task performance, it was usually difficult to accurately match perceived level of task difficulty as well as the quality of performance between healthy controls and patients with dystonia during task. Therefore, it has been claimed that the observed differences between healthy subjects and patients may be caused only by the differences in their motor performances. However, this is basically a "which came first, chicken or egg" type of problem. It is questionable whether it is possible at all to study physiologic mechanisms behind symptoms of movement disorders without evoking symptoms and differences in performance themselves.

Although the issue is not unequivocally resolved yet, there is some evidence to suggest that the overactivation is not merely compensatory. Based on the data from regional metabolic covariation analysis, the relative overactivity of the basal ganglia–thalamocortical network, including the PMC, has been suggested to be present even at rest (4). The reduction of dystonic contractions and easing of writing in patients with writer's cramp following botulinum toxin injection was not accompanied by comparable changes in PMC activation (10). Finally, the PMC overactivation has not been observed during performance of various tasks, including the free-selection joystick movements, in patients with other diseases associated with impaired motor performance such as amyotrophic lateral sclerosis (11), cerebellar degeneration (12), and Huntington's disease (13). In this regard, it has to be noted that while in studies of dystonia that detected an overactivation in PMC (6,7) a random selection of joystick movements was used as a task, all studies that failed to detect this overactivation (8,9) used simple motor tasks such as tapping and tonic contraction as well as repeated writing of a simple sentence/word (i.e., stereotyped writing). It is reasonable to assume that predominantly automatic and overlearned tasks such as stereotyped writing, which usually do not activate premotor and prefrontal structures too much (14), most probably are not able to activate these cortical regions to the level necessary for displaying abnormalities (10). In addition, in one of the studies that did not detect significant PMC overactivation in writer's cramp patients during writing (8), a significant correlation between duration and increased difficulty of writing and increase in PMC perfusion was nonetheless detected. Furthermore, a recent functional magnetic resonance imaging (fMRI) study (15) found significantly increased activation of the PMC, together with thalamus (nucleus ventralis lateralis) and cerebellar vermis, during writing in comparison to rest in writer's cramp patients, which was not present in healthy controls. However, the magnitude of this difference seemed not to be very large, and the difference was not significant in a direct comparison between groups (15).

Whatever is the case regarding proposed PMC overactivation in dystonia, it remains true that the area is one of the principal "nodes" within the complex basal ganglia–thalamocortical network for fine movement control. The relative insufficiency of inhibitory mechanisms within this network is thought to be a principal physiologic impairment in dystonia (16,17). The fact that the PMC is close to the scalp makes this area a valid candidate for any attempts to accomplish transcranial modulation of the network activity.

MODULATION OF BRAIN ACTIVITY BY REPETITIVE TRANSCRANIAL MAGNETIC STIMULATION (RTMS)

Transcranial Magnetic Stimulation

Transcranial magnetic stimulation (TMS) is a noninvasive technique for painless transcutaneous and transcranial excitation of the neural structures underlying the stimulating magnetic coil. It is based on the phenomenon that a short but powerful magnetic pulse delivered at the surface of the scalp is able to induce electrical currents in the nearby neural tissue (18). At a sufficient strength of the stimulation, single TMS pulses are able to induce both excitatory (e.g., muscle twitch if appropriate area of motor cortex is stimulated) and inhibitory (e.g., short arrest in ongoing muscle contraction) effects. The relative ease of application and ability to generate relatively robust data have made TMS an indispensable tool in clinical neuroscience research (19).

Repetitive application of TMS stimuli over the same area (repetitive TMS, rTMS) has been shown to be able to modulate the excitability of the motor cortex beyond the period of stimulation (20). Increased excitability usually occurs if higher frequencies (above 5 Hz) are used (21). By contrast, a decrease in excitability has been shown if low frequency (≤1 Hz) trains are given for 5 minutes or more. This has been

shown not only for the motor cortex (22–24), but for the visual cortex also (25).[2] The mechanism involved is not known, but the stimulation rate is similar to that producing long-term depression in animal studies (26). These observations of effects of rTMS have formed the basis for several studies that demonstrated the potential therapeutic effect of rTMS in depression and obsessive-compulsive disorders that was able to outlast stimulation for up to several weeks (27,28).

Effects of Repetitive Transcranial Magnetic Stimulation

Transcranial Doppler Studies

The ability of rTMS to induce hemisphere and large-intracranial-vessel specific changes in blood flow velocity (BFV) has been documented in several studies using transcranial Doppler measurements. Single trains of high-frequency rTMS applied over motor (29,30), frontal (31), or occipital (32) cortices were able to induce transient but significant BFV increases in respective large intracranial blood vessels with latency that was consistently around only 3.5 seconds after the onset of the rTMS train. The effect was clearly literalized and was not associated with change in any of the global hemodynamic parameters, thus suggesting local intracerebral vasodilation due to increased metabolic demand as the main cause. The opposite has been shown for low-frequency rTMS. The short (5 minutes) train of the 0.9-Hz rTMS over DLPFC induced a significant reduction of BFV in the ipsilateral middle cerebral artery (33).

Functional Imaging Studies

Functional imaging studies of the after-effects of rTMS by either single photon emission computed tomography (SPECT) or PET

---

[2]Besides from frequency of stimulus delivery, the net effect on the excitability of the targeted neural tissue is also dependent on strength and the number of the stimuli, as well as on the pattern of their delivery (e.g., number and duration of the stimuli trains, the length of the intertrain intervals) (27).

were predominantly concerned with elucidating the mechanisms behind potential therapeutic effects of rTMS over DLPFC in depression. Nevertheless, together with rare studies dedicated to the analysis of effects in healthy subjects, they have provided valuable data that allowed further descriptions of rTMS effects on brain metabolism and blood flow in general. For example, following 6 minutes of subthreshold 5-Hz rTMS over the left motor cortex, brain metabolism (FDG-PET) significantly increased in the stimulated area (34). A short (500 stimuli long) train of 5-, 10-, or 20-Hz subthreshold rTMS over the left DLPFC induced a significant increase in SPECT-derived scores of functional connectivity in the DLPFC–caudate nucleus loop on the left (35). However, a significant blood flow increase (SPECT) in the stimulated cortical region was found when high-frequency rTMS had been delivered for 5 days or more over the left DLPFC (36,37). Moreover, an $H_2^{15}O$ PET study has found a significant increase in blood flow of the PFC even 3 days after ten daily treatments with 20-Hz threshold rTMS (1,600 stimuli per session) (38). The aforementioned effects of high-frequency rTMS were mainly evaluated in studies of depressed patients (35–38), but some of them were carried on in normal subjects as well (34).

The effect of low-frequency rTMS has been studied proportionally rarely, and only in depressed patients. From the results of the neurophysiologic studies, effects opposite those of the high-frequency rTMS were expected. However, following 30 minutes of 1-Hz subthreshold rTMS over the left DLPFC, a significant reduction of metabolic activation (FGD-PET) was not found in the targeted area but only in the nearby left superior frontal gyrus (39). Similarly, 3 days after ten daily treatments with 1-Hz threshold rTMS (1,600 stimuli per session) over the left DLPFC, a significant decrease in blood flow (measured by $H_2^{15}O$ PET) was not found in the stimulated cortical area but contralaterally in the right DLPFC (38). The slightly disappointing results of low-frequency rTMS in comparison to the high-frequency rTMS regarding modulating cerebral blood flow (CBF) and metabolism in the targeted area may be partially explained by the fact that all low-frequency rTMS studies so far were carried out on depressed patients. Depressed patients generally tend to have relative hypoperfusion and hypometabolism in the targeted DLPFC (40), thus leaving rTMS reduced room for action.

It is of interest that in all PET studies, the rTMS effects were not restricted to the stimulated area only. During short trains of 10-Hz rTMS over the frontal eye field, a significant regional CBF (rCBF) increase not only in the targeted area but also in the functionally connected areas of the parieto-occipital cortex ipsilaterally and superior parietal cortex bilaterally has been found (41). Moreover, the metabolic effects in remote areas were found to persist even beyond the time of stimulation. Six minutes of high-frequency stimulation of the motor cortex elicited an increase of activation in the contralateral motor cortex and the supplementary motor area also (34). Similarly, ten daily treatments with high-frequency stimulation of the DLPFC induced an additional increase of activation in several other brain areas including the contralateral DLPFC, cingulate gyrus, amygdala, insula, basal ganglia, uncus, hippocampus, parahippocampus, thalamus, and cerebellum (38). Moreover, a unique ligand-PET study of rTMS effect on the brain dopaminergic activity has detected an increase in raclopride binding (an indicator of increased dopamine release) in the ipsilateral anterior caudate after high-frequency rTMS over the DLPFC (42). On the other hand, a single session of low-frequency rTMS over the left DLPFC induced a decrease of activation not only in the right DLPFC, but also in the bilateral anterior cingulate, basal ganglia (more ipsi- than contralaterally), hypothalamus, midbrain, and cerebellum (39). Three days after ten daily treatments with 1-Hz rTMS over the left DLPFC, a significant decrease in blood flow was found not only in the contralateral DLPFC, but also in the ipsilateral medial temporal cortex, basal ganglia, and amygdala (38).

USE OF REPETITIVE TRANSCRANIAL MAGNETIC STIMULATION IN DYSTONIA

Recently, low-frequency rTMS of the left motor cortex has been shown to improve symptoms of writer's cramp (43). Twenty minutes after 1-Hz subthreshold rTMS delivered for 30 minutes, half of the 16 patients studied reported marked or moderate improvement that lasted more than 3 hours. Nothing similar has been observed after "sham" rTMS used as a form of placebo. In addition, objective improvement in several physiologic parameters of motor cortex excitability as well as in quantitative parameters of writing was demonstrated (43). In a companion study, the authors applied the same rTMS intervention while patients scribbled with their right hand (44). This approach resulted in a more consistent clinical improvement, presumably because the network involved in task-specific dystonia was more susceptible to rTMS during scribbling.

The rationale for using rTMS on the motor cortex was that values of several neurophysiologic parameters of cortical excitability in dystonia point toward the existence of abnormally increased excitation and/or reduced inhibition in the motor cortex in this disorder (16). The probable consequence of this net hyperexcitability is that motor commands are no longer focused appropriately on muscles involved in a task, resulting in excessive involuntary activity during attempted movement. Since slow-frequency rTMS appears to reduce cortical excitability, and if this is accomplished by increasing the activity of inhibitory systems, it should be able to boost cortical inhibition in dystonia and thereby improve its symptoms. Indeed, the neurophysiologic parameters of cortical inhibition did improve following 30 minutes of low-frequency rTMS over the motor cortex (43).

However, the functional imaging data suggest that, besides the primary sensorimotor cortex, there may be other potential targets for rTMS. The metabolic abnormalities in the PMC make this area a potentially interesting target as well. Moreover, it is conceivable that in previous rTMS studies, some of the effects of rTMS delivered over the motor cortex may have been produced by a spread of effective stimulation toward the PMC. This notion is supported by a recent study that has shown that low-frequency rTMS delivered over dorsal PMC (DPMC) seems to be more effective in inducing a decrease of corticospinal excitability than rTMS delivered directly over the motor cortex itself (45).

A PET activation study that explored this option was recently completed and published in abstract form (46,47). The modulation of cortical activity induced by low-frequency rTMS delivered over the left DPMC in a group of patients with primary arm dystonia and healthy subjects was evaluated. This was a single-blinded placebo-controlled crossover study. Intervention ("real" rTMS) was 30 minutes of the subthreshold low-frequency (1-Hz) rTMS over the left DPMC. Placebo ("sham" rTMS) was done using the same parameters but with a specially designed sham coil that induced no magnetic field but evoked a comparable acoustic artifact. The aftereffects of rTMS were assessed by consecutive H_2O^{15} PET measurements of rCBF at rest and during a motor task. Data were analyzed using a general linear model and was based on a $2 \times 2 \times 2$ factorial study design that included covariates for disease *group* (patient vs. control), *task* (active vs. rest), and *rTMS* (real vs. sham). During the "active" *task* condition, subjects were required to randomly press one of the four button-keys corresponding to the fingers II to V of their right hand. Patients with dystonia did not differ significantly from controls in terms of motor performance and movement-related functional brain activation. However, the main contrast of "real" versus "sham" rTMS revealed that real rTMS significantly reduced rCBF in both active and rest conditions in the stimulated area (i.e., the left DPMC). Moreover, the effect was much greater in dystonic patients than controls, which was confirmed by a significant *group* by *rTMS* interaction.

Results of this study (46,47) provided the strongest proof so far of the ability of low-frequency rTMS to induce significant and sustained reduction of blood flow in the targeted cortical area. Several factors may have contributed to the greater strength of this study. First, instead of exclusively depressed patients, healthy subjects, together with patients with dystonia, were studied. Most probably, this allowed more room for a potential suppressive effect of low-frequency rTMS to be expressed. Second, DPMC as a target for rTMS has some important methodologic advantages over the DLPFC that has been so far targeted in all functional imaging studies of low-frequency rTMS. Due to the lack of easily observable and measurable direct output from the DLPFC, it is difficult to define physiologically the exact target spot for rTMS, as well as the appropriate values for the intensity and the number of stimulations.[3] This is not the case for DPMC. Due to the area's proximity and direct functional links with M1, it can be easily, quickly, and consistently identified in every subject. In addition, due to functional and structural similarities between M1 and PMC, the stimulus intensity can be determined using the motor cortex thresholds as a guide.

Similarly to previous rTMS-PET studies, in the latest study (47), besides the targeted area, a significant decrease of rCBF was also found in functionally interconnected cortical areas including the contralateral PMC as well as the SMA and primary sensorimotor cortex bilaterally. However, perhaps the most exciting part of the results was the finding that the rTMS induced a significant decrease of rCBF in subcortical areas, namely the ipsilateral thalamus and putamen as well. These results provide further support for the theory that rTMS physiologic and clinical effects are caused not only by modulation of activity in the directly stimulated areas, but also by modulation of activity within functional networks in which the targeted area has an active role.

Moreover, the fact that a significantly larger suppressive effect of low-frequency rTMS has been found in dystonia patients than in healthy subjects suggests that more active networks are more prone to modulation by rTMS (17).

USE OF REPETITIVE TRANSCRANIAL MAGNETIC STIMULATION IN DYSTONIA TREATMENT

Regarding the potential use of low-frequency rTMS as a treatment for dystonia, several factors have to be borne in mind. The experience with another, clinically proven, therapeutic procedure, based on physiologic modulation within the same neuronal network (i.e., deep-brain stimulation of the pallidus), has shown that it may take several days, weeks, or even months for any clear clinical benefit to appear in patients with dystonia (49). It is therefore of no surprise that following a single, comparatively short exposure to rTMS, the observable clinical benefits were absent or only partially present and short-lasting, despite a pronounced physiologic effect (43,47). Likewise, in the other diseases where rTMS has demonstrated some sustainable clinical effect (such as major depression, obsessive-compulsive disorders, epilepsy, and myoclonus), repeated application over several days has been needed (27). There is also physiologic evidence for a buildup of the effect over consecutive days of application, even in normal subjects (50). Given our lack of precise understanding of a link between measurable neurophysiologic changes and clinical phenomenology of dystonia (16), to determine the potential clinical usefulness and effectiveness of rTMS it may be necessary to deliver it over several consecutive days.

CONCLUSION

There is a substantial body of evidence showing that rTMS is able to induce sustainable plastic changes in central nervous system functional networks and that low-frequency

[3]There are no objective measures of threshold for other cortical areas than motor and visual cortex, nor is there any correlation between thresholds of the two (48).

rTMS potentially may be able to modulate the activity within the basal ganglia–thalamocortical motor networks in patients with dystonia. Although the duration of effects of rTMS remains uncertain, rTMS offers an exciting new perspective for possible therapeutic intervention in dystonia and other movement disorders.

REFERENCES

1. Gilman S, Junck L, Young AB, et al. Cerebral metabolic activity in idiopathic dystonia studied with positron emission tomography. In: Fahn S, Marsden CD, Calne DB, eds. *Dystonia 2. Advances in neurology,* vol 50. New York: Raven Press, 1988:231–236.
2. Lang AE, Garnett ES, Firnau G, et al. Positron tomography in dystonia. In: Fahn S, Marsden CD, Calne DB, eds. *Dystonia 2. Advances in neurology,* vol 50. New York: Raven Press, 1988:249–253.
3. Martin WRW, Stoessl AJ, Palmer A, et al. PET scanning in dystonia. In: Fahn S, Marsden CD, Calne DB, eds. *Dystonia 2. Advances in neurology,* vol 50. New York: Raven Press, 1988:223–229.
4. Eidelberg D, Moeller JR, Ishikawa T, et al. The metabolic topography of idiopathic torsion dystonia. *Brain* 1995;118:1473–1484.
5. Galardi G, Perani D, Grassi F, et al. Basal ganglia and thalamo-cortical hypermetabolism in patients with spasmodic torticollis. *Acta Neurol Scand* 1996;94: 172–176.
6. Ceballos-Baumann AO, Passingham RE, Warner T, et al. Overactive prefrontal and underactive motor cortical areas in idiopathic dystonia. *Ann Neurol* 1995;37: 363–372.
7. Playford ED, Passingham RE, Marsden CD, et al. Increased activation of frontal areas during arm movement in idiopathic torsion dystonia. *Mov Disord* 1998; 13:309–318.
8. Odergren T, Stone-Elander S, Ingvar M. Cerebral and cerebellar activation in correlation to the action-induced dystonia in writer's cramp. *Mov Disord* 1998;13: 497–508.
9. Ibañez V, Sadato N, Karp B, et al. Deficient activation of the motor cortical network in patients with writer's cramp. *Neurology* 1999;53:96–105.
10. Ceballos-Baumann AO, Sheean G, Passingham RE, et al. Botulinum toxin does not reverse the cortical dysfunction associated with writer's cramp. A PET study. *Brain* 1997;120:571–582.
11. Kew JJ, Leigh PN, Playford ED, et al. Cortical function in amyotrophic lateral sclerosis. A positron emission tomography study. *Brain* 1993;116:655–680.
12. Wessel K, Zeffiro T, Lou JS, et al. Regional cerebral blood flow during a self-paced sequential finger opposition task in patients with cerebellar degeneration. *Brain* 1995;118:379–393.
13. Weeks RA, Ceballos-Baumann A, Piccini P, et al. Cortical control of movement in Huntington's disease. A PET activation study. *Brain* 1997;120:1569–1578.
14. Siebner HR, Limmer C, Peinemann A, et al. Brain correlates of fast and slow handwriting in humans: a PET-performance correlation analysis. *Eur J Neurosci* 2001;14:726–736.
15. Preibisch C, Berg D, Hofmann E, et al. Cerebral activation patterns in patients with writer's cramp: a functional magnetic resonance imaging study. *J Neurol* 2001;248:10–17.
16. Berardelli A, Rothwell JC, Hallett M, et al. The pathophysiology of primary dystonia. *Brain* 1998;121: 1195–1212.
17. Vitek JL. Pathophysiology of dystonia: a neuronal model. *Mov Disord* 2002;17:S49–62.
18. Rothwell JC. Techniques and mechanisms of action of transcranial stimulation of the human motor cortex. *J Neurosci Meth* 1997;74:113–122.
19. Pascual-Leone A, Walsh V, Rothwell JC. Transcranial magnetic stimulation in cognitive neuroscience—virtual lesion, chronometry, and functional connectivity. *Curr Opin Neurobiol* 2000;10:232–237.
20. Pascual-Leone A, Tormos JM, Keenan J, et al. Study and modulation of human cortical excitability with transcranial magnetic stimulation. *J Clin Neurophysiol* 1998;15:333–343.
21. Pascual-Leone A, Valls-Sole J, Wassermann EM, et al. Responses to rapid-rate transcranial magnetic stimulation of the human motor cortex. *Brain* 1994;117: 847–858.
22. Chen R, Classen J, Gerloff C, et al. Depression of motor cortex excitability by low-frequency transcranial magnetic stimulation. *Neurology* 1997;48:1398–1403.
23. Maeda F, Keenan JP, Tormos JM, et al. Modulation of corticospinal excitability by repetitive transcranial magnetic stimulation. *Clin Neurophysiol* 2000;111: 800–805.
24. Muellbacher W, Ziemann U, Boroojerdi B, et al. Effects of low-frequency transcranial magnetic stimulation on motor excitability and basic motor behaviour. *Clin Neurophysiol* 2000;111:1002–1007.
25. Boroojerdi B, Prager A, Muellbacher W, et al. Reduction of human visual cortex excitability using 1-Hz transcranial magnetic stimulation. *Neurology* 2000;54: 1529–1531.
26. Post RM, Kimbrell T, Frye M, et al. Implications of kindling and quenching for the possible frequency dependence of rTMS. *CNS Spectrum* 1997;2:54–60.
27. Wassermann EM, Lisanby SH. Therapeutic application of repetitive transcranial magnetic stimulation: a review. *Clin Neurophysiol* 2001;112:1367–1377.
28. George MS, Lisanby SH, Sackeim HA. Transcranial magnetic stimulation. Applications in neuropsychiatry. *Arch Gen Psychiatry* 1999;56:300–311.
29. Sander D, Meyer BU, Röricht S, et al. Effect of hemisphere-selective magnetic brain stimulation on middle cerebral artery blood flow velocity. *Electroencephalogr Clin Neurophysiol* 1995;97:43–48.
30. Niehaus L, Röricht S, Scholz U, et al. Hemodynamic response to repetitive magnetic stimulation of the motor and visual cortex. In: Paulus W, Hallet M, Rossini PM, et al., eds. *Transcranial magnetic stimulation.* (EEG suppl 51.) Amsterdam: Elsevier Science, 1999:41–47.
31. Pecuch PW, Evers S, Folkerts HV, et al. The cerebral hemodynamics of repetitive transcranial magnetic stimulation. *Eur Arch Psychiatry Clin Neurosci* 2000;250: 320–324.
32. Sander D, Meyer BU, Röricht S, et al. Increase of posterior cerebral artery blood flow velocity during thre-

shold repetitive magnetic stimulation of the human visual cortex: hints for neuronal activation without cortical phosphens. *Electroencephalogr Clin Neurophysiol* 1996;99:473–478.

33. Rollnik JD, Dïsterhöft A, Däuper J, et al. Decrease of middle cerebral artery blood flow velocity after low-frequency repetitive transcranial magnetic stimulation of the dorsolateral prefrontal cortex. *Clin Neurophysiol* 2002;113:951–955.

34. Siebner HR, Peller M, Willoch F, et al. Lasting cortical activation after repetitive TMS of the motor cortex: a glucose metabolic study. *Neurology* 2000;54:956–963.

35. Shajahan PM, Glabus MF, Steele JD, et al. Left dorsolateral repetitive transcranial magnetic stimulation affects cortical excitability and functional connectivity, but does not impair cognition in major depression. *Prog Neuropsychopharmacol Biol Psychiatry* 2002;26: 945–954.

36. Nahas Z, Tenebeck CC, Kozel A, et al. Brain effects of TMS delivered over prefrontal cortex in depressed adults: role of stimulation frequency and coil-cortex distance. *Neuropsychiatry Clin Neurosci* 2001;13: 459–470.

37. Catafau AM, Perez V, Gironell A, et al. SPECT mapping of cerebral activity changes induced by repetitive transcranial magnetic stimulation in depressed patients. A pilot study. *Psychiatry Res Neuroimaging* 2001;106: 151–160.

38. Speer AM, Kimbrell TA, Wassermann EM, et al. Opposite effects of high and low frequency rTMS on regional brain activity in depressed patients. *Biol Psychiatry* 2000;48:1133–1141.

39. Kimbrell TA, Dunn RT, George MS, et al. Left prefrontal-repetitive transcranial magnetic stimulation (rTMS) and regional cerebral glucose metabolism in normal volunteers. *Psychiatry Res Neuroimaging* 2002; 115:101–113.

40. Mayberg HS. Depression. In: Mazziotta JC, Toga AW, Frackowiak RSJ, eds. *Brain mapping: the disorders.* San Diego: Academic Press, 2000:485–507.

41. Paus T, Jech R, Thompson CJ, et al. Transcranial magnetic stimulation during positron emission tomography: a new method for studying connectivity of the human cerebral cortex. *J Neurosci* 1997;17:3178–3184.

42. Strafella AP, Paus T, Barrett J, et al. Repetitive transcranial magnetic stimulation of the human prefrontal cortex induces dopamine release in the caudate nucleus. *J Neurosci* 2001;21:RC157.

43. Siebner HR, Tormos JM, Ceballos-Baumann AO, et al. Low-frequency repetitive transcranial magnetic stimulation of the motor cortex in writer's cramp. *Neurology* 1999;52:529–537.

44. Siebner HR, Auer C, Ceballos-Baumann AO, et al. Has repetitive transcranial magnetic stimulation of the primary motor hand area a therapeutic application in writer's cramp? In: Paulus W, Hallett M, Rossini PM, et al., eds. *Transcranial magnetic stimulation.* (EEG suppl. 51.) Amsterdam: Elsevier, 1999:265–275.

45. Gerschlager W, Siebner HR, Rothwell JC. Decreased corticospinal excitability after subthreshold 1 Hz rTMS over lateral premotor cortex. *Neurology* 2001;57: 449–455.

46. Filipovic SR, Siebner HR, Rowe JB, et al. Lasting suppression of the premotor cortical overactivity in arm dystonia by repetitive transcranial magnetic stimulation: a clinical and PET activation study. Preliminary data. *Mov Dis* 2002;17:1118–1119.

47. Siebner HR, Rowe JB, Filipovic SR, et al. Enhanced metabolic suppression of frontal motor areas after inhibitory repetitive TMS of the lateral premotor cortex in primary dystonia. *Mov Disord* 2002;17(suppl 5):S287.

48. Stewart LM, Walsh V, Rothwell JC. Motor and phosphene thresholds: a transcranial magnetic stimulation correlation study. *Neuropsychologia* 2001;39:415–419.

49. Krack P, Vercueil L. Review of the functional surgical treatment of dystonia. *Eur J Neurol* 2001;8:389–399.

50. Maeda F, Keenan JP, Tormos JM, et al. Interindividual variability of the modulatory effects of repetitive transcranial magnetic stimulation on cortical excitability. *Exp Brain Res* 2000;133:425–430.

Dystonia 4: Advances in Neurology, Vol. 94. Edited by Stanley Fahn, Mark Hallett, and Mahlon R. DeLong. Lippincott Williams & Wilkins, Philadelphia © 2004.

7

Dopamine Transmission in DYT1 Dystonia

*Sarah J. Augood, *Z. Hollingsworth, ††David S. Albers, ††Lichuan Yang, †Joanne Leung, †Xandra O. Breakefield, and *David G. Standaert

Center for Aging, Genetics, and Neurodegeneration, Massachusetts General Hospital, Charlestown, Massachusetts. †Molecular Neurogenetics Unit, Department of Neurology, Massachusetts General Hospital, Charlestown, Massachusetts; and Program in Neuroscience, Harvard Medical School, Boston, Massachusetts. ††Department of Neurology and Neurosciences, Weill Medical College of Cornell University, New York, New York

Most cases of early-onset generalized dystonia (Oppenheim's dystonia) are associated with the deletion of a glutamic acid residue within the protein coding region of the *TOR1A (DYT1)* gene (1). This gene encodes a novel protein termed torsinA. This 3 base-pair deletion in exon 5 of *TOR1A* is inherited as an autosomal-dominant condition with a low clinical penetrance, such that only approximately 30% of people carrying the *DYT1* deletion develop motor symptoms (2). The function of torsinA is currently unknown, although sequence homology studies have revealed a similarity with the AAA+ family of adenosine triphosphatases (ATPases) that perform chaperone-like functions and assist in protein trafficking and membrane fusion (see ref. 3 for review).

In general, the primary dystonias are not associated with overt neuronal degeneration or a prevalence of reactive gliosis, hampering the search for the anatomic foci for these neurologic disorders. However, genetics coupled with pharmacologic studies have led to the hypothesis that at least some forms of dystonia may arise from disturbances in dopamine signaling in the striatum. First, mutations within the tyrosine hydroxylase (TH) gene (4), and the guanosine triphosphate (GTP) cyclohydrolase gene (5), both of which limit dopamine synthesis, and within the dopamine D_2 receptor gene (6) result in a dystonic phenotype in humans. Second, polymorphisms within the dopamine D_5 receptor gene have been associated with cervical dystonia (7). Third, mechanical or ischemic lesions of the striatum and administration of pharmacologic agents that block dopamine D_2 receptors *in vivo* can result in a dystonic phenotype (8). Together, these studies provide compelling data in support of a dopamine (DA) dysfunction in dystonia, in particular that a perturbation in striatal DA transmission is an etiologic component of the phenotype. To address this hypothesis directly, we have examined comprehensively markers of DA signaling within the striatum of four genotypically confirmed *DYT1* brains—three cases of clinical *DYT1* dystonia and one case of parkinsonism. Biochemical indices of DA transmission were examined by measuring the tissue content of DA and its metabolites 3,4-dihydroxyphenyl-acetic acid (DOPAC) and homovanillic acid (HVA), whereas markers of DA transmission were examined by quantitative autoradiography using tritiated ligands for the dopamine and vesicular transporters (presynaptic) and DA D_1 and DA D_2 receptors (postsynaptic).

METHODS

Human Tissue

Postmortem fresh-frozen tissue blocks were provided by the Harvard Brain Tissue Resource Center (Belmont, MA) and the University of Maryland Brain Bank for Developmental Disorders (Baltimore, MD). Striatal tissue was available from six controls, three typical *DYT1* dystonia cases and one case of parkinsonism with a family history of *DYT1* dystonia. Tissue had been either passive-frozen or quick-frozen in liquid nitrogen vapor. All cases were genotyped for the GAG deletion within exon 5 of the *TOR1A* gene (1) as described previously (9). Limited clinical history was available for the three *DYT1* dystonia cases; all had a family history of dystonia and presented with early-onset childhood dystonia, a classic *DYT1* phenotype. One case of asymmetric parkinsonism, with a family history of

dystonia, was also studied. By contrast, the control cases had no known history of neurologic disease. Brain postmortem intervals did not exceed 30 hours (Table 7-1).

Striatal Content of Dopamine and Its Metabolites

Fresh-frozen striatal tissue (20–80 mg) was homogenized (1:10) in chilled 0.1 M perchloric acid, and DA and its metabolites DOPAC and HVA were measured by high-performance liquid chromatography (HPLC) with electrochemical detection (10). Concentrations of DA, DOPAC, and HVA were standardized to protein content and expressed as nanograms per milligram of protein. Protein concentrations were measured using the Bio-Rad Dc protein assay (Hercules, CA).

Dopamine D_1 and D_2 Receptor Binding and Dopamine Uptake Sites

Striatal tissue sections from the control and the four *DYT1* cases were processed for [³H]-SCH23390 (DA D_1-like), [³H]-YM-09151-2 (DA D_2-like), [³H]-mazindol (DA uptake), and [³H]-dihydrotetrabenazine (DHTB; VMAT2) ligand binding using standardized protocols as reported previously (11–14). All [³H]-ligands were obtained from New England Nuclear (Boston, MA). In brief, assay buffer contained 25 mM Tris-HCl (pH 7.5), 100 mM NaCl, 1 mM MgCl₂, 1 µM pargyline, and 0.001% ascorbate. For D_1-like binding, slides were incubated in the dark with 1.54 nM [³H]-SCH-23390 [specific activity (s.a.) 75.5 Ci/mmol] for 2.5 hours at room temperature. Nonspecific binding was defined in the presence of 1 µM cis-flupentixol. For D_2-like binding, slides were incubated in the dark with 187 pM [³H]-YM-09151-2 (s.a. 85 Ci/mmol) for 3 hours at room temperature. Nonspecific binding was defined in the presence of 100 µM DA. For DA uptake, slides were prewashed in ice-cold binding buffer (50 mM Tris-HCl, 5 mM KCl, and 300 mM NaCl, pH 7.9) for 5 minutes and

TABLE 7-1. *Demographics of the postmortem human cases used in this study*

Case	Diagnosis	Freezing method	GAG deletion in *DYT1*
B3229	Control	Liquid N₂	No
B4571	Control	Liquid N₂	No
B3956	Control	Liquid N₂	No
B3423	Control	Unknown	No
m96017	Control	Liquid N₂	No
B4635	Control	Passive	No
B4646	Control	Passive	No
B4596	Control	Passive	No
1	Dystonia	Passive	Yes
6	Dystonia	Passive	Yes
8	Dystonia	Passive	Yes
7	Parkinsonism	Passive	Yes

then incubated with 5.5 nM [³H]-mazindol (s.a. 23.5 Ci/mmol) in the presence of 300 nM desipramine for 1 hour at 4°C. Nonspecific binding was defined in the presence of 10 μM nomifensine. For VMAT2 binding, slides were warmed to room temperature, prewashed in buffer, and then incubated with 5 nM [³H]-DHTB (s.a. 20 Ci/mmol) for 40 minutes at room temperature. Nonspecific binding was defined in the presence of 2 μM tetrabenazine. After incubation with [³H]-ligand, slides were rinsed in cold assay buffer for 10 minutes, rinsed quickly in cold distilled water, dried under a stream of cool air, and apposed to tritium-sensitive film (Hyperfilm ³H, Amersham [Piscataway, New Jersey]) with calibrated ¹⁴C-standards (ARC, Inc., St. Louis, MO) for 2 to 4 weeks. Films were analyzed using computer-assisted image analysis (M1, Imaging Research, St. Catherine's, Ontario, Canada) and the density of the image converted to fmol/mg protein by automated extrapolation from the calibrated standards. Each case was assayed in duplicate, and the specific binding was determined by subtraction of the nonspecific value from the total binding value. All tissue sections were assayed in parallel.

Statistical Analysis

Statistical analyses were performed using a commercial software program (InStat 2.01), and significance levels were determined using an unpaired t-test.

RESULTS

Of the 12 brains used in this study, four were found to be positive for the GAG deletion in exon 5 of the *TOR1A* gene. Of these four, three had a clinical history of early-onset generalized dystonia and one had a clinical and pathologic diagnosis of parkinsonism (Table 7-1). None of the eight control brains used in this study were positive for the GAG deletion, demonstrating that they were not nonmanifesting gene carriers. Further, none

of the eight controls had any pathologic abnormality.

Tissue Content of DA and Its Metabolites

Striatal DA tissue content was measured in samples from control cases that had been either passive-frozen or quick-frozen in liquid nitrogen vapor, as previous reports have suggested that the method of tissue processing can impact significantly on the content of catecholamines measured (15,16). We measured a marked, and statistically significant increase in tissue DA content in slow, passive-frozen striatal tissue (34.37 ± 3.19 ng/mg protein) compared to rapid, quick frozen (6.35 ± 1.20 ng/mg protein) blocks. DOPAC and HVA values (ng/mg protein) were more consistent between the quick frozen (DOPAC, 2.29 ± 1.13; HVA 37.21 ± 3.44) and passive frozen (DOPAC, 2.26 ± 0.27; HVA, 60.02 ± 6.85) samples. The striatal tissue content of DA and its metabolites, DOPAC and HVA, measured here for control passive frozen tissue, is consistent with the reports of others (17,18) and underscores the importance of matching postmortem variables, particularly freezing methods, when using human tissue, as recently reviewed by Hornykiewicz (18).

All of the available *DYT1* cases used in this study had been passively frozen. In the *DYT1* dystonia group (*n* = 3), striatal DA tissue content was decreased (−23%) when compared to passive-frozen controls, and striatal DOPAC content was elevated (+48%) in the same cases, resulting in a significant increase in striatal DOPAC/DA ratio in *DYT1* dystonia (Table 7-2). In contrast, striatal HVA content was consistent between the two groups, resulting in an increase in the HVA/DA ratio, although this was not significant (Table 7-2). These findings were in marked contrast to the parkinsonism case bearing the *DYT1* deletion, where a marked reduction (>85%) in striatal DA, DOPAC, and HVA levels was measured (Table 7-2), consistent with the degeneration of the DAergic nigrostriatal pathway.

TABLE 7-2. *Tissue content of dopamine (DA), 3,4-dihydroxyphenylacetic acid (DOPAC), and homovanillic acid (HVA), in the passive-frozen control and DYT1 striatum*

Case	n	DA	DOPAC	DOPAC/DA	HVA	HVA/DA
Control	3	34.37 ± 3.19	2.26 ± 0.27	0.07 ± 0.01	60.02 ± 6.85	1.75 ± 0.17
Dystonia	3	26.36 ± 8.53	3.34 ± 1.16	0.12 ± 0.01*	53.66 ± 7.49	2.54 ± 1.33
		$p = 0.47$	$p = 0.46$	$p = 0.01$	$p = 0.58$	$p = 0.42$
Parkinsonism	1	0.44	0.33	0.75	5.63	12.80

Data are mean ± standard error of the mean (SEM) and are expressed in ng/mg protein.
*Significantly different from control striatum.

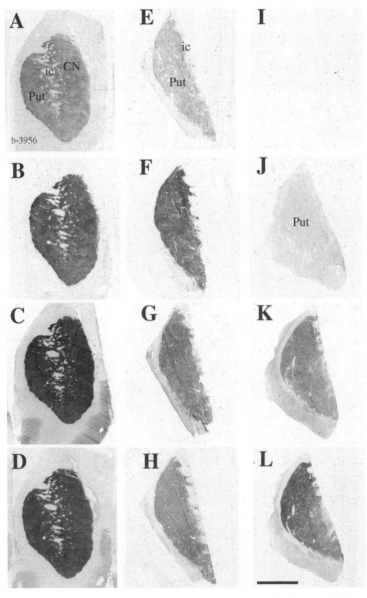

FIG. 7-1. Autoradiographic images illustrating specific binding for [³H]-mazindol **(A,E,I)**, [³H]-DHTB **(B,F,J)**, [³H]-SCH-23390 **(C,G,K)**, and [³H]-YM-09151-2 **(D,H,L)** in the striatum of a control **(A–D)**, *DYT1* dystonia **(E–H)**, and one case of *DYT1*-positive parkinsonism **(I–L)**. CN, caudate nucleus; Put, putamen; ic, internal capsule. Scale bar = 1 cm.

Dopamine Receptor Autoradiography

Quantitative receptor autoradiography was used to assay DA D_1-like, D_2-like, DA uptake, and vesicular uptake binding sites (Fig. 7-1). Levels of specific binding were determined by subtracting nonspecific binding from total binding. In the control striata, a robust and reproducible signal was measured for each of the four radioligands (Fig. 7-1A–D). Of note, DA (^{3}H-mazindol) and vesicular (^{3}H-DHTB) uptake sites were distributed in a distinct mosaic pattern (Fig. 7-1A,B) throughout the caudate-putamen, consistent with the findings of others (17). Examination of striatal sections of the three *DYT1* dystonia brains revealed no alteration in ^{3}H-mazindol or ^{3}H-DHTB binding compared to controls (compare Fig. 7-1A with Fig. 7-1E, and Fig. 7-1B with Fig. 7-1F). By contrast, there was a marked reduction in both D_1-like (^{3}H-SCH23390) and D_2-like (^{3}H-YM-09151-2) binding, although neither decrease was quite significant (Table 7-3). By contrast, examination of the *DYT1*-positive parkinsonism case revealed an almost complete absence of DA (Fig. 7-1I) and vesicular (Fig. 7-1J) uptake sites (Fig. 7-1I) coupled with a reduction in postsynaptic D_1 (Fig. 7-1K) and D_2 (Fig. 7-1L) binding sites, as expected in cases of nigrostriatal degeneration. These data are summarized in Table 7-3.

DISCUSSION

The present study provides a comprehensive examination of markers of DA transmission in the postmortem *DYT1* striatum. We found a 23% reduction in striatal DA content and a 48% increase in striatal DOPAC content in *DYT1* dystonia. Although neither of the changes alone was statistically significant, these absolute values translated into a significant increase (+71%) in striatal DOPAC/DA ratio in *DYT1* dystonia. This pattern of biochemical indices of DA transmission is consistent with an intact dopaminergic nigrostriatal system in dystonia (19,20), but the increased DOPAC/DA and HVA/DA ratios are suggestive of increased DA turnover when compared to controls. Biochemical evaluation of one other genotypically confirmed brain of *DYT1* dystonia exists in the literature (21), in addition to several other putative cases with a positive family history (22). In these cases striatal DOPAC content was not measured; however, low striatal DA content is reported, particularly in the rostral striatum (21), consistent with our biochemical findings.

Examination of markers of postsynaptic DA transmission revealed a similar picture to the biochemical data. Dopamine D_1 and D_2 receptor binding were decreased in the *DYT1* dystonic striata, although in neither case did the mean reduction achieve significance. In particular, a 29% reduction in D_1-like and a 40% reduction in D_2-like binding were measured (Fig. 7-1G and 7-1H and Table 7-3). These reductions in ligand binding are similar to those observed in the *DYT1*-positive parkinsonism striatum (Fig. 7-1K and 7-1L) and are consistent with the reductions reported by positron emission tomography (PET), in other dystonias (23,24). Whether the reductions in postsynaptic D_1 and D_2 receptor binding we report herein reflect a reduction in receptor number or affinity is un-

TABLE 7-3. *Specific binding of markers of pre- and postsynaptic DA transmission in the control and DYT1 striatum*

Case	n	DA uptake ^{3}H-mazindol	VMAT2 ^{3}H-DHTB	D_1-like binding ^{3}H-SCH23390	D_2-like binding ^{3}H-YM-09151-2
Control	5	168.10 ± 25.88	751.35 ± 115.32	266.09 ± 40.15	305.14 ± 52.31
Dystonia	3	158.14 ± 39.49	794.14 ± 38.51	225.40 ± 18.44	183.62 ± 47.32
		$p = 0.85$	$p = 0.74$	$p = 0.15$	$p = 0.15$
Parkinsonism	1	0.00	95.05	95.58	160.25

Data are mean ± SEM and expressed in fmol/mg protein.

clear, and was not possible to evaluate due to the scarcity of available *DYT1* tissue. Nevertheless, our biochemical data coupled with the receptor autoradiography are suggestive of an imbalance in DA signaling within the dystonic striatum, in particular an increase in DA turnover. Interestingly, markedly different patterns of striatal DA transmission were observed in the one parkinsonian case compared with the three dystonia striata, despite all four brains being heterozygous for the *DYT1* mutation. In the parkinsonian case, a marked reduction in striatal DA, DOPAC, and HVA content were measured, coupled with an almost complete absence of DAT and VMAT binding, consistent with the degeneration of the DAergic nigrostriatal pathway, observed postmortem, and with the parkinsonian phenotype observed clinically. The marked reduction in postsynaptic D_2 receptor binding in this one index case is consistent with *in vivo* PET data in cases of atypical parkinsonian patients (25). Whether the heterozygous *DYT1* deletion impacted on the phenotype or/and pathophysiology of this case is unclear, although the lack of cytoplasmic nigral Lewy bodies postmortem suggests that this cases may represent an atypical variant of Parkinson's disease (PD), as has been reported for familial cases of PD with mutations in the parkin gene (see ref. 26 for review). Thus, despite the positive history of *DYT1* dystonia in this family, coupled with the low clinical penetrance of the GAG deletion in *TOR1A*, it would appear that the clinical expression of this deletion, early onset generalized dystonia, was silent, although the physiologic expression may have been penetrant as suggested by Eidelberg and colleagues (27) in nonmanifesting *DYT1* gene carriers.

Increased DA turnover can be due to several factors including increased DA release, decreased vesicular packaging of DA, decreased VMAT2 activity/levels, and/or increased monoamine oxidase-B (MAO-B) activity. Impaired DA packaging or uptake, and/or compromised VMAT2 levels are possible, although the intensity of $[^3H]$-mazindol and $[^3H]$-DHTB binding were comparable in the *DYT1* dystonia and control striata (Table 7-3 and Fig. 7-1). Similarly, *in vivo*, in idiopathic dystonias patients, no abnormality in presynaptic DA binding (^{125}I-B-CIT) has been detected by single photon emission computed tomography (SPECT) (24), although a significant decrease in postsynaptic D_2 binding has been observed in the striata of the same patients, suggesting that the activity of DAT, at least, may not be compromised functionally. Indeed, Playford and colleagues (28) have reported on 11 idiopathic torsion dystonia patients with a positive family history of dystonia and found reductions in striatal $[^{18}F]$-dihydroxyphenylalanine (DOPA) uptake *in vivo*, suggestive of a reduction in DOPA decarboxylase activity. Thus, abnormal intraneuronal DA metabolism is possible, as is increased striatal MAO-B activity. Of interest pargyline, a nonspecific MAO-B inhibitor, has been reported to significantly attenuate neuroleptic-induced dystonia in primates (29), presumably by increasing brain monoamine levels, suggesting an indirect link between MAO overactivity and dystonia. However, mice transgenic for human MAO-B do not exhibit compromised striatal DA content or a dystonic phenotype despite a threefold increase in MAO-B activity (30,31). The therapeutic efficacy of MAO inhibitors in *DYT1* dystonia is unknown, and toxicity associated with MAO-A inhibitors greatly limits their clinical use. However, the efficacy of selegiline, a selective MAO-B inhibitor, has not been studied systematically in *DYT1* dystonia and may be of some benefit.

In contrast to a **hypodopaminergic** hypothesis of dystonia, Kolbe and colleagues (32) have hypothesized that neuroleptic-induced dystonia, a secondary dystonia, may be due to a **hyperdopaminergic** state associated with increased DA release onto supersensitive postsynaptic DA receptors. While we were not able to examine D_1 or D_2 B_{max} or dissociation constant (K_d) values in this study, postsynaptic receptor supersensitivity seems unlikely as *DYT1* patients do not gain any therapeutic benefit from DA receptor agonists, nor do they exhibit a stereotypic locomotor response. Nevertheless, tetrabenazine, which acts to deplete catecholamine vesicles, has been shown to be of therapeutic benefit in generalized dystonia (33).

When interpreting human postmortem biochemical studies, there are several factors that must be taken into account. First, the method of block preparation can significantly influence tissue integrity (34). Our biochemical data comparing striatal tissue DA content in passive-frozen versus quick-frozen tissue clearly demonstrate that method of freezing must be considered. Second, it is now well-documented that both pre- and postmortem variables can impact significantly on catecholamine content, and postmortem delay has been reported to negatively impact on striatal DA content (18). In this study the postmortem interval of our passive-frozen control group (26.77 ± 2.3 hours) was significantly longer than the *DYT1* dystonia group (12.37 ± 1.0 hours), suggesting that the actual difference in striatal DA content premortem in the *DYT1* cases may have been greater than is represented by the data here. Third, small group sizes can be problematic due to the inherent variability between human cases. In this study we report on three *DYT1* dystonia cases that, to our knowledge, is the total number of cases available in U.S. federally funded brain banks. We have genotyped in excess of 50 dystonia brains from three of these brain banks (Harvard Brain Tissue Resource Center, Belmont, MA; University of Maryland Brain Bank for Developmental Disorders, Baltimore, MD; and National Neurological Research Specimen Bank, Los Angeles, CA), and have identified only the cases reported herein. Thus, additional fresh-frozen postmortem brain tissue from symptomatic *DYT1* dystonia cases is not currently available.

THE NEURAL MECHANISM OF DYSTONIA

Despite the recent progress in understanding how movements are controlled, the neural mechanism of dystonia remains largely a mystery, and an adequate model is lacking. The search for the mechanisms of dystonia has been difficult because of the lack of clear abnormalities in the brain. In both primary dystonias (including *DYT1*) as well as primary-plus dystonia, routine neuropathologic examination is normal. Only relatively limited direct studies of the electrical activity of brain neurons in human dystonia have been conducted, and these have revealed in many cases abnormal activity of output neurons in the basal ganglia (35,36). Lesions and deep brain stimulators (both of which produce a local inhibitory effect) in the globus pallidus internus, the target of striatal efferents, have been successful in treating some cases of *DYT1* dystonia (37), adding credence to abnormal striatal signaling being the pathophysiologic basis for the dystonic phenotype. While the etiologic basis for this abnormal signaling in unknown, it is possible that it may have a strong developmental component, which would account for the lack of degenerative pathology postmortem. Thus mutant torsinA may impact on neurogenesis and result in "aberrant wiring" of the developing basal ganglia.

Clinically, *DYT1* dystonia is a progressive hypokinetic disorder; thus, torsinA may be considered as a member of the "parkinsonian" family of proteins, including α-synuclein, UCHL-1 (ubiquitin carboxy-terminal hydrolase L1), and parkin. Indeed, their patterns of expression in the postmortem human brain are strikingly similar, with each of these four transcripts being enriched within nigral DA neurons (38–40). Further, at the protein level, α-synuclein (41,42), torsinA (43), and parkin (44,45) have all been localized to vesicles within the presynaptic nerve terminal. Of interest, α-synuclein knockout (syn−/−) mice have been generated that display normal brain architecture, including an intact nigrostriatal DA pathway; however, they display subtle perturbations in DA homeostasis (46), including increased striatal DA release in response to electrical or elevated Ca^{2+} challenge and reduced activity in response to amphetamine, compared to wild-type mice. Baseline tissue DA content is selectively reduced in the striatum but unaffected in the ventral mesencephalon. Striatal DOPAC levels are similarly comparable, although a nonsignificant increase in the DOPAC/DA ratio is observed. These perturbations in DA homeostasis are strikingly similar to the biochemical data presented here in the striata of human *DYT1* dystonia cases. As torsinA has recently been found to interact with α-synuclein (47), it is tempting to speculate that mutant torsinA may similarly affect presynaptic DA release in the striatum, leading to increased striatal DA turnover, which may underlie the pathophysiology of *DYT1* dystonia. These studies have recently been reported in *Neurology* (2002;59: 445–448).

ACKNOWLEDGMENTS

Human postmortem brain tissue was provided by the Harvard Brain Tissue Resource Center (HBTRC), which is supported in part by U.S. Public Health Service (PHS) grant MH/NS 31862; the University of Maryland Brain Bank (UMB), which is funded in part by NICHD (National Institute of Child Health and Human Development) contract NO1-HD-8-3283, and Dr. Jean-Paul Vonsattel. The enthusiasm and support of Dr. Ron Zielke and Mr. Robert Vigorrito at the UMB, and Dr. Stephen Vincent and Mr. George Tejada at the HBTRC are gratefully acknowledged. This study was supported by NINDS (National Institute of Neurological Disorders and Stroke) NS28384 and NS37409. This study is dedicated to the fond memory of the late Dr. John B. Penney, Jr.

REFERENCES

1. Ozelius L, Hewett J, Page C, et al. *Nature Genet* 1997; 17:40–48.
2. Bressman SB, deLeon D, Brin MF, et al. *Adv Neurol* 1988;50:45–56.
3. Breakefield X, Kamm C, Hanson P. *Neuron* 2001;31: 9–12.
4. Knappskog P, Flatmark T, Mallet J, et al. *Hum Mol Genet* 1995;4;1209–1212.
5. Ichinose H, Ohye T, Takahashi E, et al. *Nat Genet* 1994; 8:236–242.
6. Klein C, Brin MF, Kramer P, et al. *Proc Natl Acad Sci USA* 1999;96:5173–5176.
7. Placzek MR, Misbahuddin A, Chaudhuri KR, et al. *J Neurol Neurosurg Psychiatry* 2001;71:262–264.
8. Rupniak N, Jenner P, Marsden C. *Psychopharmacology (Berl)* 1986;88:403–419.
9. Klein C, Pramstaller P, Castellan C, et al. *Ann Neurol* 1998;44:394–398.
10. Beal MF, Matson WR, Swartz KJ, et al. *J Neurochem* 1990;55:1327–1339.
11. Augood SJ, Hollingsworth ZR, Standaert DG, et al. *J Comp Neurol* 2000;421:247–255.
12. Thibaut F, Faucheux BA, Marquez J, et al. *Brain Res* 1995;692:233–243.
13. Scherman D, Raisman R, Ploska A, et al. *J Neurochem* 1988;50:1131–1136.
14. Arregui A, Hollingsworth Z, Penney JB, et al. *Neurosci Lett* 1994;167:195–197.
15. Spokes E. *Brain* 1979;102:333–346.
16. Kontur PJ, al-Tikriti M, Innis RB, et al. *J Neurochem* 1994;62:282–290.
17. Piggott MA, Marshall EF, Thomas N, et al. *Neuroscience* 1999;90:433–445.
18. Hornykiewicz O. *J Chem Neuroanat* 2001;22:3–12.
19. Hedreen JC, Zweig RM, DeLong MR, et al. *Adv Neurol* 1988;50:123–132.
20. Rostasy K, Augood S, Hewett J, et al. 2003;12(1):11–24.
21. Furukawa Y, Hornykiewicz O, Fahn S, et al. *Neurology* 2000;54:1193–1195.
22. Hornykiewicz O, Kish SJ, Becker LE, et al. *N Engl J Med* 1986;315:347–353.
23. Perlmutter J, Stambuk M, Markham J, et al. In: *Dystonia 3: advances in neurology*. 1998;78:161–168.
24. Naumann M, Pirker W, Reiners K, et al. *Mov Disord* 1998;13:319–323.
25. Hilker R, Klein C, Ghaemi M, et al. *Ann Neurol* 2001; 49:367–376.
26. Bonifati V, De Michele G, Lucking CB, et al. *Neurol Sci* 2001;22:51–52.
27. Eidelberg D, Moeller J, Antonini A, et al. *Ann Neurol* 1998;44:303–312.
28. Playford ED, Fletcher NA, Sawle GV, et al. *Brain* 1993; 116:1191–1199.
29. Heintz R, Casey DE. *Psychopharmacology* 1987;93: 207–213.
30. Andersen JK, Frim DM, Isacson O, et al. *Brain Res* 1994;656:108–114.
31. Shih JC, Chen K, Ridd MJ. *Annu Rev Neurosci* 1999; 22:197–217.
32. Kolbe H, Clow A, Jenner P, et al. *Neurology* 1981;31: 434–439.
33. Jankovic J, Orman J. *Neurology* 1988;38:391–394.
34. Vonsattel JP, Aizawa H, Ge P, et al. *J Neuropathol Exp Neurol* 1995;54:42–56.
35. Vitek J, Chockkan V, Zhang J-Y, et al. *Ann Neurol* 1999; 46:22–35.
36. Vitek JL, Giroux M. *Ann Neurol* 2000;47:S131–140.
37. Coubes P, Roubertie A, Vayssiere N, et al. *Lancet* 2000; 355:2220–2221.
38. Augood S, Penney J, Friberg I, et al. *Ann Neurol* 1998; 43:669–673.
39. Augood SJ, Martin DM, Ozelius LJ, et al. *Ann Neurol* 1999;46:761–769.
40. Solano S, Miller D, Augood S, et al. *Ann Neurol* 2000; 47:201–210.
41. Kahle PJ, Neumann M, Ozmen L, et al. *J Neurosci* 2000;20:6365–6373.
42. Maroteaux L, Campanelli J, Scheller R. *J Neurosci* 1988;8:2804–2815.
43. Augood S, Keller-McGandy C, Dunah A, et al. *Soc Neurosci* 2003; in press.
44. Mouatt-Prigent A, Muriel M, Gu W, et al. In: *14th International Congress on Parkinson's Disease,* Helsinki, vol P-MO-006, 2001.
45. Kubo S, Hattori N, Mizuno Y. In: *14th International Congress on Parkinson's Disease,* Helsinki, vol P-MO-015, 2001.
46. Abeliovich A, Schmitz Y, Farinas I, et al. *Neuron* 2000;25:239–252.
47. Sharma N, Hewett J, Ozelius LJ, et al. *Am J Pathol* 2001;159:339–344.

Dystonia 4: Advances in Neurology, Vol. 94. Edited
by Stanley Fahn, Mark Hallett, and Mahlon R.
DeLong. Lippincott Williams & Wilkins,
Philadelphia © 2004.

8

Development and Anatomic Localization of TorsinA

*Shelley R. Oberlin, †Marina Konakova, ‡Stefan Pulst, and
§Marie-Françoise Chesselet

*Department of Neurology, David Geffen School of Medicine at UCLA, Los Angeles, California.
†Department of Medicine, Division of Neurology, Cedars Sinai Medical Center, Los Angeles,
California. ‡Department of Neurology, David Geffen School of Medicine at UCLA, Los Angeles,
California; Ross Moss Laboratory for Parkinson and Neurodegenerative Diseases, Cedars-Sinai
Medical Center, Burns and Allen Research Institute, Division of Neurology, Cedars Sinai Medical
Center, Los Angeles, California. §Departments of Neurology and Neurobiology, David Geffen
School of Medicine at UCLA, Los Angeles, California*

A deletion of a GAG codon, encoding glutamate, in the gene coding for torsinA causes a large proportion of hereditary onset dystonia (1). Because symptoms occur during childhood or adolescence in patients carrying the mutation, it is likely that mutation-induced alterations in the function or expression of torsinA in brain during development lead to the irreversible symptoms of the disease. Therefore, it is important to know where and when torsinA is expressed when symptoms usually occur.

Rats and humans share a prolonged period of postnatal brain development. However, there is no consensus regarding the exact correspondence between postnatal development in rats and humans. Myelination occurs in rats during the third postnatal week and puberty occurs around 6 weeks of age. Therefore, it is usually considered that the first postnatal month in rats corresponds to childhood in humans. Accordingly, we have examined the distribution of torsinA between postnatal days 7 and 28 and compared the results with torsin labeling seen in adult rat brain. Two different antibodies were generated against human torsinA and were used for immunohistochemical detection of torsinA in brain sections.

METHODS

Polyclonal antibody TR1 was generated against amino acid residues 51 to 63 of torsinA and antibody TR2 against amino acid residues 224 to 237. Both antibodies have been extensively characterized (2). Immunohistochemical studies were performed on tissue sections (35 µm thick) cut from brains of rats that were perfused through the heart with 4% paraformaldehyde under deep anesthesia with equithesin (prepared as per instructions of Jansen-Saltbury laboratories). Sprague-Dawley rat pups (of both genders) were sacrificed at postnatal days 7, 14, 21, or 28, and adults (males) were 2 to 3 months olds. Brains from at least four different litters were examined at each time-point. Immunohistochemistry was performed essentially as described in Konakova and Pulst (3). Briefly, sections were successively washed in phosphate-buffered saline (PBS) (0.1M, pH 7.2) and potassium phosphate-buffered saline (KPBS)

(0.1M, pH 7.2), and processed in 3% H_2O_2 in PBS for 10 minutes at room temperature followed by washes in PBS. Sections were then incubated in 5% normal goat serum (NGS) 0.01% Triton X-100 and KPBS (Triton/KPBS) for 1 hour at room temperature and subsequently incubated overnight at 4°C in anti–torsinA antibodies (TR1 and TR2, 1:50 dilution) diluted in 0.05% Na Azide, 2.5% NGS, and Triton/KPBS. After washing in Triton/KPBS, the sections were incubated for 1 hour at room temperature in goat anti–rabbit immunoglobulin G (IgG) (Elite ABC kit, Vector Laboratories, Burlingame, CA), diluted in Triton/KPBS with 1% NGS, washed in Triton/KPBS, and processed for 45 minutes in an avidin/biotin complex (EliteABC Kit, Vector Laboratories). Following rinses in KPBS and tris-buffered saline (TBS; 0.1M, pH 7.6), sections were incubated in 0.5% 3,3′-diaminobenzidine tetrahydrochloride and 0.006% H_2O_2 until visible staining was observed. Localization of torsinA in cholinergic neurons of the striatum was identified by double-label fluorescence immunohistochemistry with an anticholinesterase antibody (Chemicon, Temecula, CA), and rhodamine and fluorescein-conjugated secondary antibodies (4).

RESULTS

Labeling for torsinA was found in the cytoplasm of neurons, with often intense labeling of neuronal processes. Already at P7, all brains showed immunostaining in the striatum, subthalamic nucleus, red nucleus, amygdala, brainstem, inferior and superior colliculus, and the cerebellum. In general, immunostaining tended to increase with age. For example, in the substantia nigra, staining was only found in a subset of brains at P7, but was present in all brains later on. In some areas, however, the pattern of staining showed marked variation with age. These are described in more detail below.

Cerebral Cortex

Intense torsinA immunoreactivity was detected in the prefrontal cortex at postnatal day 7 (P7), whereas more moderate staining was found in the entorhinal and piriform cortices. Staining in other cortical areas was highly heterogeneous and only present in half the brains examined. At P14, staining was now present in pyramidal cells of all cortical areas, including the prefrontal cortex in which staining in nonpyramidal cells decreased. Staining continued to decrease slightly in this region at P21 and P28 when it reached its adult level.

Thalamus

Only weak labeling of the thalamus was found at P7, and only in some of the brains examined. Immunostaining in this region remained weak and heterogeneous at P14. In contrast, all thalamic nuclei were clearly labeled by P21, a pattern that continued at P28 and in the adult.

Hippocampus

Staining in the hippocampus showed marked differences at the ages examined. At P7, the pyramidal cell layer of CA1, CA2, and CA3 was intensely labeled, with some staining in the stratum radiatum, stratum oriens, and stratum lucidum. A large number of cells was observed in the granular layer and the hilus of the dentate gyrus of most brains examined at that age. The staining in the dentate gyrus, particularly in the polymorphic layer, decreased dramatically at P14, whereas staining in the other regions remained unchanged. At P21, the number of labeled cells decreased in the granular cell layer, whereas the intensity of staining increased in large cells of the stratum radiatum, oriens, and lucidum as well as the polymorphic layers of the dentate gyrus. This pattern remained constant at P28 and the adult, except for a further decline in the number of labeled cells in the granular cell layer.

Striatum

Immunostaining was present in the striatum at P7. At that age, both medium-sized and large neurons were equally labeled, and most labeled cells were located in the dorsal striatum, with an occasional densely labeled large cell in the ventral striatum. Surprisingly, the labeling intensity of large neurons increased dramatically at P14. In most of the brains examined at that age, the intensely labeled large cells stood up in sharp contrast with the much more weakly labeled medium-sized cells. The intensely labeled large cells were most conspicuous in the medial striatum and were more abundant rostrally and ventrally. This striking difference in level of labeling between large and medium-sized neurons was transient. By day 21, both types of cells were equally labeled in the dorsal striatum of the majority of brains. However, densely labeled large neurons were still observed in the ventral striatum. This intense ventral immunostaining subsided by P28, when both cell types showed moderate labeling in all striatal regions. This pattern persisted in some adult brains. In others, however, medium-sized cells showed almost no immunostaining, whereas large neurons remained labeled, primarily in the ventral striatum. Double-label immunohistochemistry with choline acetyltransferase confirmed that the densely labeled large neurons observed at P14 were indeed cholinergic interneurons (5,6).

DISCUSSION

We have examined the distribution of immunostaining for torsinA in rat brain during development and in the adult. Although the staining pattern in the adult largely confirms previous observations (7–9), immunostaining during development revealed unexpected changes in the pattern of expression of torsinA between P7 and P28.

Immunostaining for torsinA was present in most brain regions at P7 and its intensity increased with age. The most conspicuous differences during development occurred in cerebral cortex, thalamus, hippocampus, and striatum. What regulates these changes in torsin expression and their functional relevance remain unclear, as little is known about the function of the protein. However, one may speculate that torsin serves a more critical function at times when its expression is increased. Accordingly, increased levels of torsin expression in normal brains may signal those times and regions that may be most affected by the torsin mutation that causes early-onset dystonia.

In the cerebral cortex, torsin expression predominates in the prefrontal cortex early in development, whereas it increases in other regions of the cortex later on. The cellular distribution of the staining changed as well, with a shift from homogeneous labeling in prefrontal cortex at P7, followed by a restricted labeling to pyramidal cells in all cortical areas, including the prefrontal cortex at later ages. Accordingly, a mutation in torsin is likely to begin to affect pyramidal neurons in the motor cortex after P7 in the rat. In the thalamus, immunostaining remains weak and heterogeneous until P21, suggesting that a torsin mutation would most likely affect neurons in this region during late postnatal development only. Conversely, torsin expression was intense in the dentate gyrus early on but decreased with age, while remaining high in other parts of the hippocampus

Extrapolation to human development is complicated by the fact that there is no consensus as to what period of human development corresponds to the first three postnatal weeks in rats. Although this period has been proposed to correspond to the third trimester of pregnancy in humans, this is unlikely to be the case for forebrain development. Indeed, myelination, which begins toward the end of the first year in humans, occurs during the third postnatal week in rats. Furthermore, if puberty is taken as a developmental landmark, then the fourth to sixth postnatal weeks should be considered the equivalent of preadolescence in humans. With this in mind, increases in torsin expression during the second and third postnatal week in rats are compatible with an onset of the effect of the mutation during childhood and early adolescence, as usually observed in humans.

The pattern of immunostaining in the striatum was of particular interest. Indeed, a role for the basal ganglia in early-onset dystonia has been postulated based on the frequent occurrence of dystonia as a symptom of lesions or of neurodegenerative diseases affecting these regions, such as Parkinson's or Huntington's disease. Interestingly, immunolabeling of the main cell type of the striatum, the medium-sized striatal efferent neurons, was moderate during development and in the adult. In contrast, large cells, identified as cholinergic interneurons based on their size and the presence of choline acetyltransferase (5) show a transient increase in torsin expression during a critical period of their development. The increase in torsin expression was conspicuous at P14, when it was observed in cholinergic interneurons throughout the striatum, but rapidly subsided in most of the region by P21, although some densely labeled cells were still observed in the ventral striatum at later ages and even in adults.

The period of intense torsinA expression in the large cholinergic interneurons of the striatum coincides with a time of intense synaptogenesis in the striatum. Between P14 and P18, the number of asymmetric synapses between cortical inputs and medium-sized striatal efferent neurons increases threefold (10). Whether cortical inputs to the cholinergic interneurons develop at the same time is unknown. However, immunohistochemical studies have revealed an increase in dendritic arborization of these neurons at the time of increased torsin expression (5). What function torsin plays in these cells, and why its expression remains high only in cholinergic interneurons located in the ventral striatum remains unknown. The hypothesis of an effect of the torsin mutation in cholinergic interneurons is attractive because evidence suggests that, in contrast to other forms of dystonia (11–13), dopamine deficits do not play a primary role in *DYT1* dystonia. Indeed, dopaminergic therapy is not effective in these patients (14,15), whereas some benefit can be gained from the use of anticholinergic agents (14,16). Because cholinergic neurons are innervated by dopaminergic terminals in the striatum, these pharmacologic data suggest that the torsin mutation may exert its primary effects downstream of the dopaminergic neurons.

CONCLUSION

The present data provide information on the pattern of expression of torsinA during postnatal development in rats. The data clearly indicate that torsinA expression is developmentally regulated during a time that is likely to correspond to the onset of symptoms in patients with the *DYT1* mutation. The dramatic changes in expression observed in brain regions that play a key role in motor control such as the cerebral cortex, thalamus, and striatum suggest that torsin may play a critical role in these regions during defined periods of development. The present data provide a framework for further defining this function and determine how the torsin mutation acts during development to cause the dramatic symptoms of early DYT1 dystonia.

SUMMARY

We have mapped the distribution of torsinA, the protein that is mutated in dystonia type 1 (DYT1), during postnatal development in rat brain. TorsinA was expressed in most brain regions at postnatal day 7, and its expression became more intense and widespread with age. The distribution of torsinA, however, showed marked age-dependent differences among regions of the cerebral cortex and hippocampus. Notably, large cholinergic interneurons of the striatum displayed intense torsin labeling between postnatal days 14 and 21, a period of intense synaptogenesis in this region.

REFERENCES

1. Ozelius LJ, Hewett JW, Page CE, et al. The early-onset torsion dystonia gene (DYT1) encodes an ATP-binding protein. *Nat Genet* 1997;17:40–48.
2. Konakova M, Huynh DP, Yong W, et al. Cellular distribution of torsin A and torsin B in normal human brain. *Arch Neurol* 2001a;58:921–927.
3. Konakova M, Pulst SM. Immunocytochemical characterization of torsin proteins in mouse brain. *Brain Res* 2001;922:1–8.

4. Soghomonian J-J, Gonzales C, Chesselet M-F. Messenger RNAs encoding glutamate decarboxylases are differentially affected by nigrostriatal lesions in subpopulations of striatal neurons. *Brain Res* 1992;576:68–79.
5. Phelps PE, Brady DR, Vaughn JE. The generation and differentiation of cholinergic neurons in rat caudateputamen. *Brain Res Dev Brain Res* 1989;46:47–60.
6. Kawaguchi Y, Wilson CJ, Augood SJ, et al. Striatal interneurons: chemical, physiological and morphological characterization. *Trends Neurosci* 1995;18:527–535.
7. Augood SJ, Martin DM, Ozelius LJ, et al. Distribution of the mRNAs encoding torsinA and torsinB in the normal adult human brain. *Ann Neurol* 1999;46:761–769.
8. Shashidharan P, Kramer BC, Walker RH, et al. Immunohistochemical localization and distribution of torsinA in normal human and rat brain. *Brain Res* 2000;853:197–206.
9. Walker RH, Brin MF, Sandu D, et al. Distribution and immunohistochemical characterization of torsinA immunoreactivity in rat brain. *Brain Res* 2001;900:348–354.
10. Uryu K, Butler AK, Chesselet MF. Synaptogenesis and ultrastructural localization of the polysialylated neural cell adhesion molecule in the developing striatum. *J Comp Neurol* 1999;405:216–232.
11. Ishikawa A, Miyatake T. A family with hereditary juvenile dystonia-parkinsonism. *Mov Disord* 1995;10:482–488.
12. Bandmann O, Valente EM, Holmans P, et al. Dopa-responsive dystonia: a clinical and molecular genetic study. *Ann Neurol* 1998;44:649–656.
13. Brashear A, Butler IJ, Hyland K, et al. Cerebrospinal fluid homovanillic acid levels in rapid-onset dystonia-parkinsonism. *Ann Neurol* 1998;43:521–526.
14. Burke RE, Fahn S, Marsden CD. Torsion dystonia: a double-blind, prospective trial of high-dosage trihexyphenidyl. *Neurology* 1986;36:160–164.
15. Roubertie A, Echenne B, Cif L, et al. Treatment of early-onset dystonia: update and a new perspective. *Childs Nerv Syst* 2000;16:334–340.
16. Greene P, Shale H, Fahn S. Analysis of open-label trials in torsion dystonia using high dosages of anticholinergics and other drugs. *Mov Disord* 1988;3:46–60.

Dystonia 4: Advances in Neurology, Vol. 94. Edited by Stanley Fahn, Mark Hallett, and Mahlon R. DeLong. Lippincott Williams & Wilkins, Philadelphia © 2004.

9

Mouse Models of TorsinA Dysfunction

*William Dauer and †Rose Goodchild

*Departments of Neurology and Pharmacology, Columbia University, New York, New York.
†Department of Neurology, Columbia University, New York, New York

Primary dystonia research has been hampered by the lack of an etiologically specific animal model of the disease. Although a number of interesting lines of mutant rodents that display abnormal motor behavior have been identified and extensively studied (1), it is unclear which human disease these animals model. The discovery that dystonia type 1 (DYT1) (Oppenheim's) is caused by a mutation in the *TOR1A* gene encoding torsinA, however, has provided investigators with the opportunity to generate genetically modified mice of definite relevance to a specific form of human primary dystonia. This chapter briefly reviews the genetics and pathophysiology of primary dystonia, and then focuses on the recent findings regarding the biology of torsinA, including a summary of our work on the generation and characterization of torsinA null mice.

PATHOPHYSIOLOGY OF PRIMARY DYSTONIA

No consistent biochemical abnormalities have been identified in primary dystonia patients, although clues from causes of secondary dystonia implicate dysfunction of the dopaminergic system (2–4), and abnormalities of dopamine (DA) metabolism have been reported from postmortem DYT1 brains (5). Primary dystonia is believed to result from abnormal function of the basal ganglia (especially putamen) or possibly thalamus because

damage to these structures is frequently associated with secondary dystonia (6–8), and metabolic studies in DYT1 patients are consistent with this localization (9). Interestingly, these metabolic studies, which measure brain glucose metabolism using fluorodeoxyglucose positron emission tomography (FDG-PET), suggest that even mutation-carrying patients who do not develop symptoms ("nonmanifesting carriers") exhibit an abnormal brain metabolic pattern. This metabolic pattern, termed "movement free" (MF), is characterized by increased metabolic activity in the lentiform nuclei, cerebellum, and supplementary motor areas (9). Manifesting carriers exhibit the MF pattern, as well as another pattern characterized by increased activity in the midbrain, cerebellum, and pons. A follow-up study of these nonmanifesting carriers suggests that that the metabolic abnormalities have a functional consequence, as these individuals are impaired in motor sequence learning, and utilize a different brain network to accomplish the task (10). This suggests that DYT1 brains perform motor (and perhaps other) tasks differently from normal ones.

Animal studies (11) and surgical recordings from patients (12–14) suggest that reduced activity in the thalamic afferents from the basal ganglia (i.e., basal ganglia output) causes dystonia, a view consistent with the classical model of basal ganglia organization (15). However, recent results of neurosurgical treatment of patients with dystonia and

Parkinson's disease (PD) are not consistent with the model that a decreased firing rate of basal ganglia efferents produces dystonia [see Vitek (16) for review]. Indeed, pallidal ablation can clearly *improve* dystonia, including in patients with DYT1, and PD patients who undergo pallidotomy do not develop dystonia. Thus an abnormal *pattern* of pallidal firing, rather than the decrease in absolute rate, may provoke dystonia, and improvement after pallidotomy may reflect that the lack of a basal ganglia signal is preferable to an abnormal or "noisy" one.

How might this abnormal basal ganglia signal produce dystonia? A growing body of literature has documented abnormalities of cortical function in patients with primary dystonia that likely reflect a downstream manifestation of basal ganglia and concomitant thalamic dysfunction. Transcranial electrical and magnetic stimulation studies suggest that the gain (i.e., slope) of the cortical input-output curve is higher in dystonic brains and that deficient intracortical inhibition may be responsible for this abnormality (17–19) [reviewed in Berardelli et al. (20)]. Abnormal cortical inhibition could interfere with the ability of cortex to focus activation on desired muscles, leading to degraded cortical maps and the characteristic spread of activation to adjacent muscles and antagonists typical of dystonic movements (21). Consistent with this view, some monkeys trained to learn a rapid repetitive gripping task develop dystonic hand posturing and display a degraded somatosensory cortical hand representation (22). This dedifferentiation of sensory feedback information has been proposed to form the basis of focal dystonia (23).

TORSINA

TorsinA is a 332 amino acid protein that belongs to the AAA protein family because of the presence of a Walker box adenosine triphosphatase (ATPase) as well as other conserved motifs (24,25) (Fig. 9-1; see below for further details and refs. 26 to 29) for in-depth reviews on this family of proteins). Within this family it is most closely related to the HSP100/Clp family of proteins; many members of this family (e.g., Hsp104, ClpX) protect cells from denaturant stress (including heat and alcohol) by *unfolding* damaged proteins (30). Interestingly, mutations in other AAA proteins produce neurologic disease (31,32). The *TOR1A* gene belongs to a gene family that includes *TOR1B*, *TOR2A*, and *TOR2B*. The *TOR1B* gene encodes a protein with 70% amino acid identity to torsinA,

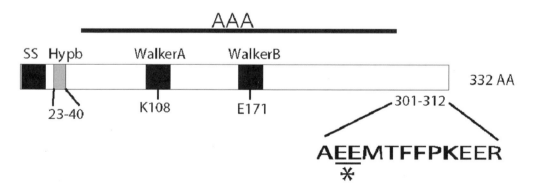

FIG. 9-1. Structure of torsinA. SS, signal sequence; Hypb, hydrophobic stretch of amino acids 23 to 40, which appears to allow torsinA to peripherally associate with membrane (NOT a transmembrane domain). The region of AAA homology is shown, including Walker motifs and site of mutations used in our studies. The C-terminal tail is unique to the torsinA family. The asterisk marks the site of the Δ302/3 deletion.

termed torsinB, while the other genes are less similar (33,34). The recently described protein ADIR [adenosine triphosphate (ATP) responsive interferon responsive gene] is 60% similar and 36% identical to torsinA (35). Furthermore, there are homologues of torsinA in *C. elegans* (Caenorhabditis elegans) (36), *D. melanogaster* (Drosophila melanogaster), and rodent as well as other species (34). TorsinA, torsinB, and ADIR are broadly expressed in both embryonic and adult tissues (24,35). *In situ* hybridization with a torsinA probe on normal human postmortem brain reveals wide expression, with the highest levels in the substantia nigra pars compacta, locus ceruleus, cerebellar Purkinje cells, dentate nucleus, ventroanterior/ventrolateral thalamus, and hippocampal formation, and moderate expression in large (presumably cholinergic) striatal neurons (37,38). An immunohistochemical study of torsinA protein confirmed widespread expression in human (and rodent) brain, as well as peripheral tissues (39).

The deleted glutamic acid of Δ302/3 torsinA normally forms one of a pair of glutamic acid residues in the C-terminus of torsinA (Fig. 9-1). This glutamic acid pair is conserved in torsinB, and the rat and mouse torsinA homologues. Three reports, using transient transfection of cell lines, have explored the subcellular localization of torsinA, and the consequences of the Δ302/3 on torsinA biology (40–42). TorsinA is a luminally oriented ER-resident glycoprotein (endoplasmic reticulum-resident glycoprotein). The Δ302/3 mutation does not appear to grossly alter torsinA protein stability or solubility (40). Further, wild-type and Δ302/3 torsinA show no difference in distribution on a sucrose gradient; both forms are found in a range of fractions, suggesting that the Δ302/3 does not grossly disturb the ability of torsinA to multimerize. Most interestingly, all groups (40–42) found that (a) wild-type torsinA is distributed throughout the cell and is extensively co-localized with ER markers, and (b) mutant torsinA concentrates in large clumps that are largely or completely segregated from ER markers. The clumps of mutant torsinA immunostaining are *not* insoluble aggregates (40) and they appear to be composed of whorled double-membrane structures (41). While these studies demonstrate an interesting effect of the Δ302/3 mutation, the mechanism underlying the abnormal behavior of torsinA remains unclear. Notably, reliable pathologic changes have not been described in specimens from DYT1 (or other primary dystonia) patients.

AAA PROTEINS

AAA proteins contain a conserved ATPase domain spanning 200 to 250 residues; these so-called AAA modules allow AAA proteins to derive energy from ATP hydrolysis and impart a mechanistic theme to AAA protein function that can provide insight into how torsinA likely acts and allow testable predictions about the possible effect of the *DYT1* mutation. However, the AAA domain is such an effective module around which to build protein function that it is used by proteins involved in an astounding array of cellular processes, including reconstitution of the ER and Golgi, mitochondrial protein import, proteasomal function, unwinding of DNA during replication, and powering molecular motors (microtubules), to list just a few examples (for extensive reviews see refs. 26 to 28). Therefore, membership in the AAA family helps to predict how the torsinA machine likely works, but provides essentially no clue about the specific biochemical pathway in which it participates.

AAA proteins assemble into ring-shaped oligomers, typically hexamers. They function via a cycle of substrate binding → noncovalent modification of substrate → substrate release, thus acting as a type of chaperone. The substrate modification typically involves unfolding of proteins or disassembling protein complexes. For example, the AAA protein NSF (*N*-ethylmaleimide sensitive factor) dissociates the SNARE (*S*oluble *N*-ethylmaleimide-sensitive factor *a*ttachment protein *r*eceptors) complex after the completion of membrane fusion (43). The same AAA protein can participate in different biochemical pathways by partnering with different adapter proteins, as exemplified by p97, which subserves distinct functions by interacting with p47 (44), Ufd1/Np14 (45), or SVIP (46) (reviewed in ref. 47). AAA proteins hydrolyze ATP at some point during the binding-action-release cycle, but the specific sequence of events and the detailed effects of ATP binding and hydrolysis are not completely clear (48–51) and may differ between AAA proteins. Nevertheless, an attractive model is illustrated by the cycle of Vps4p, for which ATP binding leads to decamerization and interaction with a membrane-associated substrate, and ATP hydrolysis is required for substrate release (and presumably modification) (52,53). Although it is not clear how the *DYT1* mutation affects this AAA catalytic cycle, one possibility is that it acts as a "dominant-negative," preventing oligomerization and leading to a loss of normal torsinA function.

TORSINA KNOCKOUT MICE

To test whether the loss of torsinA function produces a dystonic phenotype, we have used gene targeting to generate torsinA mutant mice. To address this question, we have generated torsinA knockout mice, and torsinA "knockdown" mice that express torsinA at approximately 5% of normal levels.

Breeding of mice heterozygous for the torsinA null mutation generates the different genotypes at the expected mendelian frequency. However, torsinA knockout pups fail to feed, and typically die within 24 hours of birth. The reason for the failure to feed appears to be an inability of the pup to find and latch onto the nipple because if artificially fed, their suckling appears grossly normal. In artificially fed mice milk reaches the stomach, indicating a patent esophagus and intact peristalsis. Although the knockout pups often look indistinguishable from their wild-type littermates (appearing pink, and showing normal amounts of spontaneous movement), some knockout pups appear obviously hypoactive at birth. Additionally, all knockout pups can be readily distinguished at birth by their failure to squeak in response to a nox-

ious toe pinch, although they demonstrate a clear motor response to this stimulus. The combination of the inability to feed or squeak suggests that there is an oropharyngeal abnormality in the null animals. However, no abnormal involuntary movements are present in the knockout pups, or in the adult heterozygous animals.

The gross morphology of the brain and other organs appears normal in torsinA knockout mice, although they display a trend toward a lower birth weight. To explore the cause of the lethal phenotype, we have assessed a number of defined neuronal populations in the knockout pups. The cranial nerve nuclei involved in sucking and swallowing appear grossly normal. The olfactory system and whisker innervation, the dysfunction of which could lead to feeding abnormalities, are also morphologically normal in the knockout pups. We have also verified that substantia nigra pars compacta (SNpc) dopaminergic cell bodies and their terminals are present, since a similar phenotype of failure to feed has been reported for Nurr-1 knockout mice, which lack dopaminergic neurons (56).

TORSINA KNOCKDOWN MICE

In torsinA knockdown mice, the modified allele expresses torsinA at approximately 2.5% of wild-type levels. Therefore, homozygous knockdown mice express torsinA messenger RNA (mRNA) at ~5% of normal wild-type levels. In contrast to the lethality of the knockout mice, these mice are viable and fertile, and heterozygote breeding generates the different genotypes at the expected mendelian frequency.

Importantly, torsinA knockdown mice do not display any abnormal involuntary movements. Motor function in the knockdown mice has been further evaluated by testing them in an open field apparatus and on the rotarod. The knockdown mice perform normally on the rotarod. In the initial exposure to the open field, there is a nonsignificant trend toward increased rearing in the hetero- and homozygote knockdown mice. In the second exposure to the open field, a clear gene dosage-related pattern emerges, with significant increases in both path length and rearing in the homozygote animals. When both experiments are analyzed together, there are significant increases in path length and rearing for both mutant genotypes. These findings do not appear to simply be due to increased activity of the mutants, since there are no differences in home cage activity. Rather, it appears that the mutant mice fail to normally habituate to repeated exposures to the open field. In contrast to the open field results, the mutant mice perform normally on rotarod testing of coordination. Although the behaviors observed in the open field and on the rotarod likely depend on a number of brain structures, the behavior of D_2 long receptor knockout mice suggests that some abnormalities of striatal function are detected in open field, but not on rotarod testing (54,55).

The function of the dopaminergic system has been extensively studied in the torsinA knockdown mice. The knockdown mice display a normal behavioral response when treated with the dopamine transporter (DAT) antagonist GBR-12909, suggesting that both pre- and postsynaptic elements are functioning relatively normally. A direct analysis of pre- and postsynaptic dopaminergic markers have failed to demonstrate any abnormalities in the knockdown mice. Presynaptic dopaminergic function was assessed with [^{3}H]mazindol autoradiography, and no differences in the striata of knockdown animals were observed when the data were analyzed either as an average over the entire striatum or as pattern of signal in the rostrocaudal axis. Using [^{3}H]SCH-23390, a similar type of analysis failed to demonstrate any differences in the D_1 receptor in the striatum or SNpc of the mutant animals. Dopaminergic function was further assessed in these animals using cyclic voltametry to quantify vesicular release and recycling of dopamine. This study demonstrated that the size of the readily releasable pool of dopamine, the rate of uptake by the DAT, and the rate of vesicle recycling are all normal in torsinA knockdown mice.

CONCLUSION

The phenotypes of these torsinA loss-of-function mutants do not appear to support the concept that the *DYT1* mutation produces dystonia by impairing normal torsinA function. However, these results must be interpreted cautiously as it has not yet been determined that the mouse motor system, which differs significantly from that of humans, is fully capable of generating a dystonic phenotype. It is possible that the motor abnormalities identified in the knockdown do reflect abnormal cellular function related to DYT1 dystonia. Although abnormalities of dopaminergic function are thought to be important in the pathophysiology of dystonia, the present studies do not suggest an important role for wild-type torsinA in dopaminergic function. Finally, although both mutants display clear phenotypic abnormalities, neither displays any gross morphologic abnormalities, either in the brain or other organs. This finding is consistent with the concept that abnormalities in torsinA function produce *functional* cellular disturbances, and do not lead to histopathologic changes.

ACKNOWLEDGMENTS

The authors wish to thank the generous support of the Dystonia Medical Research Foundation and the Parkinson's Disease Foundation.

REFERENCES

1. Richter A, Loscher W. Pathology of idiopathic dystonia: findings from genetic animal modls. *Prog Neurobiol* 1998;54:633–677.
2. Knappskog PM, Flatmark T, Mallet J, et al. *Hum Mol Genet* 1995;4:1209–1212.
3. Ichinose H, Ohye T, Takahashi E, et al. *Nat Genet* 1994; 8:236–242.
4. Burke RE, Fahn S, Jankovic J, et al. *Neurology* 1982; 32:1335–1346.
5. Augood SJ, Hollingsworth Z, Albers DS, et al. *Neurology* 2002;59:445–448.
6. Bhatia KP, Marsden CD. *Brain* 1994;117:859–876.
7. Lee MS, Marsden CD. *Mov Disord* 1994;9:493–507.
8. Marsden CD, Obeso JA, Zarranz JJ, et al. *Brain* 1985; 108(pt 2):463–483.
9. Eidelberg D, Moeller JR, Antonini A, et al. Functional

brain networks in DYT1 dystonia. *Ann Neurol* 1998;44: 303–312.

10. Eidelberg D, Carbon M. *7th International Congress of Parkinson's Disease and Movement Disorders.* 2002.
11. Brotchie JM, Henry B, Hille CJ, et al. *Adv Neurol* 1998; 78:41–52.
12. Vitek JL, Chockkan V, Zhang JY, et al. *Ann Neurol* 1999;46:22–35.
13. Lozano AM, Kumar R, Gross RE, et al. *Mov Disord* 1997;12:865–870.
14. Lenz FA, Suarez JI, Metman LV, et al. *J Neurol Neurosurg Psychiatry* 1998;65:767–770.
15. Wichmann T, DeLong MR. *Curr Opin Neurobiol* 1996; 6:751–758.
16. Vitek JL. *Mov Disord* 2002;17(suppl 3):S49–62.
17. Mavroudakis N, Caroyer JM, Brunko E, et al. *Neurology* 1995;45:1671–1677.
18. Ikoma K, Samii A, Mercuri B, et al. *Neurology* 1996;46: 1371–1376.
19. Ridding MC, Sheean G, Rothwell JC, et al. *J Neurol Neurosurg Psychiatry* 1995;59:493–498.
20. Berardelli A, Rothwell JC, Hallett M, et al. *Brain* 1998; 121:1195–1212.
21. Cohen LG, Hallett M. *Neurology* 1988;38:1005–1012.
22. Byl NN, Merzenich MM, Jenkins WM. *Neurology* 1996;47:508–520.
23. Pascual-Leone A. *Ann NY Acad Sci* 2001;930:315–329.
24. Ozelius LJ, Hewett JW, Page CE, et al. *Nat Genet* 1997; 17:40–48.
25. Walker JE, Saraste M, Runswick MJ, et al. *EMBO J* 1982;1:945–951.
26. Patel S, Latterich M. *Trends Cell Biol* 1998;8:65–71.
27. Vale RD. *J Cell Biol* 2000;150:F13–20.
28. Ogura T, Wilkinson AJ. *Genes Cells* 2001;6:575–597.
29. Neuwald AF, Aravind L, Spouge JL, et al. *Genome Res* 1999;9:27–43.
30. Schirmer EC, Glover JR, Singer MA, et al. *Trends Biochem Sci* 1996;21:289–296.
31. Hazan J, Fonknechten N, Mavel D, et al. *Nat Genet* 1999;23:296–303.
32. Maxwell MA, Allen T, Solly PB, et al. *Hum Mutat* 2002; 20:342–351.
33. Bressman SB, de Leon D, Raymond D, et al. *Neurology* 1997;48:1571–1577.
34. Ozelius LJ, Page CE, Klein C, et al. *Genomics* 1999; 62:377–384.
35. Dron M, Meritet JF, Dandoy-Dron F, et al. *Genomics* 2002;79:315–325.
36. Basham SE, Rose LS. *Development* 2001;128:4645–4656.
37. Augood SJ, Penney JB Jr, Friberg IK, et al. *Ann Neurol* 1998;43:669–673.
38. Augood SJ, Martin DM, Ozelius LJ, et al. *Ann Neurol* 1999;46:761–769.
39. Shashidharan P, Kramer BC, Walker RH, et al. *Brain Res* 2000;853:197–206.
40. Kustedjo K, Bracey MH, Cravatt BF. *J Biol Chem* 2000;275:27933–27939.
41. Hewett J, Gonzalez-Agosti C, Slater D, et al. *Hum Mol Genet* 2000;9:1403–1413.
42. O'Farrell C, Hernandez DG, Evey C, et al. *Neurosci Lett* 2002;327:75–78.
43. Sudhof TC. *Nature* 1995;375:645–653.
44. Kondo H, Rabouille C, Newman R, et al. *Nature* 1997; 388:75–78.
45. Meyer HH, Shorter JG, Seemann J, et al. *EMBO J* 2000; 19:2181–2192.
46. Nagahama M, Suzuki M, Hamada Y, et al. *Mol Biol Cell* 2003;14:262–273.
47. Dougan DA, Mogk A, Zeth K, et al. *FEBS Lett* 2002; 529:6–10.
48. Zhang X, Shaw A, Bates PA, et al. *Mol Cell* 2000;6: 1473–1484.
49. Rouiller I, Butel VM, Latterich M, et al. *Mol Cell* 2000; 6:1485–1490.
50. Rouiller I, DeLaBarre B, May AP, et al. *Nat Struct Biol* 2002;9:950–957.
51. Dalal S, Hanson PI. *Cell* 2001;104:5–8.
52. Babst M, Wendland B, Estepa EJ, et al. *EMBO J* 1998; 17:2982–2993.
53. Babst M, Sato TK, Banta LM, et al. *EMBO J* 1997;16: 1820–1831.
54. Kelly MA, Rubinstein M, Phillips TJ, et al. *J Neurosci* 1998;18:3470–3479.
55. Wang Y, Xu R, Sasaoka T, et al. *J Neurosci* 2000;20: 8305–8314.
56. Zetterstrom RH, Solomin L, Jansson L, et al. Dopamine neuron agenesis in Nurr1-deficient mice. *Science* 1997; 276:248–250.

Dystonia 4: Advances in Neurology, Vol. 94. Edited by Stanley Fahn, Mark Hallett, and Mahlon R. DeLong. Lippincott Williams & Wilkins, Philadelphia © 2004.

10

Dominant TorsinA Mutations in Cellular Systems

*Melisa J. Baptista, †Casey A. O'Farrell, and *Mark R. Cookson

*Laboratory of Neurogenetics, National Institute on Aging, National Institutes of Health, Bethesda,Maryland. †Neurogenetics Laboratory, Mayo Clinic Jacksonville, Jacksonville, Florida

In several of the adult-onset neurodegenerative diseases, there are rare familial forms that overlap phenotypically with the commoner, apparently sporadic disorders. For primary dystonia, there are at least 12 genes that when inherited in a mendelian (i.e., monogenic) fashion can lead to a variety of phenotypes. The first gene that was identified was *DYT1*, which usually begins in childhood or adolescence with involuntary posturing of the trunk, neck, or limbs. Dystonia type 1 (DYT1) (also known as Oppenheim's dystonia) is prevalent in Ashkenazi Jewish populations (1), though it is also found in several diverse groups (2). The disorder is inherited in an autosomal-dominant manner with a penetrance of about 30%. The gene has been cloned and named *torsinA* (2). The most common mutation is an in-frame deletion of one of a pair of glutamates (ΔE302/303), while a much rarer mutation removes six amino acids (ΔF323–Y328) (3). The family in which this larger mutation has been found also contains a mutation in the gene *SGCE*, which by itself can cause myoclonus-dystonia (4).

Many of the interesting aspects of torsinA biology are poorly understood, namely the normal function of torsin and the way in which the mutations produce a dominant disease. These aspects, and the work done in our laboratory to model the effects of torsinA on cultured cells, will be discussed here.

NORMAL FUNCTION OF TORSINA

TorsinA is expressed in various tissues of the body, including most brain regions, and is present throughout development. The encoded protein has a predicted molecular weight of 37.8 kd but is posttranslationally modified, especially by glycosylation (5). TorsinA (and its related homologue torsinB) are members of the AAA$^+$ family of adenosine triphosphate (ATP) binding proteins (2). This class of proteins has an extremely wide range of cellular functions, and include members that function in proteolysis, protein disaggregation/refolding, membrane biogenesis, DNA replication, and many other events (6). Most of these proteins are adenosine triphosphatases (ATPases), often function as multimeric protein complexes, and are usually involved in the assembly or disassembly of macromolecular complexes (7). Torsins are most closely related to the Clp ATPases (8), members of the Hsp 100 family of heat shock proteins that can unfold proteins and disaggregate protein aggregates prior to degradation (9). Whether this proves that torsins have a role in protein aggregation or clearance is not clear, especially given that the overall homology to Clp proteases is only moderate and that the AAA$^+$ family contains many other members with widely divergent functions.

Several laboratories have demonstrated that, when transfected into cells in culture, torsinA co-localizes with some endoplastic reticulum (ER) markers, such as BiP (10) or protein disulfide isomerase (5). Biochemical characterization suggests that torsinA is an integral luminal protein (10). This might be consistent with a role for torsinA in protein processing, as the ER is a major route for protein folding and degradation of misfolded proteins via retrotranslocation to the cytosol. Equally, the ER-localization of torsinA has been used to suggest that this protein may play a role in ER biogenesis, and this is equally feasible given that some AAA$^+$ proteins are involved in the generation of new organelles.

Results in intact tissue, however, have not clearly resolved the subcellular localization of the torsins. Cytoplasmic (11–14), nuclear (13, 14), and perinuclear (11,12) locations have all been reported in different laboratories using different antibodies. Subcellular fractionation experiments have been performed in culture models (10), although there are no reports of subcellular fractionation using tissue homogenates, which might clarify this important issue. Staining of pathologic structures, such as the Lewy bodies typical of Parkinson's diseases, has been reported by two independent groups (15,16).

Overall, then, there is a lack of strong evidence describing the normal function of torsinA. It may be related to chaperone and/or protein-folding functions within the cell, and the ER localization seen in some models may be relevant to this, but the lack of proof of this location brings this into question. This is not a trivial argument, as our understanding of the role of the mutations and hence our understanding of the disease process may critically depend on our ability to test how the mutations affect the normal protein function.

EFFECTS OF THE MUTATIONS IN TORSINA: WHAT ROLE DO INTRACELLULAR INCLUSIONS PLAY?

The first report of the localization of torsinA in culture models, including neuronal cell lines, demonstrated that the ΔE302/303 mutation caused the protein to form intracellular whorls apparently derived from the ER (5). Subsequent studies have been able to robustly reproduce this phenotype (17), including after stable transfections (10). The ΔE302/303 mutation produces protein that is stable, as evidenced by equivalent steady state levels in the cell, and properly folded at least at the first approximation (10). It also appears to adopt the same transluminal orientation as the wild-type protein. The continued presence of ER-derived inclusions in stable lines implies that these are not directly toxic to cells, as might be predicted for a disease in which there is little evidence of cell loss.

Despite several laboratories being able to induce these changes in various tissue culture models, there is currently no evidence that the same process occurs *in vivo* or in situations where the total torsinA expression level is similar to endogenous levels in normal cells, i.e., avoiding potential artifacts of overexpression. There is one report of staining of DYT1 brains with an antibody to torsinA (18). In this single case, there was no evidence of intracellular inclusions. However, more examples of this type of work are needed before making this statement definitively and it would be of some advantage to examine similar tissue with multiple antibodies. It should also be noted that these cases will be heterozygous and contain equal amounts of wt and ΔE302/303 proteins, and hence there may be some masking of the mislocalization of the mutant protein by wt. To date there are no published reports of mutant torsin transgenic mice, although several laboratories are making these animals. Whether intracellular whorls are seen in these tissues will be an important clarifying result. In an ideal world, such animals would be "knock-in" mice, thus avoiding the potentially confounding contribution of overexpression.

The second mutation, ΔF323-Y328, has been transfected into cells in our lab (Fig. 10-1). We failed to see any evidence for inclusions with this mutant protein. Therefore, we have the possibility that the formation of ER-derived inclusions is either specific to the

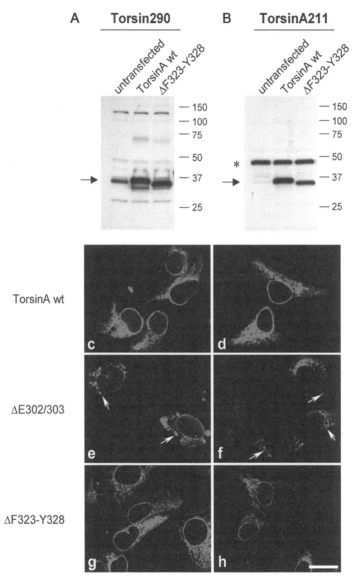

FIG. 10-1. Expression and localization of the ΔF323-Y328 mutant form of torsinA in transfected HEK cells. **A,B:** HEK293 cells were transiently transfected with wt (lane 2) or ΔF323-Y328 mutant (lane 3) torsinA (lane 1: untransfected controls). Cell extracts were blotted using rabbit polyclonal antibodies anti-torsin290 **(A)** or anti-torsinA211 **(B)**. *Arrow* shows torsinA (~37 kd). A cross-reactive band of unknown origin was seen with the torsinA211 antibody *(asterisk)*. **C–H:** Localization of torsinA. Cells were transfected and fixed and stained with polyclonal antibodies torsin290 **(C,E,G)** or torsinA211 **(D,F,H)**. Cells transfected with wild-type torsinA **(C,D)** showed relatively homogeneous staining throughout the cytoplasm. The ΔE302/303 mutation **(E,F)** formed multiple cytoplasmic inclusions, but the ΔF323-Y328 mutation **(G,H)** was distributed similarly to wild-type protein. Each transfection was performed in duplicate, and each experiment is representative of at least two experiments. Scale bar in **H** represents 20 μm and applies to all panels. (From O'Farrell CA, Hernandez DG, Evey C, et al. Normal localization of DF323-Y328 mutant torsinA in transfected cells. *Neurosci Lett* 2002;327: 75–78, with permission.)

ΔE302/303 mutation (and by inference that the two mutations produce disease by different mechanisms) or that the formation of inclusions is not the way in which mutations cause disease. Alternatively, this larger mutation may not be truly pathogenic. This seems unlikely given that it is, like DE302/303, an in-frame deletion in the C-terminal portion of the protein. The difficulty of assessing whether the ΔF323-Y328 is pathogenic has been that the family reported is rather small and contains few affected individuals. The description of the family has been extended recently (4), and the picture is perhaps now more interesting as the definitely affected individuals also have an amino acid substitution in the epsilon sarcoglycan gene (*SCGE*). A series of frameshift or truncated *SCGE* mutations are associated with myoclonus-dystonia. Therefore, the observation of myoclonus in this family may be due to inheritance of the *SGCE* allele. There is one patient who has only the ΔF323-Y328 mutation and is described as having "possible" dystonia (4). Therefore, the status of this mutation is intriguing and it is not clear whether the ΔF323-Y328 deletion is pathogenic by itself. Hence, the lack of effect of the ΔF323-Y328 deletion on the properties of the protein is also doubtful.

TorsinA mutations are inherited in a dominant fashion, albeit at reduced penetrance. Conceptually, dominant mutations at the cellular level may work by any one of several mechanisms. The mutant protein may act to reduce the net function of the wild-type protein, a dominant negative effect. This action is often seen with enzymes that act as part of a multimeric complex, such as with dominant mutations in GTPCH1 (19). This is feasible if torsinA acts as a multimer, as seen for other AAA$^+$ family proteins, but is difficult to test until we have a clear assay for function of the enzyme. A second possibility is that the mutant protein has some acquired property that is itself damaging, a so-called toxic gain of function. Proteins that tend to aggregate when mutated may fall into this category, such as the SOD1 mutations in amyotrophic lateral sclerosis (ALS), where the apparent ability of mutations to cause disease is unrelated to their effects on enzyme activity (20). It could be argued that the mislocalization of ΔE302/303 torsinA suggests a toxic gain of function directed at the ER. However, as we do not have a clear idea how these inclusions affect cells, this is difficult to test. There are important questions that one might ask along the way, such as whether wild-type protein is recruited into these aggregates. Finally, we might also consider the possibility that a reduction in the functional complement of torsinA within neurons drives the disease process (i.e., insufficiency). This is also difficult to assess without an assay for torsinA function, but could be answered by making knockout mice.

Overall, the data so far suggest that the mislocalization of ΔE302/303 is robust, but this requires confirmation in either another system or with a second mutation. It seems likely that the formation of ER-derived whorls reflects some property of the ΔE302/303 mutation. At the current time, with no functional assay of the torsin proteins, this is our best measure of the effects of the mutation on the cell. Development of animal models, and further descriptions of brain tissue from patients with DYT1 dystonia are required.

FUTURE POSSIBILITIES FOR USING CELL BIOLOGY TO MODEL DYT1 DYSTONIA

What are the next steps and how can we use what we know so far to better understand the mechanisms that lead to neuronal dysfunction in dystonia? There are several ways in which cell models might be used. We have already discussed (above) that data on the normal function are lacking: this might be addressed using a combination of different techniques.

There are many other outstanding questions related to torsinA. For example, we do not know what modifiers (genetic or otherwise) affect the penetrance of *DYT1* mutations. Also, there are few clear markers of pathology in dystonia generally, as there is no overt neuronal loss and no consistent descriptions of pathologic inclusions in surviving neurons. The ability to identify new molecular markers of disease progression would have a practical application in allowing us to refine our knowledge of neuronal dysfunction in dystonia brains. Finally, at the present time there are no studies of torsinA mutations on neuronal function. For example, does expression of mutant torsinA affect dopamine release or postsynaptic responses to dopamine?

One way in which we may be able to better understand the effects of mutant torsinA would be to define the molecular pathways that are altered in response to expression of the protein. We have used complementary DNA (cDNA) microarrays to identify the transcriptional changes induced by expression of torsinA in a heterologous cell line, HEK293 (M. J. Baptista, unpublished results). The number of genes whose expression was altered by more than 50% in either direction was very small. One of the few consistent hits that we identified was in the heat shock protein family, namely in HSP70.1, HSP70.2, HSP90, and their transcription factor HSTF-2. This work was done by pooling several clonal cell lines stably transfected with wild-type or mutant torsinA, where the inclusions previously described HSP90 was increased by about 60%, while HSP70.1 and HSP70.2 were increased twofold. When we examined protein levels of these two gene products, the protein amounts were not increased. This might represent increased turnover, in turn a possible reflection of ER stress. However, the effect of wild-type torsinA was very similar to ΔE302/303, and hence we have not uncovered an effect of the mutant protein to date, despite the continued presence of the intracellular ER-derived inclusions.

The difficulty with experiments in HEK or other heterologous cell lines is that while they may be useful in defining some of the biochemical functions of torsinA, we may well be missing out on some of the interesting effects of the mutations. There is some evidence of altered striatonigral communication in DYT1 patients, such as the recent description of decreased dopamine receptor binding in a series of postmortem brains (21). A small decrease of dopamine content in some regions of the striatum has been noted in one DYT1 patient (22). One way in which to expand current knowledge would be to examine how mutant torsinA affects the components of the dopaminergic system, either in cultured cells or in transgenic animals. For example, would expression of the mutant protein decrease dopamine levels? Alternatively, would dopamine levels remain normal while postsynaptic responsiveness was altered? The lack of responsiveness of DYT1 patients to dopamine replacement therapy [as seen in patients with tyrosine hydroxylase or guanosine triphosphate (GTP) cyclohydrolase mutations] suggests that a postsynaptic mechanism is most likely.

CONCLUSION

The best-characterized mutation in torsinA, ΔE302/303, robustly forms intracellular inclusions in transfected cell lines. These are apparently derived from the ER, where torsinA normally resides. However, there is currently insufficient *in vivo* evidence to support this as a mechanism of how mutant torsinA produces neuronal dysfunction in this disorder.

REFERENCES

1. Bressman SB, de Leon D, Kramer PL, et al. Dystonia in Ashkenazi Jews: clinical characterization of a founder mutation. *Ann Neurol* 1994;36:771–777.
2. Ozelius LJ, Hewett JW, Page CE, et al. The early-onset torsion dystonia gene (DYT1) encodes an ATP-binding protein. *Nat Genet* 1997;17:40–48.
3. Leung JC, Klein C, Friedman J, et al. Novel mutation in the TOR1A (DYT1) gene in atypical early onset dystonia and polymorphisms in dystonia and early onset parkinsonism. *Neurogenetics* 2001;3:133–143.
4. Klein C, Liu L, Doheny D, et al. e-sarcoglycan mutations found in combination with other dystonia gene mutations. *Ann Neurol* 2002 *(in press)*.
5. Hewett J, Gonzalez-Agosti C, Slater D, et al. Mutant torsinA, responsible for early-onset torsion dystonia, forms membrane inclusions in cultured neural cells. *Hum Mol Genet* 2000;9:1403–1413.
6. Ogura T, Wilkinson AJ. AAA+ superfamily ATPases:

common structure-diverse functions. *Genes to Cells* 2001;6:575–597.

7. Neuwald AF, Aravind L, Spouge JL, et al. AAA+: a class of chaperone-like ATPases associated with the assembly, operation, and disassembly of protein complexes. *Genome Res* 1999;9:27–43.

8. Schirmer EC, Glover JR, Singer MA, et al. HSP100/Clp proteins: a common mechanism explains diverse functions. *Trends Biochem Sci* 1996;21:289–296.

9. Glover JR, Tkach JM. Crowbars and ratchets: hsp100 chaperones as tools in reversing protein aggregation. *Biochem Cell Biol* 2001;79:557–568.

10. Kustedjo K, Bracey MH, Cravatt BF. TorsinA and its torsion dystonia-associated mutant forms are luminal glycoproteins that exhibit distinct subcellular localizations. *J Biol Chem* 2000;275:27933–27939.

11. Konakova M, Huynh DP, Yong W, et al. Cellular distribution of torsinA and torsinB in normal human brain. *Arch Neurol* 2001;58:921–927.

12. Konakova M, Pulst SM. Immunocytochemical characterization of torsin proteins in mouse brain. *Brain Res* 2001;922:1–8.

13. Shashidharan P, Kramer BC, Walker RH, et al. Immunohistochemical localization and distribution of torsinA in normal human and rat brain. *Brain Res* 2000; 853:197–206.

14. Walker RH, Brin MF, Sandu D, et al. Distribution and immunohistochemical characterization of torsinA immunoreactivity in rat brain. *Brain Res* 2001;900: 348–354.

15. Shashidharan P, Good PF, Hsu A, et al. TorsinA accumulation in Lewy bodies in sporadic Parkinson's disease. *Brain Res* 2000;877:379–381.

16. Sharma N, Hewett J, Ozelius LJ, et al. A close association of torsinA and alpha-synuclein in Lewy bodies: a fluorescence resonance energy transfer study. *Am J Pathol* 2001;159:339–344.

17. O'Farrell CA, Hernandez DG, Evey C, et al. Normal localization of DF323-Y328 mutant torsinA in transfected cells. *Neurosci Lett* 2002;327:75–78.

18. Walker RH, Brin MF, Sandu D, et al. TorsinA immunoreactivity in brains of patients with DYT1 and non-DYT1 dystonia. *Neurology* 2002;58:120–124.

19. Hwu WL, Chiou YW, Lai SY, et al. Dopa-responsive dystonia is induced by a dominant-negative mechanism. *Ann Neurol* 2000;48:609–613.

20. Cleveland DW. From Charcot to SOD1: mechanisms of selective motor neuron death in ALS. *Neuron* 1999;24: 515–520.

21. Baptista MJ, O'Farrell C, Hardy J, Cookson MR. Microarray analysis reveals induction of HSP mRNAs by DYT1 torsion dystonia protein, TorsinA. *Neurosci Letts* 2003;343:5–8.

22. Augood SJ, Hollingsworth Z, Albers DS, et al. Dopamine transmission in DYT1 dystonia: a biochemical and autoradiographical study. *Neurology* 2002;59: 445–448.

23. Furukawa Y, Hornykiewicz O, Fahn S, et al. Striatal dopamine in early-onset primary torsion dystonia with the DYT1 mutation. *Neurology* 2000;54:1193–1195.

Dystonia 4: Advances in Neurology, Vol. 94. Edited by Stanley Fahn, Mark Hallett, and Mahlon R. DeLong. Lippincott Williams & Wilkins, Philadelphia © 2004.

11

An Animal Model to Discern Torsin Function: Suppression of Protein Aggregation in *C. elegans*

Guy A. Caldwell, Songsong Cao, Christopher C. Gelwix, Elaina G. Sexton, and Kim A. Caldwell

The University of Alabama, Department of Biological Sciences, Tuscaloosa, Alabama

Dystonia is a movement disorder characterized by sustained muscle contractions that frequently cause twisting or repetitive movements or abnormal postures (1). Oppenheim's dystonia, the most severe early-onset form of this disorder, is transmitted in an autosomal-dominant manner with reduced penetrance (30% to 40%) and has been linked to specific deletions in the human *DYT1 (TOR1A)* gene that encodes a protein of unknown function termed torsinA (2–4). These breakthroughs have established the groundwork for subsequent investigation of the cellular mechanisms responsible for dystonia using the comparative genomics of model organisms.

The nematode, *Caenorhabditis elegans,* is a genetically tractable organism for which a wealth of molecular markers and defined cell lineage is available. This microscopic worm grows from embryo to adult in 3 days and has a transparent anatomy, facilitating examination of developmental and cellular change over time in an intact animal. Whereas the human brain contains over 100 billion neurons, *C. elegans* has exactly 302. Moreover, the complete neuronal connectivity of this animal has been determined and diagrammed by electron microscopy (5). Despite its simplicity, this nematode shares many of the hallmarks of human neuronal function including ion channels, neurotransmitters (dopamine, serotonin, acetylcholine) and axon pathfinding cues, among other molecules (6). The *C. elegans* genome contains many predicted proteins that exhibit a high degree of similarity with gene products implicated in human diseases and this model system has been exploited to gain insights into sensory and neurologic mechanisms underlying a variety of disorders (7,8).

The genomic sequence of *C. elegans* predicts three gene products that share significant amino acid similarity to torsins (9). The identification of a nematode torsin-like protein was first reported in the original paper on positional cloning of the human *DYT1* gene (2). This protein has been shown to be encoded by the *ooc-5* gene (9). The *C. elegans* OOC-5 protein has not been shown to function neuronally but is involved in the establishment of embryonic asymmetry and oogenesis in *C. elegans* (9,10). Two additional torsin-related genes have been since identified within the completed genome sequence of *C. elegans,* and we named these *tor-1* and *tor-2.*

Although strides toward discerning sites of torsin expression and localization have been made, a precise cellular activity for members of this protein family has not been determined (11–13). Torsins share amino acid sequence similarity with the diverse AAA+ family of adenosine triphosphatase (ATPase) proteins that includes heat shock proteins, proteosome subunits, proteases, and dynein (14). A recurrent theme in neurologic disease is the evidence of aberrant protein folding (15–17). Overexpression of molecular chaperones has been shown to suppress formation of protein inclusions in cells and decrease neurotoxicity (18,19). In this regard, mutations in neuroprotective molecules that function in a capacity to monitor protein folding may also be responsible for the symptomatic features of dystonia. We hypothesize that torsins function in a capacity similar to molecular chaperones in facilitating the proper cellular management of misfolded proteins. To experimentally test this hypothesis, we utilized an *in vivo* assay for examining states of intracellular protein aggregation in living nematodes (20). These experiments serve to simultaneously define a cellular activity for torsin proteins while establishing *C. elegans* as a model system for the analysis of torsin function.

RESULTS AND DISCUSSION

Suppression of Protein Aggregation by Torsins

While all human and nematode torsin-like gene products contain adenosine triphosphate (ATP)-binding and other sequence motifs common to AAA$^+$ proteins (9,14), a functional role for torsins in mediating protein folding has not been previously demonstrated. We isolated a complementary DNA (cDNA) corresponding to the worm *tor-2* gene product, the nematode torsin homologue that shares highest global sequence identity to human torsinA. The 1.3-kilobase (kb) *tor-2* cDNA encodes a protein of 412 amino acids that is detected in *C. elegans* extracts by TOR-2–specific peptide antisera (not shown). This cDNA corresponds precisely to *C. elegans* open reading frame Y37A1B.13 in GenBank;

all predicted splice junctions and amino acids have been verified by DNA sequencing.

Differential states of protein solubility were generated *in vivo* by ectopic expression of gene fusions between variable lengths of CAG codons (encoding polyglutamine repeats) fused to the green fluorescent protein (GFP) in *C. elegans* using the *unc-54* body wall muscle promoter (20). Direct comparison between transgenic animals expressing either a fusion of 19 glutamines to GFP (Q19::GFP) or 82 glutamines fused to GFP (Q82::GFP) demonstrated that fluorescent protein aggregation could be induced by polyglutamine expansion and readily visualized in these transparent animals. The evenly distributed and diffuse GFP localization associated with Q19::GFP (Fig. 11-1A) was dramatically transformed into a pattern of distinct fluorescent cellular aggregates in Q82::GFP animals (Fig. 11-1B). In contrast, coexpression of wild-type TOR-2 protein dramatically reduced GFP-containing aggregates in animals containing Q82::GFP (Fig. 11-1C), even partially restoring diffuse body wall muscle GFP fluorescence. Torsin suppression of polyglutamine-induced protein aggregation persisted over time as these animals aged post-adulthood. Coexpression of TOR-2 with Q19::GFP did not alter the normal cytoplasmic distribution of GFP in these animals (not shown).

Specific amino acid deletions in torsinA have been linked to Oppenheim's dystonia, implicating the carboxy-terminus of this protein as being essential for torsin function (2–4). Although the glutamic acid residue deleted in patients with early-onset torsion dystonia (ΔE302/303) is not strictly conserved across species, it is found within a stretch of overall high-sequence identity at the C-terminus (14). We used site-directed mutagenesis to examine the consequences of altering this portion of the worm TOR-2 protein. To putatively mimic the effects of aberrant torsin activity associated with dystonia, we generated a mutant *tor-2* gene that encoded a protein lacking a serine at position 368 of TOR-2 [TOR-2(Δ368)]. Coexpression of the TOR-2(Δ368)

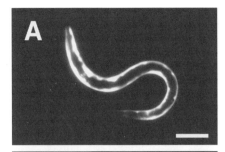
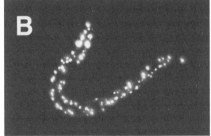
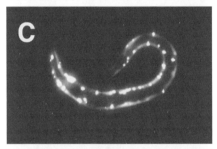
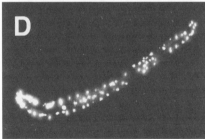
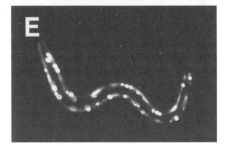

mutation with Q82::GFP protein was incapable of ameliorating protein aggregation and did not restore the diffuse body-wall fluorescence to these animals (Fig. 11-1D). Interestingly, coexpression of TOR-2(Δ368) with Q19::GFP did not alter the general cytoplasmic expression of GFP from what is found in Q19::GFP animals alone (data not shown). Immunoblotting of *C. elegans* extracts indicated that the various lines of transgenic animals, including TOR-2(Δ368), all contained equivalent levels of TOR-2 protein (not shown). Therefore, these data are indicative of a loss of torsin activity that is associated with the TOR-2(Δ368) mutation rather than a change in protein stability.

To test if the sequence homology shared between torsin proteins extended to functional homology, we obtained a human *DYT1* cDNA encoding torsinA and placed it under control of the *C. elegans unc-54* promoter. As was previously determined for nematode TOR-2, the human gene product was capable of suppressing protein aggregate formation and restoring diffuse body wall fluorescence in transgenic animals when coexpressed with Q82::GFP protein (Fig. 11-1E). This indicates that conservation of torsin protein activity is maintained across species boundaries and among members of this medically significant protein family.

FIG. 11-1. *C. elegans* lines containing transgenes expressing polyglutamine-GFP fusions and torsin proteins under the control of the *unc-54* body wall muscle specific promoter. **A:** Transgenic nematodes expressing a Q19::GFP protein fusion exhibit a normal diffuse green fluorescent protein (GFP) expression pattern, in comparison to animals expressing a Q82::GFP fusion in either the absence of TOR-2 **(B)** in the presence of TOR-2 **(C)**, or the presence of TOR-2(Δ368) mutant protein **(D)**. Suppression of polyglutamine-induced protein aggregation is evident in the presence of wild-type TOR-2 protein **(C)**, whereas the TOR-2(Δ368) mutant has lost this activity **(D)**. Likewise, coexpression of human torsinA in the presence of Q82::GFP also results in a clear reduction in protein aggregation **(E)**. The anterior of all animals is on the left of each panel. Scale bar represents 50 μM.

Overexpression of human torsinA ΔE302/303 has been shown to alter the subcellular distribution of this protein and result in the formation of membranous whorls in culture (21,22). In contrast, O'Farrell et al. (23) have shown in transfected human cell cultures that expression of an altered torsinA protein, lacking the 18 base pair (bp) (ΔF323-Y328) clinically linked to early-onset dystonia, does not change the localization of torsinA or result in the formation of membranous inclusions. Our data indicate that deletion of one specific C-terminal residue in the nematode TOR-2 protein (serine 368) results in a loss of this protein's ability to suppress protein aggregation without an apparent change in either TOR-2 localization or cellular morphology (see below). Further experimentation will be needed to clarify the significance, or lack thereof, of aberrant membrane inclusions on torsin activity and dystonia. Systematic structure-function analyses of torsin activity using this *C. elegans* assay system will allow for changes in cytoplasmic architecture to be directly coordinated with protein function.

TOR-2 Localizes to the Sites of Protein Aggregation

We examined the localization of wild-type and mutant TOR-2 in animals containing Q82::GFP aggregates by immunofluorescence microscopy using a TOR-2–specific affinity-purified antibody. Figure 11-2(A,B) depicts TOR-2 localization to the sites of polyglutamine-induced protein aggregation in a tight ring-like pattern completely surrounding the fluorescent protein aggregates. Immunolocalization of TOR-2 in animals overexpressing TOR-2(Δ368) did not lead to a discernible change in the cellular distribution of this protein (Fig. 11-2C,D). Thus, although this mutant torsin appeared to be localized to protein aggregates, it was incapable of functionally altering their solubility.

The distinctive localization of *C. elegans* TOR-2 to sites of protein aggregation is overtly reminiscent of cellular bodies called aggresomes (24). These inclusions, which also contain ubiquitinated proteins, proteosome subunits, and chaperones, are formed in response to excess misfolded proteins. Likewise, human torsinA has been shown to be in abundance at sites of α-synuclein aggregation termed Lewy bodies, a clinical characteristic in the brains of patients with Parkinson's disease (25). Interestingly, we have also shown that the sites of TOR-2/polyglutamine association are also sites of concentrated ubiquitin staining (Fig. 11-2E,F). Coupled with a report that heat shock proteins can suppress neurotoxicity associated with misfolding of α-synuclein in *Drosophila* (19), these combined data represent an exciting insight into the relationship between Parkinson's disease and dystonia at a molecular level.

Toxic misfolded protein intermediates are being heavily scrutinized as potential causative agents in a variety of neurologic disorders (15–17). The failure of intracellular quality control mechanisms can result in aberrant protein aggregation and associated disease states. Studies in yeast have identified numerous proteins involved in the cellular response to misfolded proteins; however, metazoan counterparts to these mechanisms still remain poorly defined (26). Our combined data implicating torsins in protein folding and co-localizing with ubiquitin at sites of protein aggregation are suggestive of a possible role for this exclusively metazoan family of proteins in the ATP-dependent retrotranslocation of misfolded proteins at the endoplasmic reticulum. Deficits in this mechanism may have significant consequences on neuronal activity, and dystonia may be a clinical manifestation of subtle changes in the ability of torsins to properly manage malformed protein structures in response to cellular stress.

Continued investigation of torsin function in *C. elegans* and other animal models will provide further insights into the molecular mechanism underlying dystonia. For example, the effect of structural alterations to torsin proteins may be evaluated for their functional consequences on chaperone-like activity and

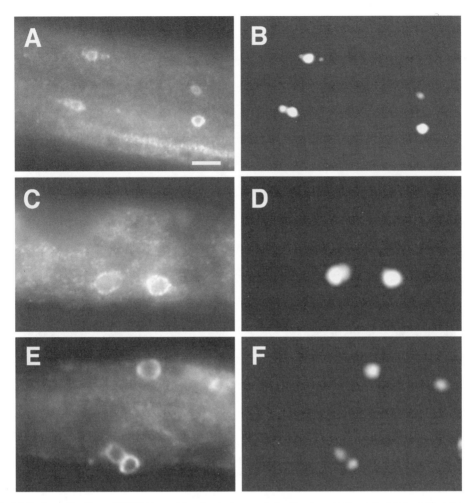

FIG. 11-2. Localization of TOR-2 or ubiquitin in transgenic *C. elegans* lines by immunofluorescence microscopy. Using an affinity purified TOR-2 specific antibody, both wild-type TOR-2 **(A)** or mutant TOR-2(Δ368) protein **(C)** are found to be highly localized to sites of Q82::GFP protein aggregation in body wall muscles **(B,D)**. Transgenic animals stained with an affinity purified antiubiquitin antibody exhibit a very similar pattern of localization **(E)** around fluorescent Q82::GFP protein aggregates **(F)**. The scale bar represents 5 μM.

then subsequently transferred to neuronal cells (i.e., dopaminergic) for examination of putative dominant negative phenotypes. As *C. elegans* is amenable to both traditional genetic and large-scale genomic screening methods such as RNAi (double-stranded RNA-mediated interference), the strengths of this system may be further exploited to facilitate functional characterization of genes influencing torsin activity. Screens for putative suppressors and enhancers of torsin activity using isogenic lines of mutagenized animals containing torsin and polyglutamine::GFP transgenes will yield effectors of torsin function (Fig. 11-3). Such studies may concurrently interface with ongoing human genetic mapping efforts to more rapidly discern genetic loci corresponding to other dystonias.

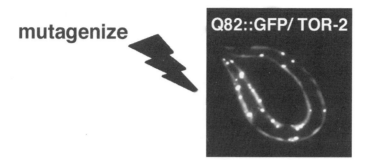

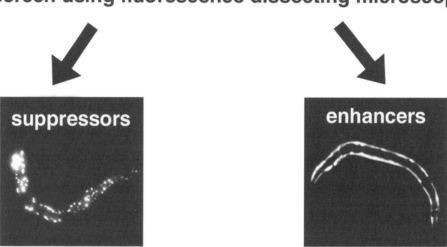

FIG. 11-3. Use of *C. elegans* to identify putative effectors of torsin activity by genetic screening. An isogenic line of transgenic *C. elegans* expressing a torsin protein that exhibits partial suppression of protein aggregate formation may be mutagenized. Progeny from these hermaphrodites can be rapidly screened under a fluorescence dissecting microscope for candidate genes that enhance or suppress protein aggregation when mutated.

ACKNOWLEDGMENTS

Special thanks go to Rick Morimoto for generously providing polyglutamine vectors and strains and to Ben Cravatt for the human *DYT1* cDNA. Funding for this work came from the Dystonia Medical Research Foundation and an Undergraduate Science Program Grant from the Howard Hughes Medical Institute to The University of Alabama. G.A.C. is a Basil O'Connor Scholar of the March of Dimes.

REFERENCES

1. Fahn S, Bressman SB, Marsden CD. Classification of dystonia. In: Fahn S, Marsden CD, DeLong M, eds. *Dystonia 3: advances in neurology.* Philadelphia: Lippincott-Raven, 1998:1–10.
2. Ozelius LJ, Hewett JW, Page CE, et al. The early-onset torsion dystonia gene *(DYT1)* encodes an ATP-binding protein. *Nat Genet* 1997;17:40–48.
3. Ozelius LJ, Page C, Klein C, et al. The *TOR1A (DYT1)* gene family and its role in early-onset torsion dystonia. *Genomics* 1999;62:377–384.
4. Leung JC, Klein C, Friedman J, et al. Novel mutation in the *TOR1A (DYT1)* gene in atypical early-onset dystonia and polymorphisms in dystonia and early-onset parkinsonism. *Neurogenetics* 2001;3:133–143.
5. White JG, Southgate E, Thomson JN, et al. The structure of the ventral nerve cord of *Caenorhabditis elegans. Philos Trans R Soc Lond B Biol Sci* 1976;275:327–348.
6. Bargmann CI. Neurobiology of the *Caenorhabditis elegans* Genome. *Science* 1998;282:2028–2033.
7. Culetto E, Sattelle DB. A role for *Caenorhabditis ele-*

gans in understanding the function and interactions of human disease genes. *Hum Mol Genet* 2000;9:869–877.

8. Dawe AL, Caldwell KA, Harris PM, et al. Evolutionarily conserved nuclear migration genes required for early embryonic development in *Caenorhabditis elegans*. *Dev Genes Evol* 2001;211:434–441.

9. Basham SE, Rose LS. The *Caenorhabditis elegans* polarity gene *ooc-5* encodes a torsin-related protein of the AAA+ ATPase superfamily. *Development* 2001;28:4645–4656.

10. Basham SE, Rose LS. Mutations in *ooc-5* and *ooc-3* disrupt oocyte formation and the reestablishment of asymmetric PAR protein localization in two-cell *Caenorhabditis elegans* embryos. *Dev Biol* 1999;215:253–263.

11. Shashidharan P, Good PF, Hsu A, et al. TorsinA accumulation in Lewy bodies in sporadic Parkinson's disease. *Brain Res* 2000;877:379–381.

12. Augood SJ, Martin DM, Ozelius LJ, et al. Distribution of the mRNAs encoding torsinA and torsinB in the normal adult human brain. *Ann Neurol* 1999;46:761–769.

13. Shashidharan P, Kramer BC, Walker RH, et al. Immunohistochemical localization and distribution of torsinA in normal human and rat brain. *Brain Res* 2000;853:197–206.

14. Neuwald AF, Aravind L, Spouge JL, et al. AAA+: a class of chaperone-like ATPases associated with the assembly, operation, and disassembly of protein complexes. *Genome Res* 1999;9:27–43.

15. Sherman MY, Goldberg AL. Cellular defenses against unfolded proteins: a cell biologist thinks about neurodegenerative diseases. *Neuron* 2000;29:15–32.

16. Muchowski PJ. Protein misfolding, amyloid formation, and neurodegeneration: A critical role for molecular chaperones? *Neuron* 2002;35:9–12.

17. Taylor JP, Hardy J, Fischbeck KH. Toxic proteins in neurodegenerative disease. *Science* 2002;296:1991–1995.

18. Warrick JM, Chan HY, Gray-Board GL, et al. Suppression of polyglutamine-mediated neurodegeneration in *Drosophila* by the molecular chaperone HSP70. *Nat Genet* 1999;23:425–428.

19. Auluck PK, Chan HY, Trojanowski JQ, et al. Chaperone suppression of alpha-synuclein toxicity in a *Drosophila* model for Parkinson's disease. *Science* 2002;295:865–868.

20. Satyal S, Schmidt E, Kitagaya K, et al. Polyglutamine aggregates alter protein folding homeostasis in *Caenorhabditis elegans*. *Proc Natl Acad Sci USA* 2000;97:5750–5755.

21. Kustedjo K, Bracey MH, Cravatt BF. TorsinA and its torsion dystonia-associated mutant forms are luminal glycoproteins that exhibit distinct subcellular localizations. *J Biol Chem* 2000;275:27933–27939.

22. Hewett J, Gonzalez-Agosti C, Slater D, et al. Mutant torsinA, responsible for early-onset torsion dystonia, forms membrane inclusions in cultured neural cells. *Hum Mol Gen* 2000;9:1203–1313.

23. O'Farrell CO, Hernandez DG, Evey C, et al. Normal localization of ΔF323-Y328 mutant torsinA in transfected human cells. *Neurosci Lett* 2002;327:75–78.

24. Bence NF, Sampat RM, Kopito RR. Impairment of the ubiquitin-proteasome system by protein aggregation. *Science* 2001;292:1552–1555.

25. Sharma N, Hewett J, Ozelius LJ, et al. A close association of torsinA and alpha-synuclein in Lewy bodies: a fluorescence resonance energy transfer study. *Am J Pathol* 2001;159:339–344.

26. Travers KJ, Patil CK, Wodicka L, et al. Functional and genomic analyses reveal an essential coordination between the unfolded protein response and ER-associated degradation. *Cell* 2000;101:249–258.

Dystonia 4: Advances in Neurology, Vol. 94. Edited
by Stanley Fahn, Mark Hallett, and Mahlon R.
DeLong. Lippincott Williams & Wilkins,
Philadelphia © 2004.

12

TorsinA and Early-Onset Torsion Dystonia

D. Cristopher Bragg, Damien J. Slater, and Xandra O. Breakefield

*Molecular Neurogenetics Unit, Department of Neurology, Massachusetts General
Hospital, and Program in Neuroscience, Harvard Medical School,
Boston, Massachusetts*

EARLY-ONSET TORSION DYSTONIA: FROM GENE TO PROTEIN

The past 6 years have witnessed a significant shift in the focus of research efforts devoted to understanding the pathophysiology of early-onset torsion dystonia: from the genetic linkage analyses, which bore fruit in 1997 with the identification of the *DYT1 (TOR1A)* gene and the 3-base-pair deletion associated with most cases of disease [for review, see Ozelius et al. (1)], to the more recent biochemical and cell biologic studies of the *DYT1* gene product, torsinA. The torsins represent newly discovered members of the AAA+ superfamily, a broad class of adenosine triphosphatases (ATPases) that typically form six-membered oligomeric rings and function as molecular chaperones in a diverse spectrum of intracellular activities (2,3). Four mammalian torsins have been identified to date: torsins A and B, which share approximately 70% homology, and the torsin-related proteins, torp2A and torp3A, which are approximately 50% identical to torsinA and torsinB (4). TorsinA is a 332 amino acid protein of approximately 37 kd molecular weight, with N-linked carbohydrates and potential sites for phosphorylation (5). The mutation responsible for most cases of early-onset torsion dystonia consists of a single codon (GAG) deletion that results in the loss of a glutamic acid residue near the carboxy terminus of torsinA. How this loss of a single amino acid ultimately translates into the severe loss of motor control characteristic of dystonia remains unclear. This chapter summarizes the recent investigations into the localization and function of torsinA, as well as the current efforts to determine the functional consequences of the mutation that underlies the disease.

TorsinA IN NEURAL CELLS

Since the initial identification of torsinA, multiple investigators have described its expression within the human and rodent central nervous system (CNS) by *in situ* hybridization and immunohistochemistry. Early attempts to map the distribution of torsinA protein were often complicated by antibodies that could not distinguish torsinA and torsinB. Despite some variations, however, these studies have provided largely consistent demonstrations of torsin in numerous regions, with particularly high expression levels in cortical layers III and V (6,7), multiple hippocampal subfields (6–13), cerebellar Purkinje cells (7–11,13), and diverse cell populations within the basal ganglia (7,10,11,13). In each case, torsin was detected primarily in neurons, with no evidence of significant expression in glia. The pattern of immunoreactivity suggests that torsin may be localized within both neuronal cell bodies and fiber tracts. Yet perhaps the most striking finding was the demonstration of robust torsinA messenger RNA (mRNA) expression in the dopaminergic neurons of the substantia nigra pars compacta (SNc) (8,9,12), since multiple lines of evidence have implicated this neurotransmitter system in dystonia pathogenesis (14,15). Overall, torsin appears to be widely distributed throughout all levels of the neuraxis, in association with regions and transmitter systems that have not all been linked to the clinical manifestation of disease.

Two recent studies have compared torsin immunoreactivity in brains collected from patients with a history of early-onset torsion dystonia bearing the GAG deletion and other forms of dystonia, as well as controls with no clinically relevant neurologic disease (13,16). These comparisons detected no obvious difference in torsin protein expression, nor was there any evidence of neurodegeneration within the brains of affected individuals positive for the *DYT1* mutation. These findings support the contention that the motor deficits associated with early-onset torsion dystonia do not develop due to frank neuronal loss but may instead represent a functional impairment within specific neural systems. Rostasy et al. (13) conducted a morphometric analysis of the pigmented SNc neurons and observed that, although neuron number in dystonia type 1 (DYT1) and control brains was not apparently different, the average size of neuronal cell bodies was increased. In addition, dopaminergic SNc neurons were arranged in much closer apposition to each other than was observed in control tissue. The mechanisms underlying these alterations, as well as their functional consequences, remain unclear, and future studies are required to determine what relationship, if any, these subtle abnormalities bear to clinical disease.

Studies of cultured cells have provided further details regarding the intracellular localization of wild-type and mutant torsinA, using antibodies reactive to both torsins (17,18) as well as those specific to torsinA (19). These data have collectively indicated that torsinA is localized primarily in the lumen of the endoplasmic reticulum (ER), based on (a)

subcellular fractionation and protease resistance in the absence of detergent (18,19); (b) glycosylation state (17–19); (c) cleavage of the predicted N-terminal signal sequence (19); and (d) pattern of torsinA immunoreactivity, which overlaps significantly with labeling for the ER resident proteins, protein disulfide isomerase (PDI) (17) and BiP (18). Biochemical analysis of overexpressed mutant and wild-type proteins did not detect differences in the respective patterns of subcellular fractionation, protease sensitivity, and glycosylation (18), although a prominent distinction in the subcellular localizations of mutant and wild-type torsinA was observed by immunocytochemistry (17,18). Overexpressed wild-type torsinA was diffusely distributed throughout the cell cytoplasm, in a pattern characteristic of ER proteins (17,18). In contrast, overexpressed mutant torsinA immunoreactivity was restricted to large, spheroid inclusions that frequently flanked the nucleus and displayed only partial overlap with PDI (17) and no colocalization with BiP (18). This same pattern of intracellular localization has been subsequently detected in neural cells following infection with herpes simplex virus (HSV) amplicon vectors bearing the coding sequence for either wild-type or mutant torsinA (Fig. 12-1).

Ultrastructural analysis revealed these mutant torsinA-positive inclusions to be whorled, multilamellar membrane structures within the cytoplasm (Fig. 12-2A) or surrounding the nucleus (Fig. 12–2B) (17). Inclusions were frequently enriched in PDI and appeared to derive from a compartment of the ER and/or nuclear membrane. These structures closely resembled the inducible membrane arrays, known as karmellae, that have been observed in the yeast *Saccharomyces cerevisiae*. Karmellae biogenesis in *S. cerevisiae* has been linked to the unfolded protein response (UPR) (20,21), a signal transduction pathway activated by the accumulation of misfolded proteins in the ER (22). Activation of the UPR results in increased transcription of genes encoding the cellular machinery to decrease protein syn-

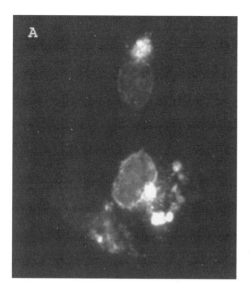
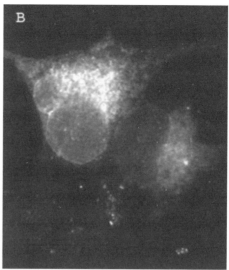

FIG. 12-1. Immunofluorescence for torsinA in human glioma cells (Gli36) following overexpression of mutant or wild-type torsinA by herpes simplex virus (HSV) amplicon vector-mediated gene transfer. Gli36 cells were infected with amplicon vectors bearing the full length coding sequence of either wild-type or mutant torsinA. Cells were washed after 24 hours and maintained in culture for an additional 24 hours prior to fixation and processing for immunofluorescence. TorsinA was detected via labeling with the monoclonal antibody, DMG10 (17), followed by reaction with a secondary antibody [goat-anti-mouse immunoglobulin G (IgG)] conjugated to Cy3. **A:** Mutant torsinA in Gli36 cells was localized primarily within discrete spheroid structures that frequently flank the nucleus. Faint immunoreactivity was also observed directly surrounding the nucleus in most cells. **B:** Overexpression of wild-type torsinA resulted in a diffuse cytoplasmic distribution characteristic of ER resident proteins.

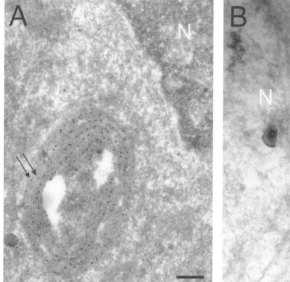
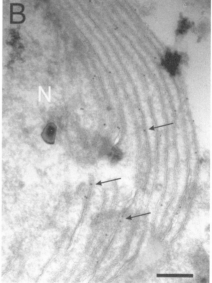

FIG. 12-2. Ultrastructural analysis of membrane inclusions in CAD cells following overexpression of mutant torsinA by transient DNA transfection. Cells were collected via centrifugation at 3 days post-transfection and sectioned for immunogold labeling/electron microscopic examination using a poly-clonal antibody to torsin (TAB1) (17) and protein A-conjugated to colloidal gold. **A:** Gold particles indicate torsin immunoreactivity associated with lipid bilayer membranes in whorled inclusions. N, nucleus. Scale bar = 200 nm. **B:** Torsin immunoreactivity associated with lipid bilayer of lamellar membranes surrounding the nucleus. N, nucleus. Scale bar = 100 nm.

thesis, remove accumulated proteins, and expand the processing capacity of the ER via de novo membrane proliferation. These observations suggest a simple possibility—that mutant torsinA is itself a misfolded protein and produces an overproliferation of ER membranes by triggering the UPR. Although this hypothesis has not been rigorously tested, it seems unlikely given that mutant torsinA within these inclusions did not form protein aggregates, as determined by electron microscopy (17). In addition, biochemical analysis of overexpressed mutant and wild-type torsinA showed that both forms could be readily solubilized to completion in nonionic detergent and displayed similar migration patterns in sucrose gradients (18). These data argue against mutant torsinA existing as a grossly misfolded protein. Furthermore, overexpression of mutant torsinA in cultured cells did not result in increased expression of the ER chaperone, BiP, which is typically upregulated during UPR activation (D. C. Bragg, unpublished data).

While membrane inclusions remain one of the most distinctive consequences of mutant torsinA expression characterized to date, relatively little is known about the mechanisms governing their formation or their effects on cellular physiology. Although these studies detected no evidence of enhanced cytotoxicity in cultures following overexpression of mutant torsinA, it is possible that some of the numerous cellular functions conducted within the ER could be compromised. Moreover, torsinA-positive inclusions have not been demonstrated in the limited number of postmortem DYT1 brain samples examined to date (13,16), which could indicate that these structures form only at high expression levels achieved in cultured cells by DNA transfection or viral vector-mediated gene transfer. Thus future studies are required to determine whether these aberrant membrane structures represent a key component of dystonia pathogenesis or an enhanced phenotype in cell culture that points to other cellular consequences of mutant torsinA expression.

FUNCTIONAL STUDIES OF TorsinA: CHAPERONE ACTIVITY AND RESPONSE TO STRESS

Members of the AAA+ superfamily often function as chaperone proteins, using adenosine triphosphate (ATP) hydrolysis for proper folding of target proteins, degradation of misfolded proteins, and trafficking of membranes and newly assembled organelles (2,3). Torsin's membership in this family suggests that it may participate in some aspect of cellular quality control, and empirical evidence supporting this hypothesis has recently emerged. Immunohistochemical analysis of brain sections from patients with Parkinson's disease (PD) revealed intense torsinA immunoreactivity within Lewy bodies (23) and a strong association with another Lewy body component, α-synuclein as determined by fluorescence resonance energy transfer (FRET) (24). McLean et al. (25) subsequently tested the hypothesis that torsinA might function as a molecular chaperone for α-synuclein by cotransfecting human neuroglioma cells with expression constructs for torsinA and a C-terminally modified α-synuclein that forms aggregates. Overexpression of wild-type torsinA dramatically reduced the number of transfected cells containing α-synuclein aggregates. In contrast, mutant torsinA failed to suppress α-synuclein aggregation, and the inclusions produced by these two proteins represented distinct, nonoverlapping cytoplasmic structures.

Additional support for torsin-related chaperone activity in the nematode *Caenorhabditis elegans* was recently provided by Caldwell et al. (26). The torsinA orthologue in *C. elegans*, TOR-2, also appears to be a resident ER protein based on the presence of a putative ER retention signal and co-localization with the nematode ER marker, TRAM. Overexpression of either TOR-2 or human wild-type torsinA significantly suppressed the aggregation of a fusion protein consisting of extended polyglutamine repeats and green fluorescent protein (GFP). These GFP-polyglutamine aggregates were highly immunoreactive for

TOR-2, similar to the association observed between torsinA and α-synuclein in Lewy bodies (23,24). Furthermore, a mutant form of TOR-2, lacking a serine residue in a position closely aligned to the glutamic acid that is deleted in human torsinA, failed to reduce protein aggregation. Thus the data that emerge from these two model systems display clear parallels and point to a possible chaperone function of torsinA, in that it appears to be recruited to intracellular sites of aberrant protein deposition and, at least at high expression levels, can suppress or resolve aggregates.

Studies of the endogenous torsinA in PC12 cells have offered further clues regarding its function. Hewett et al. (19) exposed cells to a diverse range of sublethal cellular stresses, followed by Western blot analysis to monitor changes in torsinA expression. Only oxidative stress induced by micromolar concentrations of hydrogen peroxide (H_2O_2) exerted a marked effect, consisting of an increase in the apparent molecular weight of torsinA that did not appear to reflect either glycosylation or phosphorylation. Exposure to H_2O_2 also shifted the intracellular localization of torsinA: from a diffuse cytoplasmic distribution in the absence of H_2O_2 to intense labeling of "bleb"-like projections from the cell surface after exposure to 5 μM H_2O_2 for 1 hour. TorsinA immunoreactivity in these blebs did not appear to co-localize with PDI, in contrast to the overlapping staining patterns observed in untreated cells. The demonstration that torsinA may display a dynamic intracellular distribution under different conditions could help explain its apparent association with aggregated proteins like α-synuclein that are not thought to enter the lumen of the ER.

The effects of H_2O_2 on torsinA state and localization in PC12 cells are intriguing, although it is unclear if torsinA is damaged and/or modified during exposure to oxidative insults or if it directly participates in the cellular signaling response to oxidative stress. The latter possibility is an attractive hypothesis given that (a) the dopaminergic neurons of the SNc have been hypothesized to play a key role in the development of dystonia-related motor deficits (14,15); (b) these cells experience endogenous oxidative stress due to dopamine metabolism (27); and (c) they express high levels of torsinA (8,9,12). It remains to be determined whether torsinA confers protection to dopaminergic neurons during oxidative insults and whether this protection is somehow compromised as a result of the GAG deletion. As new disease models, such as mutant mice and primary cell culture systems, become available, these hypotheses can eventually be tested.

Although the investigations summarized above provide compelling insight into possible functions for torsinA, additional possibilities have been suggested by studies of torsin-related proteins in diverse species [recently reviewed in Breakefield et al. (28)]. These proteins include (a) OOC-5, a *C. elegans* protein involved in positioning of the nuclear-centrosome complex during embryogenesis and establishing cell polarity (29); (b) SKD3, a nuclear-encoded mitochondrial protein in mice that is upregulated during conditions of energy deficiency (30); and (c) ADIR, a recently identified ER protein in mice, equivalent to torp3A (4), that is upregulated by α-interferon and viral infection (31). Although seemingly disparate, these related proteins exhibit the common functional themes of membrane/organelle trafficking and responses to cellular stress that are characteristic of many AAA+ superfamily members. Further characterization of torsin relatives in their respective hosts remains an important goal in the efforts to understand torsinA function.

EARLY-ONSET TORSION DYSTONIA: FROM PROTEIN TO GENES

Efforts to unravel the molecular etiology of early-onset torsion dystonia have indeed expanded beyond molecular genetics to involve new arenas of cell biology and neuroscience as investigators now attempt to characterize the function of torsinA and the effects of the GAG deletion. Yet genetic analyses still hold an important place in dystonia research. *DYT1* is one of over 12 genes currently associated with some form of dystonia (32). Although the GAG deletion in *DYT1* has been linked to most cases of early-onset dystonia (33), the recent discoveries of novel deletions in *DYT1* (34,35) highlight the prospect that other mutations may still exist. Such analyses may be effectively complemented by the identification of proteins that functionally interact with torsinA, some of which may be encoded by other dystonia genes. With the development of commercial gene array technologies, it is now possible to rapidly conduct global transcript screens to identify genes that respond to wild-type and mutant torsinA expression; such studies can potentially illuminate intracellular pathways in which torsinA participates, as well as possible novel functions assumed by the mutant protein. Armed with such powerful new tools, the search for dystonia-related genes and the function of torsinA continues.

ACKNOWLEDGMENTS

The authors thank Dr. Christoph Kamm and Jeffrey Hewett, both of Massachusetts General Hospital, and Dr. Caroline Shamu of Harvard Medical School for offering valuable insight and advice. This work was supported the Jack Fasciana Fund for Support of Dystonia Research (X.O.B.) and NINDS (National Institute of Neurological Disorders and Stroke) grants NS28384. Dr. Bragg was a recipient of a postdoctoral fellowship funded by an institutional National Research Service Award (NRSA) to the Program in Neuroscience at Harvard Medical School.

REFERENCES

1. Ozelius LJ, Hewett JW, et al. The gene (DYT1) for early-onset torsion dystonia encodes a novel protein related to the Clp protease/heat shock family. In: Fahn S, Marsden CD, DeLong M, eds. *Dystonia 3: advances in neurology,* vol 78. Philadelphia: Lippincott-Raven, 1998:95–105.
2. Neuwald AF, Aravind L, Spouge JL, et al. AAA+: a class of chaperone-like ATPases associated with the assembly, operation, and disassembly of protein complexes. *Genome Res* 1999;9:27–43.
3. Vale RD. AAA proteins: lords of the ring. *J Cell Biol* 2000;150:F13–F19.
4. Ozelius LJ, Page CE, Klein C, et al. The TOR1A (DYT1) gene family and its role in early onset torsion dystonia. *Genomics* 1999;62:377–384.
5. Ozelius LJ, Hewett J, Page C, et al. The early-onset torsion dystonia gene (DYT1) encodes an ATP-binding protein. *Nat Genet* 1997;17:40–48.
6. Shashidharan P, Kramer BC, Walker RH, et al. Immunohistochemical localization and distribution of torsinA in normal human and rat brain. *Brain Res* 2000; 853:197–206.
7. Konakova M, Huynh DP, Yong W, et al. Cellular distribution of torsin A and torsin B in normal human brain. *Arch Neurol* 2001;58:921–927.
8. Augood SJ, Penney JB, Friberg IK, et al. Expression of the early-onset torsion dystonia gene (DYT1) in human brain. *Ann Neurol* 1998;43:669–673.
9. Augood SJ, Martin DM, Ozelius LJ, et al. Distribution of the mRNAs encoding torsinA and torsinB in the normal adult human brain. *Ann Neurol* 1999;46:761–769.
10. Konakova M, Pulst SM. Immunocytochemical characterization of torsin proteins in mouse brain. *Brain Res* 2001;922:1–8.
11. Walker RH, Brin MF, Sandu D, et al. Distribution and immunohistochemical characterization of torsinA immunoreactivity in rat brain. *Brain Res* 2001;900:348–354.
12. Ziefer P, Leung J, Razzano T, et al. Molecular cloning and expression of rat torsinA in the normal and genetically dystonic (dt) rat. *Mol Brain Res* 2002;132–135.
13. Rostasy K, Augood SJ, Hewett JW, et al. TorsinA protein and neuropathology in early onset generalized dystonia with GAG deletion. *Neurobiol Dis* 2003;101:12:11–24.
14. Todd RD, Perlmutter JS. Mutational and biochemical analysis of dopamine in dystonia. *Mol Neurobiol* 1998; 16(2):135–147.
15. Augood SJ, Hollingsworth Z, Albers DS, et al. Dopamine transmission in DYT1 dystonia: a biochemical and autoradiographical study. *Neurology* 2002;59:445–448.
16. Walker RH, Brin MF, Sandu D, et al. TorsinA immunoreactivity in brains of patients with DYT1 and non-DYT1 dystonia. *Neurology* 2002;58:120–124.
17. Hewett J, Gonzalez-Agosti C, Slater D, et al. Mutant torsinA, responsible for early-onset torsion dystonia, forms membrane inclusions in cultured neural cells. *Hum Mol Genet* 2000;9(9):1403–1413.
18. Kustedjo K, Bracey MH, Cravatt BF. Torsin A and its torsion dystonia-associated mutant forms are luminal glycoproteins that exhibit distinct subcellular localizations. *J Biol Chem* 2000;275(36):27933–27939.
19. Hewett J, Ziefer P, Bergeron D, et al. TorsinA in PC12 cells: localization in the endoplasmic reticulum and response to stress. *J Neurosci Res* 2003;72:158–168.
20. Cox JS, Chapman RE, Walter P. The unfolded protein response coordinates the production of endoplasmic reticulum protein and endoplasmic reticulum membrane. *Mol Biol Cell* 1997;8:1805–1814.
21. Menzel R, Vogel F, Kargel E, et al. Inducible membranes in yeast: relation to the unfolded-protein-response pathway. *Yeast* 1997;13:1211–1229.
22. Kaufman RJ. Stress signaling from the lumen of the endoplasmic reticulum: coordination of gene transcriptional and translational controls. *Genes Dev* 1999;13: 1211–1233.

23. Shashidharan P, Good PF, Hsu A, et al. TorsinA accumulation in Lewy bodies in sporadic Parkinson's disease. *Brain Res* 2000;877:379–381.

24. Sharma N, Hewett J, Ozelius LJ, et al. TorsinA has a tight intermolecular association with alpha synuclein in Lewy bodies: a fluorescence resonance energy transfer study. *Am J Pathol* 2001;159(1):339–344.

25. McLean PJ, Kawamata H, Shariff S, et al. TorsinA and heat shock proteins act as molecular chaperones: suppression of α-synuclein aggregation. *J Neurochem* 2002;83:846–854.

26. Caldwell GA, Cao S, Sexton EG, et al. Suppression of polyglutamine-induced protein aggregation in *Caenorhabditis elegans* by torsin proteins. *Hum Mol Genet* 2003;12(3):307–319.

27. Olanow CW. Oxidation reactions in Parkinson's disease. *Neurology* 1990;40(suppl 3):S32–37.

28. Breakefield XO, Kamm C, Hanson PI. TorsinA: movement at many levels. *Neuron* 2001;31:9–12.

29. Basham SE, Rose LS. Mutations in *ooc-5* and *ooc-3* disrupt oocyte formation and the reestablishment of asymmetric PAR protein localization in two-cell *Caenorhabditis elegans* embryos. *Dev Biol* 1999;215(253):253–263.

30. Murdock DG, Boone BE, Esposito LA, et al. Up-regulation of nuclear and mitochondrial genes in the skeletal muscle of mice lacking the heart/muscle isoform of the adenine nucleotide translocator. *J Biol Chem* 1999; 13:14429–14433.

31. Dron M, Meritet JF, Dandoy-Dron F, et al. Molecular cloning of *ADIR*, a novel interferon responsive gene encoding a protein related to the torsins. *Genomics* 2002; 79(3):315–325.

32. Klein C, Breakefield XO, Ozelius LJ. Genetics of primary dystonia. *Semin Neurol* 1999;19(3):271–280.

33. Bressman SB, Sabatti C, Raymond D, et al. The DYT1 phenotype and guidelines for diagnostic testing. *Neurology* 2000;54:1746–1752.

34. Leung JC, Klein C, Friedman J, et al. Novel mutation in the *TOR1A* (*DYT1*) gene in atypical, early onset dystonia and polymorphisms in dystonia and early onset parkinsonism. *Neurogenetics* 2001;3:133–143.

35. Kabakci K, Pramstaller PP, Hedrich K, et al. Screening of a large cohort of movement disorder patients and controls for the GAG deletion in the DYT1 gene and detection of a novel mutation. In: *Movement Disorders* 2002;17(55):S928.

Dystonia 4: Advances in Neurology, Vol. 94. Edited by Stanley Fahn, Mark Hallett, and Mahlon R. DeLong. Lippincott Williams & Wilkins, Philadelphia © 2004.

13

An Epidemiologic Survey of Dystonia Within the Entire Population of Northeast England Over the Past Nine Years

*Anthony G. Butler, †Philip O. F. Duffey, ‡Maurice R. Hawthorne, and §Michael P. Barnes

*Dystonia Epidemiologist, Durham, United Kingdom. †York District Hospital, York, United Kingdom. ‡The North Riding Infirmary, Middlesbrough, United Kingdom. §Department of Neurological Rehabilitation, University of Newcastle, Hunters Moor Rehabilitation Centre, Newcastle-upon-Tyne, United Kingdom

The Epidemiological Survey of Dystonia (ESD) began on May 6, 1993, with just 143 people known to have dystonia in the northeast of England and Cumbria. By the time of the 3rd International Dystonia Conference held in Florida in June 1996, that is, just 3 years later, there were a total of 641 cases that had been positively diagnosed (1). As of November 1, 2002, the total number of patients with dystonias within this same geographic region was 1,339. This research has proven that dystonia is the third most prevalent movement disorder in the United Kingdom after Parkinson's disease and benign essential tremor.

Although there have been a number of epidemiologic studies of dystonia published throughout the world in the last 20 years (2–11), there is very little published data giving the prevalence of dystonia in the UK (12,13). This study is due to be completed on May 6, 2003, thus giving a comprehensive, longitudinal, and continuous survey over a 10-year period.

This will be the first time that an epidemiologic study has attempted to identify *all* cases of dystonia within a well-defined population. All other previous dystonia epidemiologies either have taken medical referral centers as the basis for their statistics or have been flawed in that ascertainment of the diagnosis was incomplete or the nature of the diagnostic criteria was limited in some way. In this case, a definite geographic region has been taken and as far as possible everyone known to have dystonia who lives in or is treated within that region has been included. Over 12.1% of these people were not registered at any hospital or medical treatment center at the time of their ascertainment.

Darlington, a small town in the northeast of England, with a known population of 101,766 individuals within 45,383 households, was the subject of an intensive epidemiologic study undertaken in 1996. This town had just 39 people with dystonia within it at the time of the last publication (12). The study has continued to date, and currently this town has exactly 53 people within the same boundaries with a form of dystonia, thus indicating a prevalence of 1 in 2,000 people (precisely 1 in 1,850). A detailed analysis has not been done on any of these statistics, as there is less than

9 months to run before the entire survey will be completed after 10 years.

METHODOLOGY

The methodology has not changed since it was previously reported in 1998 (12). The catchment area for this study comprises the counties of Northumberland, Tyne and Wear, Durham, Cleveland, Cumbria, and parts of North Yorkshire. The region contains both rural and urban areas with major conurbations existing around the cities of Newcastle, Middlesbrough, Sunderland, and York. This area measures approximately 80 miles by 120 miles (130 km by 200 km)—very small in world terms, but it nevertheless contains the world's largest regional database on dystonia.

There are certain advantages of performing an epidemiologic survey of dystonia in this area. It is relatively insular and is served by a relatively small number of neurologists operating from just four main centers. However, since the last publication in 1998, there has been a vast increase in the various methods of treating people with dystonia in this area.

This is entirely due to the establishment of a total of eight dystonia nurses now giving injections of botulinum toxin therapy in a total of six different clinics throughout the region, and one of these nurses is the world's first outreach dystonia nurse practitioner, injecting over 150 patients in their own homes on a regular basis. This development is due to the tremendous increase in dystonia patients demanding treatment, in part due to the success of the ESD. The ESD is inclusive of all types of dystonia movement, whether primary, dystonia-plus, secondary, or heredodegenerative. Each case is clinically verified to ensure complete authenticity and has been examined by a qualified neurologist. Each person is personally interviewed. After the initial methodology trial was completed in 1993, prior to the start of the ESD, it was vitally important that none of the methods used be changed or modified in any way. The exception to this rule is that a number of additional questions have been asked of each person, as new technology and developments have come on stream, particularly related to genetics.

INTERIM RESULTS

The earliest onset date was 1924, with the earliest recorded diagnosis in 1942. There were 330 people diagnosed between 1980 and 1992 before we started this research program, averaging just 25.7 per year or less than 0.5 persons per week. Prior to that date there were just 42 diagnoses within 37 years, i.e., 1.1 per year. Table 13-1 shows the 1,338 people currently diagnosed and their onset dates.

Since the start of the ESD, the average rate of detection is 101.3 patients per year over the 9<fr1/2> years the ESD has been running to date. This averages out at 1.95 new patients discovered each and every week. As no one

TABLE 13-1. *Onset vs. diagnosis in each year*

Year	Onset in the year	Diagnosis in the year	Notes
2002	2	38	Data to end of October
2001	22	89	
2000	50	134	
1999	48	85	
1998	76	90	
1997	53	128	
1996	69	91	
1995	58	113	
1994	92	96	
1993	87	98	Project started on May 6
1992	67	71	
1991	69	59	
1990	76	50	
1980	—	—	
1989	348	154	
1970	—	—	
1979	128	27	
1960	—	—	
1969	56	11	
1950	—	—	
1959	16	2	
1940	—	—	
1949	11	2	
1930	—	—	
1939	7	0	
1920	—	—	
1929	3	0	
Total	1,338	1,338	+ 1 patient— no information

dies from dystonia and as our detection rates improve, we shall see this rate be maintained and even increase. The natural death rate has been at an average of 8.63 persons per annum. Only two people have died unnatural deaths, one from a heroin overdose and another from suicide, as previously reported (1).

Based on the Darlington statistics, the current *undetected* dystonic population within the northeast could be between 300 and 400 people, assuming an average 6.2 years between onset and diagnosis and an average age of 39.4 years at onset (both statistics taken from the interim results of the ESD) and using life tables (14), which show male life expectancy at birth to be 72.7 years (78.3 years for females) and at 40 years (the closest to 39.4) male life expectancy is 74.8 years (79.6 years for females). This means between 22.4% and 29.9% of the local dystonic population still remains undetected.

An alternative method of calculating the undetected population would be to extrapolate the various study figures for the entire region. The population of the four northern counties was 2,605,100 (UK Office for National Statistics, estimated residential population) in mid-1995. The best set of prevalence data yet known in the region are the Darlington study figures deduced at 1 in 1,850, which gives a dystonic population for the four northern counties of the northeast of 1,408. Based on the Darlington figures, a total of 1,044 dystonias are already known in this immediate geographic area (as of October 31, 2002), thus the deduced number remaining still undetected is 364 people.

One of the most rewarding results of the research to date is that there has been a positive identification that 28.7% of all these cases have a proven member of the family with a form of dystonia, i.e., with a definite and genetic connection within the dystonic family, thus increasing the present known incidence of familial dystonia. Based on interviews in which patients have described relations not positively identified but thought to have had a form of dystonia, there are a further 94 people who have come to light, thus potentially in-

creasing the genetic connection to 35.7%. Our plans for proving this genetic connection are discussed in greater detail later.

The detection rates have improved tremendously since the start of the ESD. Currently 10.7% of patients are diagnosed within the first 12 months of onset, 19.1% within the second year, 17.4% within the third year, and 9.8% within the fourth year. Therefore, exactly 57% of patients are being diagnosed and treated within 4 years from the initial onset, 37% have taken between 4 and 19 years to get diagnosed, and only 6% have taken over 20 years to get a correct diagnosis. The longest time taken for a correct diagnosis has been 66 years for spasmodic torticollis, 40 years for blepharospasm, 29 years for spasmodic dysphonia, and 25 years for writer's cramp.

Table 13-2 lists all secondary and heredo-degenerative patients. All of these statistics are interim, as there is less than 9 months to go before the entire 10-year survey has been completed. This shows that the majority of patients seen at any one of the botulinum toxin dystonia clinics are afflicted with drug-induced dystonia. The vast majority of these patients have or had no specific indication that the cause of their dystonic spasm was due to this potential cause. The number of tardive

TABLE 13-2. *Secondary and heredodegenerative patients*

Description	Number of patients
Psychogenic	3
Benign essential tremor	3
Meningitis	4
Stroke	5
Metabolic?	6
Tardive dyskinesia	6
Multiple sclerosis	9
Cerebral palsy	11
Cardiovascular accident (CVA) or aneurysm	14
Heredodegenerative	18
Drug-induced	26

Note: Apart from the three patients who are psychogenic, the remainder are classified according to their main condition. They have been collected as they attended a local botulinum toxin dystonia clinic. No specific details have been sought of other secondary cases through other areas to gain potential numbers.

TABLE 13-3. *Statistics about the dystonias*

Type of dystonia	Prevalence per 100,000	Average age at onset (years)	Time for diagnosis (years)	Ratio (M:F)
Spasmodic torticollis	18.31 or 1/4,500	42.1	6.9	1:2.1
Blepharospasm	8.14 or 1/12,300	54.7	4.7	1:2.8
Spasmodic dystonia	4.26 or 1/23,500	47.4	8.8	1:4.6
Writer's cramp	2.69 or 1/37,000	37.1	6.2	1.4:1
Focal dystonia totals:	38.08 or 1/2,626	48.3	5.5	1:2.2
Generalized	3.92 or 1/25,500	22.2	12.5	1:1.6
Segmental	3.99 or 1/25,000	42.6	8.6	1:1.9
Hemidystonia	1.57 or 1/64,000	29.4	6.2	1:1.7
Multifocal	1.15 or 1/87,000	40.3	10.2	1:2.0

dyskinesias is as defined and classified by the medical profession, as opposed to tardive dystonias.

The overall distribution, shown on Table 13-3, above, is as follows: 78.2% have focal dystonia, 8.3% segmental, 8.0% generalized, 3.2% hemidystonia (most of which are secondary), and 2.3% have multifocal dystonia. Of the segmental dystonias, 36 people have craniocervical, 34 cranial, 16 brachial, 10 axial, and 10 crural. Of the focal dystonias, 566 have cervical dystonia, which is the most common form; 345 have peripheral dystonia, with 178 being in the leg and 167 in the arm; 219 have blepharospasm; 129 laryngeal dystonia (spasmodic dysphonia); 93 action-induced writer's cramp; 73 oromandibular; and 53 people have dystonia in their trunk. This leaves 21 people with facial, 18 with dystonia of the mouth, and 10 with dystonia in a lingual form. A number of the above definitions are included under segmental, multifocal, or generalized forms of dystonia; thus the numbers do not correlate exactly with the previous figures.

We also have in the study a total of 227 people with hemifacial spasm (HFS), which is assumed not to be dystonia, being caused by a blood vessel in contact with a nerve behind the ear on the side of the face affected. HFS is defined as a dystonic-type spasm affecting one side of the face only. It has been argued that all cases of HFS should not be classified as being a focal dystonia (15). The results of the above research have brought this definition into dispute, and it could be argued that this is a false assumption and that a number of so-called HFSs are in fact a focal dystonia of one side of the face, or in particular one set of eyelids. In the ESD, the statistics work out that we have 116 people with HFS on the left side of their face and a further 111 people with HFS on the right side.

However, to satisfy current medical opinion the term *unilateral blepharospasm* should be used to differentiate between the two definitions. We currently have 186 people with blepharospasm (BL), i.e., both eyelids shutting involuntarily. However, we also have 19 people with BL in the right eye and a further 14 people with BL in the left eye. This is definitely classed as unilateral blepharospasm.

DISCUSSION

Recent research undertaken by Jabusch and Altenmueller in musicians in Germany (see Chapter 32) has shown that the prevalence of dystonia could be as high as 1 in 200. The reason for this may be that musicians, almost more than any other occupation, make very fine repetitive movements of the fingers and hands and that very small dystonic tremors or postures, which are not noticeable and do not cause a problem in others, can be devastating to them.

Dystonia is not a rare disorder, but it does remain little known or recognized, even within medical circles. Research, such as the above, has proven it has a known prevalence of less than 1 in 2,000 people in the general population and even higher in specialist groups. However, the most recent advances in the genetics of dystonia have given the above research study an opportunity to advance the knowledge of dystonia greatly. It is proposed, indeed it is already happening, that every one of the 1,250+ people, currently alive, in the above study will have the opportunity to volunteer to give a 10-mL sample of their blood to the research team stored in ethylenediaminetetraacetic acid (EDTA) tubes. Total genomic DNA will be extrapolated within 48 hours using a nuclear DNA extraction kit and the DNA sample will be stored at −80°C.

The above development has the potential, over the next few years, to be used to determine the exact prevalence of the various genes, as they become identified, within the regional database on dystonia within the northeast of England. This unique resource can then be offered to other researchers throughout the world, eventually, it is hoped, to find the cure to this devastating disorder. In the meantime, we make the same plea that we made at the symposium: There are famous people with dystonia, but they are going to remain relatively unheard of by the general public until someone world famous comes out and says, "I have dystonia."

REFERENCES

1. Butler AG, Duffey POF, Hawthorne MR, et al. The socioeconomic implications of dystonia. *Adv Neurol* 1998;78:349–358.
2. Zilber N, Korczyn AD, Kahana E, et al. Inheritance of idiopathic torsion dystonia among Jews. *J Med Genet* 1984;21:13–20.
3. Li S, Schoenberg BS, Wang C, et al. A prevalence study of Parkinson's disease and other movement disorders in the Peoples Republic of China. *Arch Neurol* 1985; 42:655–657.
4. Nutt JG, Muenter MD, Aronson A, et al. Epidemiology of focal and generalised dystonia in Rochester, Minnesota. *Mov Disord* 1983;3:188–194.
5. Gimenez-Roldan S, Delgado G, Marin M, et al. Hereditary torsion dystonia in Gypsies. *Adv Neurol* 1988;50: 73–81.
6. Kandil MRA, Tohamy SA, Fattah HA, et al. Prevalence of chorea, dystonia and athetosis in Assiut, Egypt: a clinical and epidemiological study. *Neuroepidemiology* 1994;13:202–210.
7. Risch N, de Leon D, Ozelius L, et al. Genetic analysis of idiopathic torsion dystonia in Ashkenazi Jews and their recent descent from a smaller founder population. *Nat Genet* 1995;9:152–159.
8. Nakashima K, Kusumi M, Inoue Y, et al. Prevalence of focal dystonias in the western area of Tottori Prefecture in Japan. *Mov Disord* 1995;10:440–443.
9. Erjanti HM, Marttila RJ, Rinne UK. The prevalence and incidence of cervical dystonia in South Western Finland. *Mov Disord* 1996;11(suppl):A215(abst).
10. Defazio G, Livrea P. Epidemiology of primary blepharospasm. *Mov Disord* 2002;17(1):7–12.
11. Muller J, Kiechl S, Wenning GK, et al. The prevalence of primary dystonia in the general community. *Neurology* 2002;59:941–943.
12. Duffey POF, Butler AG, Hawthorne MR, et al. The epidemiology of the primary dystonias in the North of England. *Adv Neurol* 1998;78:121–125.
13. The Epidemiological study of Dystonia in Europe (ESDE). A prevalence study of primary dystonia in eight European countries. *J Neurol* 2000;247:787–792.
14. Life tables. In: *Annual abstract of statistics*. London. Central Statistical Office, 1993.
15. Elston JS. Hemi-facial spasm. *Dystonia Society Newsletter* 1997;27:5–6.

Dystonia 4: Advances in Neurology, Vol. 94. Edited by Stanley Fahn, Mark Hallett, and Mahlon R. DeLong. Lippincott Williams & Wilkins, Philadelphia © 2004.

14

Dystonia Genotypes, Phenotypes, and Classification

Susan B. Bressman

Department of Neurology, Beth Israel Medical Center, New York, and Albert Einstein College of Medicine, Bronx, New York

Over the last century, classification schemes and categories of dystonia have evolved, undergoing several important changes. To a great extent this evolution reflects increasing knowledge about etiology. For example, the lumping of all nondegenerative dystonia into a category of "idiopathic" dystonia has been discarded as genes and loci for this group of disorders have been discovered (1,2). This evolution, however, also reflects a continuing effort to refine clinical syndromes and terminology, with the ultimate goal of clarifying etiology. Spearheaded by Marsden et al. (3) and Fahn (4), classification schemes have been formulated and promoted because they provide a crucial aid for organizing thinking about the heterogeneity of dystonia. Rather than simply mirroring progress, classification facilitates the clinical approach to patient evaluation and treatment; more importantly it acts as a guide for investigating dystonia pathogenesis. For example, the identifications of *DYT1*-torsinA, *DYT5*-GCH1, and *DYT11*-ε-sarcoglycan were all dependent on careful clinical observation and classification of dystonia subtypes.

In the context of this introduction and justification for continuing the process of classification, and also a warning that the process is ever changing, this chapter reviews one current proposal for classification (Tables 14-1 and 14-2) with special emphasis on the DYT1

and genetic forms of the nondegenerative dystonias.

CLASSIFICATION

Age at Onset and Distribution

Since Marsden and colleagues' (3,5) hallmark clinical descriptions, three basic approaches to classification have been employed: age at onset, body regions or distribution affected, and etiology. The categories of age at onset and affected body distribution have undergone some refinements over the years, but they are substantively unchanged. They are also intimately related. In their seminal descriptions of clinical features, Marsden and colleagues (3,5) stressed age at onset as the single most important feature in determining outcome; the earlier the age at onset, the more likely symptoms will be severe, with dystonia spreading to involve multiple regions. Based on these observations, they proposed categories for age at onset and body regions or distribution. An ad hoc committee convened in 1984 expanded these categories, recommending three age-at-onset subclasses: childhood (age 0 to 12 years), adolescent (13 to 20 years) and adult (≥21 years), and five subclasses of distribution (focal, segmental, generalized, multifocal, and hemidystonia). Subsequent analysis of the

TABLE 14-1. *Classification of dystonia*

By age at onset
  Early (<26)
  Late
By distribution
  Focal (single body region)
  Segmental (contiguous regions)
  Multifocal (noncontiguous regions)
    Hemi (a type of multifocal–ipsilateral arm and
    leg)
  Generalized (leg + trunk + one other region or
    both legs ± trunk + one other region)
By cause
  Primary—dystonia is only sign, except tremor,
    and no acquired/exogenous cause or
    degenerative disorder
  Secondary
    Due to inherited and/or degenerative disorders—
    signs other than dystonia and/or brain
    degeneration distinguish from primary dystonia
    Due to acquired or exogenous causes
  Dystonia as a feature of another neurologic
    disorder (e.g., tics, paroxysmal dyskinesias)
  Pseudodystonia (e.g., Sandifer's, psychogenic)

distribution of ages at onset in a clinically ascertained population (6) demonstrated a bimodal distribution (with modes at 9 and 45 and a nadir at 27 years). This bimodality suggests that age at onset might be collapsed into two groups, early and late, and more recent classification schemes, including that proposed here, have followed this breakdown (2,7).

Establishing discrete groups for age at onset and affected body distributions, although not arbitrary, does not fully reflect the complex relationship between age at onset, muscles involved at onset, progression or spread of dystonia, and cause (8). It especially does not address the relationship observed in primary torsion dystonia between body region first affected and age at onset, with ascension from the legs (which overwhelmingly occurs in childhood) and arms, to neck and voice, and finally facial muscles. Nevertheless categorizing by age at onset and distribution serves as a useful guide in clinical practice and for grouping families and patients for clinical trials and genetic studies.

TABLE 14-2. *Causes of dystonia*

Primary
  Autosomal dominant
    Early limb (*DYT1,* other genes to be determined)
    Mixed (*DYT6, DYT13,* other genes to be determined)
    Late focal (*DYT7,* other genes to be determined)
  Other genetic causes
    ?Autosomal recessive, complex
Secondary
  Inherited
    Dystonia plus (nondegenerative)
      DRD (*DYT5-GCH1, DYT14,* other biopterin deficiencies, tyrosine hydroxylase deficiency)
      Myoclonus—dystonia (*DYT11*-epsilon sarcoglycan, 18p locus)
      Rapid-onset dystonia parkinsonism (*DYT12*)
    Degenerative
      Autosomal dominant (e.g., Huntington's disease, SCAs especially SCA3)
      Autosomal recessive (e.g., Wilson's, NBIA1, GM1, and GM2 gangliosidoses, *parkin*)
      X-linked (e.g., X-linked dystonia-parkinsonism/Lubag, deafness-dystonia/DDP)
      Mitochondrial
    Complex/unknown
      Parkinsonism (e.g., Parkinson's disease, multisystem atrophy, progressive supranuclear palsy,
        corticobasal degeneration)
    Acquired
      e.g., drug-induced, perinatal injury, head trauma, cervical trauma, peripheral trauma, infectious
        and postinfectious, tumor, AVM, stroke, central pontine, myelinolysis, multiple sclerosis

AVM, arteriovenous malformation; DDP, deafness dystonia peptide; DRD, dopa-responsive dystonia; GCH1, guanosine triphosphate (GTP) cyclohydrolase 1; NBIA1, neurodegeneration with brain iron accumulation; SCA, spinocerebellar ataxia.

Etiology

Historically, the causes of dystonia have been divided into two main groups: idiopathic (or primary) and symptomatic (or secondary) (4,9). Idiopathic dystonia was distinguished from the symptomatic dystonias both by its lack of known cause and the absence of consistent brain pathology. Over the past decade it has become clear that idiopathic dystonia comprises a group of clinical syndromes that are known or likely to have a genetic basis. Further, as loci for various categories of idiopathic (primary), secondary, and paroxysmal dystonias have been proposed or discovered, and assignments given by the Human Genome Organization/Genome Database (HUGO/GDB), a new classification of dystonia (DYT) loci has developed (Table 14-3), only further confusing the terminology.

One could argue, as Calne and Lang (10) did in 1988, that as genes for idiopathic dystonia are mapped and discovered, they should be moved into the symptomatic group, and idiopathic should be reserved for the remaining population awaiting a clarified etiology. But criteria for idiopathic dystonia have always rested on more than the lack of cause or consistent pathology. That is, there is a common distinguishing clinical characteristic for all id-

iopathic dystonia, i.e., dystonia is the sole abnormality directly attributable to the condition. The two other exclusionary criteria are that there are no laboratory or imaging abnormalities to suggest an acquired or degenerative cause for dystonia and no dramatic response to levodopa to suggest dopa-responsive dystonia, and historical information does not implicate a known acquired or environmental cause of dystonia (e.g., neuroleptic exposure, perinatal asphyxia).

In an attempt to incorporate genetic advances into an etiologic classification and to maintain clinical relevance and promote future research into pathogenesis, it has been proposed that (a) the term *primary (torsion) dystonia* (PTD) replace idiopathic, and (b) the three clinical criteria enumerated above be employed to distinguish primary from other nonprimary forms (1). However, even these apparently straightforward criteria have caveats. For example, tremor resembling essential tremor may accompany PTD, especially torticollis (11,12). Also, as genotype/phenotype associations are scrutinized, additional clinically covert features are being added, such as abnormalities in sequence learning, recently reported in *DYT1* carriers (13). Finally, although pathologic studies have not consistently or convincingly demonstrated abnormalities and neu-

TABLE 14-3. *Dystonia (DYT) genetic loci*

Gene	Locus	Inheritance	Phenotype	Gene product
DYT1	9q34	AD	Early limb onset	TorsinA
DYT2	Not mapped	AR	Early onset	
DYT3	Xq13.1	XR	Filipino dystonia/parkinsonism	Not identified
DYT4	Not mapped	AD	Whispering dysphonia	
DYT5	14q22.1	AD	DRD/parkinsonism	GCH1
DYT6	8p	AD	Mixed	Not identified
DYT7	18p	AD	Adult cervical	Not identified
DYT8	2q33–35	AD	PDC/PNKD	Not identified
DYT9	1p21	AD	Episodic choreoathetosis/ataxia spasticity	Not identified
DYT10	16	AD	PKC/PKD (EKD1&2)	Not identified
DYT11	7q21	AD	Myoclonus dystonia	Epsilon-sarcoglycan
DYT12	19q	AD	Rapid-onset dystonia/parkinsonism	Not identified
DYT13	1p36.13=p36.32	AD	Cervical/cranial/brachial	Not identified
DYT14	14q13	AD	DRD	Not identified

AD, autosomal dominant; AR, autosomal recessive; DRD, dopa responsive dystonia; GCH1, GTP gyclohydrolase 1; PDC, paroxysmal dystonic choreoathetosis; PKC, paroxysmal kinesigenic choreoathetosis or dyskinesia; PNKD, paroxysmal non-kinesigenic dyskinesia; XR, x-linked recessive.

rodegeneration does not appear to occur in primary dystonia, functional or other pathologic markers for the primary dystonias are being sought and may also have impact on future criteria for this group. For the present, however, with the exception of tremor, the three criteria proposed appear to adequately distinguish PTD from secondary/nonprimary subtypes.

PRIMARY TORSION DYSTONIA (PTD)

Early-Onset PTD and *DYT1 (TOR1A)*

Early-onset PTD is three to five times more common in Ashkenazi Jews compared to other populations (14,15) and is transmitted in an autosomal-dominant fashion with reduced penetrance of 30% to 40% in both Ashkenazi Jews and non-Ashkenazim (6, 16–18). The difference in disease frequency is thought to be the result of a founder mutation in *DYT1* that was introduced into the Ashkenazi population at the time of a "bottleneck" in the 1600s, followed by a period of tremendous population growth (15).

The gene at locus *DYT1* (also named *TOR1A*) was identified in 1997 (19) and is responsible for a large proportion of early limb onset PTD (also known as dystonia musculorum deformans or Oppenheim's disease) across many different populations (20–25). Except for one family in which there was myoclonus and dystonia as well as a concomitant mutation in the ε-sarcoglycan *(SGCE)* gene (26–28), all PTDs due to *DYT1* have the same (recurring) mutation, a GAG deletion. Despite this single molecular basis, clinical features, even within families, range from mild focal to severe generalized PTD (29,30). However, there are common *DYT1* clinical characteristics: the great majority of people with dystonia due to *DYT1* have early onset (before 26 years) that first affects an arm or leg (23). About 65% progress to a generalized or multifocal distribution, the rest having segmental (10%) or only focal (25%) involvement. When viewed in terms of body regions ultimately involved, one or more limbs are almost always affected (over 95% have an affected arm). The trunk and neck may also be affected (about 25% to 35%), and they may be the regions producing the greatest disability (31); the cranial muscles are less likely to be involved (<15%). Rarely, affected family members have late onset (up to age 64 years) (30). Also, although the arm is the body region most commonly affected in those with focal disease, the neck or cranial muscles have been reported as isolated affected sites (23,32,33). Because of the founder effect, the *TOR1A* GAG deletion is more important in the Ashkenazi population, where it accounts for about 80% of early-onset (less than 26 years) cases (23,34); this compares with 16% to 53% in early-onset non-Jewish populations (20–23,35,36).

With identification of the *DYT1* gene it has become possible to more fully investigate the clinical features and expression of the gene, including assessing psychomotor and imaging measures. By comparing *DYT1* gene carriers, including nonmanifesting carriers, to noncarriers, gene-associated features can be distinguished. Using this paradigm and ^{18}F-fluorodeoxyglucose positron emission tomography (FDG-PET) and network analysis, Eidelberg and colleagues (37) demonstrated an abnormal pattern of glucose utilization characterized by covarying metabolic increases in the basal ganglia, cerebellum, and supplementary motor area (SMA) cortex that was present in both manifesting and nonmanifesting gene carriers (37). More recent PET studies using psychomotor testing in nonmanifesting gene carriers show subtle abnormalities in sequence learning in both the motor performance and recruitment of brain networks (13,38). These studies strongly support the presence of abnormal brain processing in gene carriers regardless of overt motor signs of dystonia, expanding the notion of penetrance and phenotype to include subclinical features or endophenotypes.

Early-Onset But Not TOR1A

There remains a large group of early-onset PTD, especially among non-Jewish populations, that is not due to the *TOR1A* GAG deletion. Two loci, *DYT6* (39) and *DYT13* (40), have been mapped in families having an average age at onset in adolescence. However, neither locus has been confirmed in other families, and they are suspected to account for only a minority of non-*DYT1* early-onset cases. Further, overall clinical features in these two families differ from *DYT1* (although features in any single family member may overlap with *DYT1*). The family phenotypes for *DYT6* and *DYT13* are marked by prominent involvement of cranial and cervical muscles with variable spread; also, compared to *DYT1*, a greater proportion of family members have later adolescent and adult onset (see Chapter 15). To distinguish this phenotype from the typical early-onset phenotype associated with *DYT1* and typical late-onset focal phenotypes, the term *mixed* has been applied (39,41).

Late-Onset PTD

Like early-onset PTD, late-onset PTD also appears to have autosomal-dominant inheritance (42–44). However, unlike early-onset dystonia, most studies show that penetrance is even more reduced (about 12% to 15% compared to 30% for early-onset); alternatively, penetrance may be higher in a subset, with the remainder sporadic. Consistent with the notion of increased penetrance in a subset of late-onset PTD, are descriptions of large families with more highly penetrant autosomal-dominant disease (12,45). One such family with adult-onset torticollis was studied, resulting in the mapping of *DYT7* (see Chapter 15) (46). Other clinically similar families have been excluded from *DYT7* (47), suggesting yet other loci for adult-onset focal PTD. Most recently a polymorphism in the D_5 dopamine receptor gene has been associated with adult-onset torticollis and blepharospasm, and the role of this gene as a susceptibility factor remains to be elucidated (48,49).

SECONDARY DYSTONIA AND DYSTONIA PLUS SYNDROMES

Etiologic subgroups for secondary dystonias include inherited causes, a group of pri-

marily parkinsonian disorders including Parkinson's disease that are thought to have complex etiologies, and the group of environmental or acquired causes. In addition, most classifications also include other movement disorders that may display dystonic phenomenology such as tics and the paroxysmal dyskinesias and the pseudodystonias; the latter are not considered true dystonia but rather muscle contractions mimicking dystonia, such as seen in Sandifer's syndrome, orthopedic conditions, and psychogenic dystonia.

Among the inherited forms of secondary dystonia, there is a relatively newly defined category of dystonia-plus syndromes consisting of three clinically defined entities: dopa-responsive dystonia (DRD), myoclonus-dystonia (M-D), and rapid-onset dystonia-parkinsonism (RDP). The dystonia-plus category was distinguished from both primary dystonia and other inherited secondary dystonias by Fahn and colleagues (1) because it shares some but not all features of both groups. That is, like primary dystonia, these three syndromes do not appear to be degenerative. Although pathology is limited, evidence to date supports genetic defects that result in functional brain changes not associated with progressive neuronal death. Further, unlike primary dystonia, but similar to the other degenerative secondary dystonias, the dystonia-plus group has as characteristic clinical features signs other than dystonia including parkinsonism for DRD and RDP and myoclonus for M-D.

As our understanding of these syndromes is expanding, the complexity of their genetic and clinical heterogeneity is being detailed. For example, for DRD there are currently several known genetic biochemical etiologies, each with protean clinical manifestations, and for M-D there appear to be at least two genetic etiologies (see Chapters 16 and 18).

CONCLUSION

Over the past 30 years there has been tremendous growth in our knowledge of the clinical and genetic complexity of dystonia, especially PTD and the dystonia-plus syndromes. Classification schemes offer an opportunity to organize this complexity and to help direct future investigation, although the classification itself is subject to the expanding knowledge base and needs to remain a fluid guide. With this in mind, it has become apparent that schemes have and probably should remain tied to the clinical realm. Beginning with Marsden's clinical approach to classification based on clustered clinical phenomenology, the application of clinical subtyping (including its use in creating and refining etiologic subgroups or syndromes) has been instrumental for investigations into cause and disease mechanism. By defining distinct primary and dystonia-plus clinical syndromes, research into genetic causes is facilitated. Also, once a genetic etiology is determined, the clinical refinement continues as the disease spectrum is redefined and the pathophysiology explored.

ACKNOWLEDGMENTS

The author is supported by National Institutes of Health grant RO1NS26656.

REFERENCES

1. Fahn S, Bressman SB, Marsden CD. Classification of dystonia. In: Fahn S, Marsden CD, DeLong MR, eds: *Advances in neurology,* vol 78. Philadelphia: Lippincott-Raven, 1998:1–10.
2. Bressman SB. Dystonia. *Curr Opin Neurol* 1998;11: 363–372.
3. Marsden CD, Harrison MJG, Bundey S. Natural history of idiopathic dystonia. *Adv Neurol* 1976;14:177–187.
4. Fahn S. Concept and classification of dystonia. *Adv Neurol* 1988;50:1–8.
5. Marsden CD, Harrison MJG. Idiopathic torsion dystonia. *Brain* 1974;97:793–810.
6. Bressman SB, de Leon D, Brin MF, et al. Idiopathic torsion dystonia among Ashkenazi Jews: evidence for autosomal dominant inheritance. *Ann Neurol* 1989;26: 612–620.
7. Jarman PR. Warner TT. The dystonias. *J Med Genet* 1998;35:314–318.
8. Greene P, Kang UJ, Fahn S. Spread of symptoms in idiopathic torsion dystonia. *Mov Disord* 1995;10: 143–152.
9. Fahn S, Marsden CD, Calne DB. Classification and investigation of dystonia. In: Marsden CD, Fahn S, eds. *Movement disorders 2.* London: Butterworth, 1987: 332–358.
10. Calne DB, Lang AE. Secondary dystonia. *Adv Neurol* 1988;50:9–33.
11. Couch J. Dystonia and tremor in spasmodic torticollis. *Adv Neurol* 1976;14:245–258.
12. Bressman SB, Warner TT, Almasy L, et al. Exclusion of the DYT1 locus in familial torticollis. *Ann Neurol* 1996; 40:681–684.
13. Ghilardi MF, Carbon M, Silvestri G, et al. Sequence learning is impaired in clinically unaffected carriers of the DYT1 mutation. *Mov Disord* 2002;17(suppl 5): S300.
14. Zeman W, Dyken P. Dystonia musculorum deformans; clinical, genetic and pathoanatomical studies. *Psychiatr Neurol Neurochir* 1967;70:77–121.
15. Risch N, de Leon D, Ozelius L, et al. Genetic analysis of idiopathic torsion dystonia in Ashkenazi Jews and their recent descent from a small founder population. *Nat Genet* 1995;9:152–159.
16. Zilber N, Korczyn AD, Kahana E, et al. Inheritance of idiopathic torsion dystonia among Jews. *J Med Genet* 1984;21:13–26.
17. Pauls DL, Korczyn AD. Complex segregation analysis of dystonia pedigrees suggests autosomal dominant inheritance. *Neurology* 1990;40:1107–1110.
18. Fletcher NA, Harding AE, Marsden CD. A genetic study of idiopathic torsion dystonia in the United Kingdom. *Brain* 1990;113:379–396.
19. Ozelius LJ, Hewett JW, Page C, et al. The early-onset torsion dystonia gene (DYT1) encodes an ATP-binding protein. *Nat Genet* 1997;17:40–48.
20. Valente EM, Warner TT, Jarman PR, et al. The role of primary torsion dystonia in Europe. *Brain* 1998;121: 2335–2339.
21. Lebre AS, Durr A, Jedtnak P, et al. DYT1 mutation in French families with idiopathic torsion dystonia. *Brain* 1999;122:41–45.
22. Slominski PA, Markova ED, Shadrina MI, et al. A common 3-bp deletion in the DYT1 gene in Russian families with early-onset torsion dystonia. *Hum Mutat* 1999; 14:269.
23. Bressman SB, Sabatti C, Raymond D, et al. The DYT1 phenotype and guidelines for diagnostic testing. *Neurology* 2000;54:1746–1752.
24. Matsumoto S, Nishimura M, Kaji R, et al. DYT1 mutation in Japanese patients with primary torsion dystonia. *Neuroreport* 2001;12:793–795.
25. Kamm C, Castelon-Konkiewitz E, Naumann M, et al. GAG deletion in the DYT1 gene in early limb-onset idiopathic torsion dystonia in Germany. *Mov Disord* 1999;14:681–683.
26. Leung J, Klein C, Friedman J, et al. Novel mutation in the TOR1A (DYT1) gene in atypical early onset dystonia and polymorphisms in dystonia and early onset parkinsonism. *Neurogenetics* 2001;3:133–143.
27. Doheny D, Danisi F, Smith C, et al. Clinical findings of a myoclonus-dystonia family with two distinct mutations. *Neurology* 2002;59:1244–1246.
28. Klein C, Liu L, Doheny D, et al. Epsilon sarcoglycan mutations found in combination with other dystonia mutations. *Ann Neurol* 2002;52:675–679.
29. Gasser T, Windgassen K, Bereznai B, et al. Phenotypic expression of the DYT1 mutation: a family with writer's cramp of juvenile onset. *Ann Neurol* 1998;44:126–128.
30. Opal P, Tintner R, Jankovic J, et al. Intrafamilial phenotypic variability of the DYT1 dystonia: from asympto-

matic TOR1A gene carrier status to dystonic storm. *Mov Disord* 2002;17(2):339–345.

31. Chinnery PF, Reading PJ, McCarthy EL, et al. Late-onset axial jerky dystonia due to the DYT1 deletion. *Mov Disord* 2002;17:196–198.

32. Leube B, Kessler KR, Ferbert A, et al. Phenotypic variability of the DYT1 mutation in German dystonia patients. *Acta Neurol Scand* 1999;99:248–251.

33. Tuffery-Giraud S, Cavalier L, Roubertie A, et al. No evidence of allelic heterogeneity in the DYT1 gene of European patients with early onset torsion dystonia. *J Med Genet* 2001;38:E35.

34. Bressman SB, de Leon D, Kramer PL, et al. Dystonia in Ashkenazi Jews: clinical characterization of a founder mutation. *Ann Neurol* 1994;35:771–777.

35. Brassat D, Camuzat A, Vidailhet M, et al. Frequency of the DYT1 mutation in primary torsion dystonia without family history. *Arch Neurol* 2000;57:333–335.

36. Zorzi G, Garavaglia B, Invernizzi F, et al. Frequency of DYT1 mutation in early onset primary dystonia in Italian patients. *Mov Disord* 2002;17:407–408.

37. Eidelberg D, Moeller JR, Antonini A, et al. Functional brain networks in DYT1 dystonia. *Ann Neurol* 1998; 44:303–312.

38. Carbon M, Ghilardi MF, Dhawan V, et al. Brain networks subserving motor sequence learning in DYT1 gene carriers. *Neurology* 2002;P03.067(abst).

39. Almasy L, Bressman SB, Kramer PL, et al. Idiopathic torsion dystonia linked to chromosome 8 in two Mennonite families. *Ann Neurol* 1997;42:670–673.

40. Valente EM, Bentivoglio AR, Cassetta E, et al. DYT13, a novel primary torsion dystonia locus, maps to chromosome 1p36.13-36.32 in an Italian family with cranial-cervical or upper limb onset. *Ann Neurol* 2001;49: 363–364.

41. Bressman SB, De Leon D, Raymond D, et al. Clinical-genetic spectrum of primary dystonia. *Adv Neurol* 1998;78:79–92.

42. Defazio G, Livrea P, Guanti G, et al. Genetic contribution to idiopathic adult-onset blepharospasm and cranial-cervical dystonia. *Eur Neurol* 1993;33:345–350.

43. Waddy HM, Fletcher NA, Harding AE, et al. A genetic study of idiopathic focal dystonias. *Ann Neurol* 1991; 29:320–324.

44. Stojanovic M, Cvetkovic D, Kostic VS. A genetic study of idiopathic focal dystonias. *J Neurol* 1995;242: 508–511.

45. Münchau A, Valente EM, Davis MB, et al. A Yorkshire family with adult-onset cranio-cervical primary torsion dystonia. *Mov Disord* 2000;15:954.

46. Leube B, Doda R, Ratzlaff T, et al. Idiopathic torsion dystonia: assignment of a gene to chromosome 18p in a German family with adult onset, autosomal inheritance and purely focal distribution. *Hum Mol Genet* 1996;5: 1673–1677.

47. Jarman P, Valente EM, Leube B, et al. Primary torsion dystonia: the search for genes is not over. *J Neurol Neurosurg Psychiatry* 1999;67:395–397.

48. Placzek MR, Misbahuddin A, Chaudhuri KR, et al. Cervical dystonia is associated with a polymorphism in the dopamine (D5) receptor gene. *J Neurol Neurosurg Psychiatry* 2001;71:262–264.

49. Misbahuddin A, Placzek MR, Chaudhuri KR, et al. A polymorphism in the dopamine receptor DRD5 is associated with blepharospasm. *Neurology* 2002;58: 124–126.

Dystonia 4: Advances in Neurology, Vol. 94. Edited by Stanley Fahn, Mark Hallett, and Mahlon R. DeLong. Lippincott Williams & Wilkins, Philadelphia © 2004.

15

Update on the Genetics of Primary Torsion Dystonia Loci *DYT6, DYT7,* and *DYT13* and the Dystonia-Plus Locus *DYT12*

Laurie J. Ozelius

Department of Molecular Genetics, Albert Einstein College of Medicine, Bronx, New York

At least 13 different loci have been identified for various forms of inherited dystonia. This chapter discusses the genetic findings relevant to the following types of primary torsin dystonia (PTD): *DYT6, DYT7, DYT13,* and a dystonia-plus form associated with parkinsonism *DYT12*. All of these forms of dystonia appear to be inherited as autosomal-dominant traits with reduced penetrance.

The *DYT6* locus was identified by linkage analysis using 15 affected members in two Swiss Mennonite families (1). Penetrance appears to be about 30% and the clinical picture is broad or "mixed" with an early age of onset (18.6 ± 11.9 years, range 5–38 years) and progression to involve multiple body regions. Most patients have their greatest disability due to involvement of muscles of the neck, larynx, or face, with common but less severe limb involvement. The PTD locus in these families maps to chromosome 8 [maximum two-point logarithm of odds (LOD) score = 5.80 at the anonymous locus D8S1797] (1) (Fig. 15-1). As initially described, the delimited region bearing the disease gene spanned 40 centimorgan (cM), with identical haplotypes segregating in both families, suggesting a common founder. Subsequent genealogic investigation revealed this common ancestor. Reevaluating these families using additional

polymorphic markers and a newly ascertained branch of the family containing two affected members revealed historical recombination events at markers D8S2323 and D8S2317, thus narrowing the obligate genetic region from 40 cM to about 23 cM (Ozelius, unpublished results).

Several studies support the idea that late-onset PTD is inherited (2–5); however, most studies suggest that penetrance is very reduced (about 12% to 15% compared to 30% for early onset). Alternatively, penetrance may be higher in a subset, with the remainder nongenetic. Consistent with this notion of increased penetrance in a subset, several large families with more highly penetrant autosomal-dominant disease have been described (6,7). One such family, from Northwest Germany, was studied, resulting in the mapping of *DYT7*. The family manifests primarily late-onset focal cervical dystonia (torticollis), although mild cranial and arm involvement was observed (8). The *DYT7* gene localizes to a 30-cM region on chromosome 18p between D18S1153 and 18pter (8) (Fig. 15-1). The same group reported allelic association for the marker D18S1098 in sporadic and familial torticollis, suggesting a founder mutation for adult-onset torticollis in the Northwest German population (9,10). However, the find-

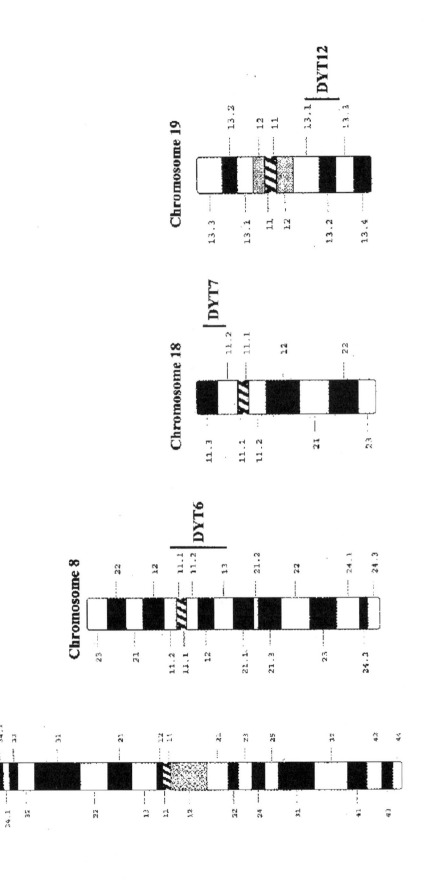

ing of allelic association could not be replicated in another group of German focal dystonia patients (11), and when Leube and Auburger (12) attempted to confirm their findings, they could not. Although a common founder of focal dystonia cases from Northern German or Central European origin has been ruled out, two findings support presence of at least one dystonia gene on chromosome 18p–. These include patients with a deletion of the short arm of chromosome 18 (18p⁻ syndrome) who exhibit dystonic symptoms (13,14), as well as a family with myoclonus-dystonia linked to markers overlapping this region on 18p (15).

A genome-wide search in a large Italian PTD family from central Italy with 11 definitely affected members resulted in the identification of a novel locus, *DYT13* (16). The phenotype in this family is characterized by prominent cervical-cranial and upper limb involvement with early onset (between 5 and 40 years, average 15.6 years) and mild severity (17). Over time, most showed progression with cervical dystonia, producing the predominant disability. The phenotype is not clearly different from *DYT6* except that leg and laryngeal involvement may be less significant for *DYT13*. Linkage and haplotype analysis placed the locus within a 22-cM interval on the short arm of chromosome 1, with a maximum LOD score of 3.44 between the disease and marker D1S2667 (16) (Fig. 15–1). In addition, the *DYT13* locus shares a 6-cM region in common with a recently identified locus for autosomal-recessive early-onset parkinsonism *(PARK7)*, raising the possibility that *DYT13* and *PARK7* might be allelic disorders, despite apparent differences in phenotype and transmission pattern (18).

It seems likely that *DYT6, DYT7,* and *DYT13* account for only a small proportion of adult- and cervical/cranial-onset PTD, as several large families with clinically similar features have been excluded by linkage analysis from these loci (6,7,19,20), supporting the presence of other as yet unmapped genes. In addition, an association between alleles at a nonfunctional polymorphic site near [about 18 kilobase (kb) upstream] the dopamine D_5 receptor and focal dystonia was reported (21,22). The authors found an overrepresentation of allele 2 in a group of 100 cervical dystonia patients and 88 blepharospasm patients as compared to controls, suggesting that this polymorphism is in linkage disequilibrium with a nearby pathogenic change. However, further studies are needed to determine the significance of this finding.

To date, four unrelated families have been reported with rapid-onset dystonia-parkinsonism (RDP, *DYT12*) (23–25; Zaremba, unpublished data). RDP is characterized by abnormal movements typical of both dystonia (twisting or repetitive movements, dystonic postures) and parkinsonism (bradykinesia and postural instability). Symptoms come on rapidly (over hours to days), or there is an episode of rapid progression from mild to severe disability generally followed by stable symptoms for years (26). Onset generally occurs late in childhood or early in adulthood, but has a wide range, between 4 and 55 years. By patients' reports, onset can be triggered by stressful events, including intense physical exertion, fever, or emotional stress. Some patients have decreased levels of homovanillic acid in the cerebral spinal fluid yet little or no response to L-dopa, while neuroimaging studies reveal no loss of dopaminergic neurons (27,28). In addition, no pathologic changes were noted in the brain from a patient with RDP (29). Using two of the families, a gene for RDP was mapped to chromosome 19q13 *(DYT12)* with the highest multipoint LOD score of 5.77 at the marker D19S198 (Fig. 15-1). Obligate recombination events at markers D19S587 and D19S900 defined a candidate

FIG. 15-1. Ideograms displaying the chromosomal location of dystonia genes described in the text. (Modified from David Adler, Department of Pathology, University of Washington: *http://www.pathology.washington.edu/research/cytopages/idiograms/human/*.)

region of approximately 8 cM (30). Both an Irish family with eight affected individuals and a family from Poland with four affected members have been linked to the same chromosome 19 locus (29; Ozelius, unpublished data), but neither shows recombination events that would refine the locus position.

ACKNOWLEDGMENTS

This work was supported by grants from the Dystonia Medical Research Foundation and NIH grants NS26656 and NS37409.

REFERENCES

1. Almasy L, Bressman SB, Raymond D, et al. Idiopathic torsion dystonia linked to chromosome 8 in two Mennonite families. *Ann Neurol* 1997;42:670–673.
2. Defazio G, Livrea P, Guanti G, et al. Genetic contribution to idiopathic adult-onset blepharospasm and cranial-cervical dystonia. *Eur Neurol* 1993;33:345–350.
3. Waddy HM, Fletcher NA, Harding AE, et al. A genetic study of idiopathic focal dystonias. *Ann Neurol* 1991; 29:320–324.
4. Stojanovic M, Cvetkovic D, Kostic VS. A genetic study of idiopathic focal dystonias. *J Neurol* 1995;242: 508–511.
5. Leube B, Kessler KR, Goecke T, et al. Frequency of familial inheritance among 488 index patients with idiopathic focal dystonia and clinical variability in a large family. *Mov Disord* 1997;12:1000–1006.
6. Jarman P, Valente EM, Leube B, et al. Primary torsion dystonia: the search for genes is not over. *J Neurol Neurosurg Psychiatry* 1999;67:395–397.
7. Münchau A, Valente EM, Davis MB, et al. A Yorkshire family with adult-onset cranio-cervical primary torsion dystonia. *Mov Disord* 2000;15:954–959.
8. Leube B, Doda R, Ratzlaff T, et al. Idiopathic torsion dystonia: assignment of a gene to chromosome 18p in a German family with adult onset, autosomal inheritance and purely focal distribution. *Hum Mol Genet* 1996;5: 1673–1677.
9. Leube B, Hendgen T, Kessler KR, et al. Sporadic focal dystonia in Northwest Germany: molecular basis on chromosome 18p. *Ann Neurol* 1997;42:111–114.
10. Leube B, Hendgen T, Kessler KR, et al. Evidence for DYT7 being a common cause of cervical dystonia (torticollis) in Central Europe. *Am J Med Genet* 1997;74: 529–532.
11. Klein C, Ozelius L, Hagenah J, et al. Search for a founder mutation in idiopathic focal dystonia from Northern Germany. *Am J Hum Genet* 1998;63: 1777–1782.
12. Leube B, Auburger G. Questionable role of adult-onset focal dystonia among sporadic dystonia patients. *Ann Neurol* 1998;44:984–985.
13. Tezzon F, Zanoni T, Passarin MG, et al. Dystonia in a patient with deletion of 18p. *Ital J Neurol Sci* 1998; 19:90–93.
14. Klein C, Page CE, LeWitt P, et al. Genetic analysis of three patients with an 18p- syndrome and dystonia. *Neurology* 1999;52:649–651.
15. Grimes D, Han F, Lang A, et al. A novel locus for inherited myoclonus-dystonia on 18p11. *Neurology* 2002; 59:1183–1186.
16. Valente EM, Bentivoglio AR, Cassetta E, et al. DYT13, a novel primary torsion dystonia locus, maps to chromosome 1p36.13-36.32 in an Italian family with cranial-cervical or upper limb onset. *Ann Neurol* 2001;49: 363–364.
17. Bentivoglio AR, Del Grosso N, Albanese A, et al. Non-DYT1 dystonia in a large Italian family. *J Neurol Neurosurg Psychiatry* 1997;62:357–360.
18. Bonifati V, Breedveld GJ, Squitieri F, et al. Localization of autosomal recessive early-onset parkinsonism to chromosome 1p36 (PARK7) in an independent data set. *Ann Neurol* 2002;51:253–256.
19. Klein C, Pramstaller PP, Castellan CC, et al. Clinical and genetic evaluation of a family with a mixed dystonia phenotype from South Tyrol. *Ann Neurol* 1998;44: 394–398.
20. Brancati F, Defazio G, Caputo V, et al. Novel Italian family supports clinical and genetic heterogeneity of primary adult-onset torsion dystonia. *Mov Disord* 2002; 17:392–397.
21. Placzec MR, Misbahuddin A, Chaudhuri KR, et al. Cervical dystonia is associated with a polymorphism in the dopamine (D5) receptor gene. *J Neurol Neurosurg Psychiatry* 2001;71:262–264.
22. Misbahuddin A, Placzec MR, Chaudhuri KR, et al. A polymorphism in the dopamine receptor DRD5 is associated with blepharospasm. *Neurology* 2002;58: 124–126.
23. Dobyns WB, Ozelius LJ, Kramer PL, et al. Rapid-onset dystonia-parkinsonism. *Neurology* 1993;43:2596–2602.
24. Brashear A, de Leon D, Bressman SB, et al. Rapid-onset dystonia-parkinsonism in a second family. *Neurology* 1997;48:1066–1069.
25. Webb DW, Broderick A, Brashear A, et al. Rapid onset dystonia-parkinsonism in a 14-year-old girl. *Eur J Paediatr Neurol* 1999;3:171–173.
26. Brashear A, Farlow MR, Butler IJ, et al. Variable phenotype of rapid-onset dystonia-parkinsonism. *Mov Disord* 1996;11:151–156.
27. Brashear A, Butler IJ, Hyland K, et al. Cerebrospinal fluid homovanillic acid levels in rapid-onset dystonia-parkinsonism. *Ann Neurol* 1998;43:521–526.
28. Brashear A, Mulholland GK, Zheng Q-H, et al. PET imaging of the pre-synaptic dopamine uptake sites in rapid-onset dystonia-parkinsonism (RDP). *Mov Disord* 1999;14:132–137.
29. Pittock SJ, Joyce C, O'Keane V, et al. Rapid-onset dystonia-parkinsonism: a clinical and genetic analysis of a new kindred. *Neurology* 2000;55:991–995.
30. Kramer PL, Mineta M, Klein C, et al. Rapid-onset dystonia-parkinsonism: linkage to chromosome 19q13. *Ann Neurol* 1999;46:176–182.

Dystonia 4: Advances in Neurology, Vol. 94. Edited by Stanley Fahn, Mark Hallett, and Mahlon R. DeLong. Lippincott Williams & Wilkins, Philadelphia © 2004.

16

Inherited Myoclonus-Dystonia

Friedrich Asmus and Thomas Gasser

Department of Neurodegenerative Disorders, Hertie-Institute for Clinical Brain Research, University of Tübingen, Tübingen, Germany

The dystonias are a common, clinically and genetically heterogeneous group of movement disorders characterized by involuntary muscle contractions, leading to sustained or repetitive movements or abnormal postures. Based on additional clinical or pharmacologic features, several "dystonia-plus" syndromes can be differentiated from primary dystonia, including dopa-responsive dystonia, the paroxysmal dystonias, or X-linked dystonia-parkinsonism (1).

Myoclonus-dystonia (M-D) is a term that has relatively recently been coined to describe one of the autosomal-dominant inherited dystonia-plus syndromes, which is characterized, in addition to dystonia, by a predominance of brief "lightning-like" myoclonic jerks affecting mostly the proximal extremities and the trunk (2–4) (Table 16-1).

Families with these clinical features have previously been described under the terms of *(familial) essential myoclonus* (5–7), *myoclonic dystonia* (8,9), and *hereditary dystonia with lightning jerks responsive to alcohol* (10). Affected patients in families from all of these categories have been found to carry mutations in the recently identified major gene for M-D, ε-sarcoglycan.

It is important to distinguish inherited M-D from inherited and sporadic primary dystonia with concomitant myoclonic jerks in the dystonic limb, a condition that has also been called myoclonic-dystonia (11), although this distinction may be difficult in some individual cases.

More than ten loci for inherited forms of dystonia have been mapped, but only four mutated genes have been identified so far: torsinA in the early-onset generalized form *(DYT1)* (12), guanosine triphosphate (GTP)-cyclohydrolase I in dominant *(DYT5)* (13), tyrosine hydroxylase in recessive dopa-responsive dystonia (14), and, most recently, ε-sarcoglycan *(SGCE)* in myoclonus-dystonia syndrome (M-D, *DYT11*) (15).

GENE MAPPING AND CLONING

In 1999, Nygaard et al. (16) mapped a locus in a previously undescribed large family with M-D to the long arm of chromosome 7 (7q21). It soon became apparent that this is a major locus for this disorder, as a number of other groups confirmed linkage to this region in several of their families (17–19). Asmus and coworkers (18) narrowed the critical region to approximately 3 centimorgan (cM). Using a classic positional cloning approach, Zimprich et al. (15) then identified five different heterozygous loss-of-function mutations in the gene for ε-sarcoglycan *(SGCE)* in six German families with M-D. Mutations co-segregated with the disease in all families, indicating that *SGCE* mutations are in fact causative for M-D. Subsequently, additional mutations were reported by several groups (3,20,21).

TABLE 16–1. *Clinical characteristics of myoclonus-dystonia*

Brief, "lightning-like" myoclonus as primary feature; focal or segmental dystonia of subtle to marked severity may be also seen but is rarely sole feature
Autosomal-dominant inheritance with incomplete penetrance and variable expressivity; in SGCE-mutation "+" cases suppression of phenotype upon maternal transmission or "pseudo-sporadic" inheritance
Onset usually in the first or second decade
Exclusion of additional neurologic features, such as cerebellar ataxia, spasticity, dementia, and seizures
No structural abnormalities in cranial imaging, normal EEG, and somatosensory evoked potentials
Usually a benign clinical course with no continuous progression of symptoms, normal life expectancy but great social stigmatization

Updated including proposed diagnostic criteria of refs. 2, 4, and 40.

This finding was unexpected, as the four other known members of the sarcoglycan family of genes (α, β, γ, and δ) so far had been implicated only in autosomal-recessive limb girdle muscular dystrophies (22). By contrast to these other sarcoglycans, however, which are almost exclusively expressed in skeletal and smooth muscle, *SGCE* expression is found in a wide variety of embryonic and adult tissues, including several brain regions (23). However, its distribution in different cell types of the central nervous system (CNS) and the subcellular localization and

function of the ε-sarcoglycan protein has not yet been investigated.

The *SGCE* gene consists of 12 exons (exon 1 to 11, plus an alternatively spliced exon 9a). The gene encodes a ubiquitously expressed 438-amino-acid protein, which has a single transmembrane domain and is 68% homologous to α-sarcoglycan. The role of the sarcoglycans has been studied in depth in skeletal muscle cells, where α-, β-, γ-, and δ-sarcoglycan are found, together with dystroglycan and other proteins, in a transmembrane complex called the dystrophin-glycoprotein complex (DGC). This complex links intracellular structural proteins, such as dystrophin, to extracellular matrix proteins (laminin). A similar complex exists in smooth muscle, where ε-sarcoglycan has been shown to replace α-sarcoglycan as an integral part of the complex (24). It is unknown whether ε-sarcoglycan forms similar complexes in nonmuscle tissue.

Up to now, 15 different mutations of the *SGCE* gene in families with M-D have been published (Fig. 16-1) (3,15,20,21), and several others have been reported in abstract form. The vast majority of mutations are typical of "loss of-function" mutations: single base pair changes that introduce stop-codons and consequently a premature termination of protein translation, small deletions or inser-

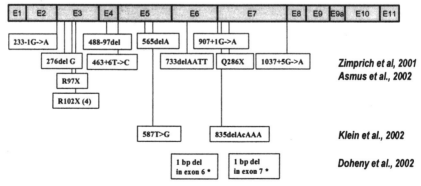

FIG. 16-1. Reported mutations in the *SGCE* gene in myoclonus-dystonia. All mutations except 587T>G are predicted to lead to a loss protein function by introducing stop codons, by out-of-frame deletions or insertions or by altering splice sites. *The precise nature of these mutations is not indicated in the original publication.

tions resulting in a shift of the reading frame, or splice site mutations. All of these mutations are predicted to lead to either a complete or near-complete loss of functional protein. However, a few mutations have been found to result in single amino acid changes only (21; Klein, personal communication). From the limited information available to date, there is no indication of a major difference in the phenotype between different types of mutations.

CLINICAL PICTURE

The spectrum of clinical manifestations associated with *SGCE* mutations can now be studied in detail, based on the analysis of patients from families with proven mutations. So far, the clinical picture closely corresponds to the diagnostic criteria that have been proposed before the identification of the gene (2).

The predominant symptom at presentation as well as during the course of the disease in most patients is myoclonic jerks, affecting mostly axial muscles (neck and trunk) but also muscles of the upper more than lower extremities, with proximal muscles being more affected than distal ones. Jerks are very brief, "lightning-like," and are precipitated or aggravated by action and psychological stress, but also occur at rest. More sustained, dys-

tonic movements are observed in about two thirds of patients, with torticollis and writer's cramp being the most common manifestations. Dystonia of the lower limbs is occasionally seen, leading to dystonic gait disturbances. This symptom may even predominate the clinical picture in a few patients, particularly in the very young. Usually, however, dystonia of the extremities has the characteristics of an action dystonia and is rarely disabling. Dystonia alone (torticollis) has been found in only a small minority of patients. A typical cross section of clinical characteristics of patients from nine pedigrees with *SGCE* mutations has been published recently (Table 16-2) (3).

Additional neurologic manifestations, such as cerebellar ataxia, spasticity, dementia, or seizures, so far have not been found in M-D patients, unless explained by additional pathology such as perinatal hypoxia.

Onset varies between 2 and 38 years of age, with a mean age at onset of 5.4 years (3). In three cases with *SGCE* nonsense mutations, the disease started very early (before age 2), resulting in marked delay of gait development caused by severe lower limb dystonia. At school age the presentation of these patients evolved into a typical M-D phenotype, with the exception of one patient, who continued to have a severe gait disorder.

TABLE 16–2. *Clinical characteristics of 24 myoclonus-dystonia syndrome (MDS) patients from nine European pedigrees*

Characteristic clinical signs	At onset		At examination	
	$n = 24$	%	$n = 24$	%
Myoclonus (%)	19	79	23	96
Distribution				
Face/voice	2/—	8/—	2/2	8/8
Neck/axial/shoulders	11	46	19	79
UL	16	67	21	88
LL	2	8	3	13
Dystonia (%)	9	38	13	54
Distribution				
Neck	9	38	11	46
Axial/shoulder	—	—	5	21
UL/writer's cramp	8	33	13	54
LL	2	8	4	16
Postural tremor (%)	2	8	4	16

UL, upper limb; LL, lower limb.

Symptoms of M-D evolve over several years into adolescence and young adulthood, but then show no further progression over many years (9).

Relief of both myoclonus and dystonia following the ingestion of alcohol has been described in many families. This finding has been confirmed in some, but not all, mutation-positive cases (19), and alcohol-responsive and -nonresponsive patients can be found in single families. Also, the dose necessary to provide relief can vary considerably, and patients can experience a heavy rebound of motor symptoms after single doses of alcohol or benzodiazepines. In contrast to cortical or posthypoxic myoclonus valproic acid, piracetam and levetiracetam provide neither significant nor lasting improvement of motor symptoms, although controlled therapeutic trials on M-D patients have not been published.

PSYCHIATRIC FEATURES OF MYOCLONUS-DYSTONIA

Many reports on families with the M-D phenotype mentioned nonmotor features like mild cognitive slowing in one pedigree (8) and psychiatric disturbances like panic attacks, personality disorders, and alcohol abuse in several others (3,16,25,26).

In a more systematic investigation of possible psychiatric manifestations of the disorder using the computerized version of the Composite International Diagnostic Interview (CIDI), Saunders-Pullman et al. (4) assessed a total of 55 individuals of three families with linkage to the 7q21 locus.

Probands were classified on the basis of motor symptoms and molecular findings as manifesting carriers (MCs; $n = 18$), nonmanifesting carriers (NMCs; $n = 11$), and noncarriers (NCs; $n = 28$) of the disease-associated haplotype.

Symptoms of obsessive-compulsive disorder (OCD) were found to be more common in carriers of the disease-associated haplotype, both with and without motor symptoms, as compared to noncarriers, suggesting that these symptoms may be a primary manifesta-

tion of the disease. By contrast, alcohol and benzodiazepine abuse appeared to be related to the presence of motor symptoms of M-D, and therefore were thought more likely to be secondary to the experience of symptomatic control of motor symptoms.

Psychiatric symptoms such as OCD, anxiety disorders, or depression may be greatly improved by selective serotonin reuptake inhibitors (SSRIs) in some cases (25). In other *SGCE*-positive M-D cases, worsening of myoclonus has been observed after administration of fluoxetine, paroxetine, and sertraline.

MATERNAL IMPRINTING OF THE *SGCE* GENE

The mechanism, by which mutations in the *SGCE* gene cause M-D is unknown. It is likely that a loss of ε-sarcoglycan function is critical, as the majority of mutations published so far appear to lead to a premature termination of protein translation (nonsense mutations resulting in a premature stop codon, or small deletions or insertions leading to a shift of the reading frame, or splice-site mutations, resulting in aberrant splicing of exons). This is unusual in a dominant disorder, as the vast majority of loss-of-function mutations cause diseases with autosomal-recessive inheritance. However, the peculiar pattern of reduced penetrance observed in M-D families appears to provide an explanation.

Pedigree analysis showed a marked difference in penetrance depending on the parental origin of the disease allele, with reduced penetrance (approximately 5–10%) occurring if the disease allele is passed on by the mother, while penetrance approaches 90% following paternal transmission. This pattern is suggestive of a differential activation or inactivation of the disease gene, depending on its parental origin (a process called "parental imprinting"). This type of differential gene expression has been well described for many genes, particularly for those involved in early embryonic development. The most common mechanism for this phenomenon is the specific inactivation of one of the parental alleles by methylation of cytosine residues in the promotor region.

Maternal imprinting of the *SGCE* gene has been demonstrated in the mouse (27), and this mechanism could in fact explain dominant inheritance and reduced penetrance in M-D: If the mutated allele is inherited from the father, inactivation of the maternal allele due to imprinting leads to complete ε-sarcoglycan deficiency, and hence to the development of clinical symptoms. If, on the other hand, the mutated allele is inherited from the mother, the intact paternal allele is sufficient to sustain ε-sarcoglycan function (as in most cases of loss-of-function mutations).

Experimental evidence could be obtained in support of this hypothesis. The differential methylation of parental alleles of the *SGCE* gene could be demonstrated by bisulfite-sequencing in cell lines with uniparental disomy of chromosome 7q21, and by analysis of DNA from blood lymphocytes and from brain tissue (28,29).

In addition, reverse-transcriptase polymerase chain reaction (rtPCR) experiments indicate that only one paternal allele appears to be expressed in blood lymphocytes (29); A. Zimprich, unpublished observations).

In some families the methylation pattern of the maternal allele appears to be incomplete, as shown by bisulfite sequencing of the maternal promotor region in a control pedigree (28).

In a small proportion of cases, inheritance does not follow the expected pattern, and symptoms of M-D develop despite maternal transmission of the mutated gene. Possible explanations could be a dominant negative effect of the mutation, or low expression of the healthy paternal allele. Quantitative assays are presently under way to determine the underlying mechanism of this phenomenon.

MOLECULAR PATHOGENESIS OF MYOCLONUS-DYSTONIA

The normal function of ε-sarcoglycan in the brain is unknown. In smooth and cardiac muscle, ε-sarcoglycan is an integral component of the dystrophin-glycoprotein complex

that also includes β-, γ-, and δ-sarcoglycan, as well as β-dystroglycan and sarcospan (22). This complex reinforces the connection between the intracellular cytoskeleton (an important component of which is, at least in muscle, the dystrophin protein) and the extracellular matrix. In smooth muscle, ε-sarcoglycan replaces α-sarcoglycan as an integral part of this complex.

In contrast to α-sarcoglycan, *SGCE* is highly expressed in the brain, but also in other nonmuscle tissues. It is interesting to speculate why clinical symptoms of *SGCE* deficiency should be restricted to the CNS. One could speculate that, in smooth muscle cells, for example, an ε-sarcoglycan deficiency could be compensated for by an upregulation of α-sarcoglycan. In a similar fashion, α-sarcoglycan is partially replaced by ε-sarcoglycan in cardiac muscle in α-sarcoglycan knockout mice (24).

Whether ε-sarcoglycan exists in CNS neurons in a dystrophin-glycoprotein complex comparable to that found in muscle tissues is unknown. If this should prove to be the case, then recent work on this complex in the CNS might provide interesting clues as to the molecular pathogenesis of M-D. It has recently been shown that dystroglycan, in the brain, co-localizes specifically with postsynaptic γ-aminobutyric acid (GABA)ergic receptors and is necessary for the maintenance of these structures. It therefore could be hypothesized that ε-sarcoglycan deficiency may lead to alterations in the architecture of GABAergic synapses, and that consequently a disturbed GABAergic inhibition in some parts of the brain could be the direct cause of the involuntary movements (and possibly also the psychiatric disturbances) observed in this disorder.

Interestingly, another component of the dystrophin-glycoprotein complex, dysbindin, has recently implicated in the pathogenesis of schizophrenia (30,31).

GENETIC HETEROGENEITY IN MYOCLONUS-DYSTONIA

Mutational screening by genomic DNA sequencing in a European sample of 39 index patients with typical M-D showed heterozygous *SGCE* mutations in 28% (*n* = 11) of all patients, whereas the prevalence of *SGCE* mutations in familial cases was 65%. Clinical presentation in *SGCE*-negative patients did not differ significantly from cases with proven mutations. In a proportion of the former cases, mutations (e.g., total exon deletions) could have been missed by the screening methods employed. In other cases, however, mutations in other genes may be responsible (3).

Prior to the identification of linkage to chromosome 7q21, Klein et al. (26) reported a missense change in the gene for the dopamine D₂-receptor *(DRD2)* in a single family with M-D. This missense change segregated with the disease in this family [logarithm of odds (LOD) score of 2.93] and led to the exchange of an amino acid (Val154Ile) in a conserved region of the protein. The change was not found on control chromosomes, but also not in other individuals or families affected with M-D. In addition, no evidence for linkage to the region on chromosome 11, which bears the *DRD2* gene, could be obtained in other families (18,32). Recently, the group that reported the original finding in the *DRD2* gene identified a mutation in the *SGCE* gene in this family, which also co-segregates with the disease. Together with the fact that cell culture studies did not show functional effects of the sequence alteration in the D₂ receptor (33), this finding raises doubts as to the functional significance of the *D2DR* variant.

TorsinA is the major gene identified to cause primary early-onset torsion dystonia (EOTD) (12). A single mutation, a GAG deletion, has been identified in cases of typical EOTD. The only other coding sequence alteration in the *TOR1A* gene was an 18-base-pair (bp) deletion, which was found in a sibling pair with an M-D phenotype (34). Interestingly, in this family an additional mutation was also identified in the *SGCE* gene (21). This mutation was inherited from the father, who had possible myoclonus with an onset of 3 years of age, i.e., a phenotype compatible

with mild M-D. The 18-bp deletion had been inherited from the mother, who showed only a mild laterocollis of unknown onset (rated as "possible dystonia"). Therefore, again, the relevance of the 18-bp deletion for the clinical phenotype in the two siblings remains uncertain.

The mapping of a second locus in a family with a typical M-D phenotype, but no *SGCE* mutations and no indication of transmission-specific reduced penetrance, was reported by Grimes et al. (35). This group provided evidence for linkage to a 18-cM region on the short arm of chromosome 18 with a LOD score of 3.96 (35). In this family, the clinical spectrum is practically identical to that reported in chromosome 7–linked pedigrees, including the early onset, predominance of myoclonus, and psychiatric abnormalities. Interestingly, this genetic region had been implicated in dystonic syndromes before: patients with a deletion of part of chromosome 18p have, among other disturbances, dystonia [18p-deletion syndrome (36)], and one form of adult-onset craniocervical dystonia *(DYT7)* was mapped to this region (37), although this finding had not been confirmed in other families.

Other conditions that may mimic M-D are dopa-responsive dystonia (38) (1 case published) and vitamin E deficiency (39).

REFERENCES

1. Fahn S, Bressman SB, Marsden CD. Classification of dystonia. *Adv Neurol* 1998;78:1–10.
2. Gasser T. Inherited myoclonus-dystonia syndrome. *Adv Neurol* 1998;78:325–334.
3. Asmus F, Zimprich A, Tezenas Du MS, et al. Myoclonus-dystonia syndrome: epsilon-sarcoglycan mutations and phenotype. *Ann Neurol* 2002;52(4):489–492.
4. Saunders-Pullman R, Ozelius L, Bressman SB. Inherited myoclonus-dystonia. *Adv Neurol* 2002;89:185–191.
5. Feldmann H, Wieser S. Klinische Studie zur essentiellen Myoklonie. *Arch Psych Z Ges Neurol* 1964;205:555–570.
6. Przuntek H, Muhr H. Essential familial myoclonus. *J Neurol* 1983;230(3):153–162.
7. Fahn S, Sjaastad O. Hereditary essential myoclonus in a large Norwegian family. *Mov Disord* 1991;6(3):237–247.
8. Kyllerman M, Forsgren L, Sanner G, et al. Alcohol-responsive myoclonic dystonia in a large family: dominant inheritance and phenotypic variation. *Mov Disord* 1990;5(4):270–279.

9. Gasser T, Bereznai B, Müller B, et al. Linkage studies in alcohol-responsive myoclonic dystonia. *Mov Disord* 1996;12:363–370.

10. Quinn NP, Rothwell JC, Thompson PD, et al. Hereditary myoclonic dystonia, hereditary torsion dystonia and hereditary essential myoclonus: an area of confusion. *Adv Neurol* 1988;50:391–401.

11. Obeso JA, Rothwell JC, Lang AE, et al. Myoclonic dystonia. *Neurology* 1983;33(7):825–830.

12. Ozelius L, Hewett JW, Page CE, et al. The early-onset torsion dystonia gene (Dyt1) encodes an ATP- binding protein. *Nat Genet* 1997;17:40–48.

13. Ichinose H, Ohye T, Takahashi E, et al. Hereditary progressive dystonia with marked diurnal fluctuation caused by mutations in the GTP cyclohydrolase I gene. *Nat Genet* 1994;8(3):236–242.

14. Knappskog PM, Flatmark T, Mallet J, et al. Recessively inherited L-DOPA-responsive dystonia caused by a point mutation (Q381K) in the tyrosine hydroxylase gene. *Hum Mol Genet* 1995;4(7):1209–1212.

15. Zimprich A, Grabowski M, Asmus F, et al. Mutations in the gene encoding epsilon-sarcoglycan cause myoclonus-dystonia syndrome. *Nat Genet* 2001;29(1):66–69.

16. Nygaard TG, Raymond D, Chen C, et al. Localization of a gene for myoclonus-dystonia to chromosome 7q21-q31. *Ann Neurol* 1999;46(5):794–798.

17. Klein C, Schilling K, Saunders-Pullman RJ, et al. A major locus for myoclonus-dystonia maps to chromosome 7q in eight families. *Am J Hum Genet* 2000;67(5):1314–1319.

18. Asmus F, Zimprich A, Naumann M, et al. Inherited myoclonus-dystonia syndrome: narrowing the 7q21-q31 locus in German families. *Ann Neurol* 2001;(5)121–124.

19. Vidailhet M, Tassin J, Durif F, et al. A major locus for several phenotypes of myoclonus-dystonia on chromosome 7q. *Neurology* 2001;56(9):1213–1216.

20. Doheny D, Brin M, Smith C, et al. Phenotypic features of myoclonic dystonia in two kindreds. *Mov Disord* 2000;15,suppl3:162.

21. Klein C, Liu L, Doheny D, et al. Epsilon-sarcoglycan mutations found in combination with other dystonia gene mutations. *Ann Neurol* 2002;52(5):675–679.

22. Lim LE, Campbell KP. The sarcoglycan complex in limb-girdle muscular dystrophy. *Curr Opin Neurol* 1998;11(5):443–452.

23. Ettinger AJ, Feng G, Sanes JR. epsilon-Sarcoglycan, a broadly expressed homologue of the gene mutated in limb-girdle muscular dystrophy 2D. *J Biol Chem* 1997;272(51):32534–32538.

24. Straub V, Ettinger AJ, Durbeej M, et al. Epsilon-sarcoglycan replaces alpha-sarcoglycan in smooth muscle to form a unique dystrophin-glycoprotein complex. *J Biol Chem* 1999;274(39):27989–27996.

25. Scheidtmann K, Muller F, Hartmann E, et al. [Familial myoclonus-dystonia syndrome associated with panic attacks]. *Nervenarzt* 2000;71(10):839–842.

26. Klein C, Brin MF, Kramer P, et al. Association of a missense change in the D2 dopamine receptor with myoclonus dystonia. *Proc Natl Acad Sci USA* 1999;96(9):5173–5176.

27. Piras G, El Kharroubi A, Kozlov S, et al. Zac1 (Lot1), a potential tumor suppressor gene, and the gene for epsilon-sarcoglycan are maternally imprinted genes: identification by a subtractive screen of novel uniparental fibroblast lines. *Mol Cell Biol* 2000;20(9):3308–3315.

28. Muller B, Hedrich K, Kock N, et al. Evidence that paternal expression of the epsilon-sarcoglycan gene accounts for reduced penetrance in myoclonus-dystonia. *Am J Hum Genet* 2002;71(6):1303–1311.

29. Grabowski M, Zimprich A, Lorenz-Depiereux B, et al. Epsilon-sarcoglycan (SGCE), the gene mutated in myoclonus-dystonia, is imprinted. *Eur J Hum Genet* 2003;(2):38–44.

30. Schwab SG, Knapp M, Mondabon S, et al. Support for association of schizophrenia with genetic variation in the 6p22.3 gene, dysbindin, in sib-pair families with linkage and in an additional sample of triad families. *Am J Hum Genet* 2003;72(1):185–190.

31. Straub RE, Jiang Y, MacLean CJ, et al. Genetic variation in the 6p22.3 gene DTNBP1, the human ortholog of the mouse dysbindin gene, is associated with schizophrenia. *Am J Hum Genet* 2002;71(2):337–348.

32. Durr A, Tassin J, Vidailhet M, et al. D2 dopamine receptor gene in myoclonic dystonia and essential myoclonus. *Ann Neurol* 2000;48(1):127–128.

33. Klein C, Gurvich N, Sena-Esteves M, et al. Evaluation of the role of the D2 dopamine receptor in myoclonus dystonia [In Process Citation]. *Ann Neurol* 2000;47(3):369–373.

34. Leung JC, Klein C, Friedman J, et al. Novel mutation in the TOR1A (DYT1) gene in atypical early onset dystonia and polymorphisms in dystonia and early onset parkinsonism. *Neurogenetics* 2001;3(3):133–143.

35. Grimes DA, Han F, Lang AE, et al. A novel locus for inherited myoclonus-dystonia on 18p11. *Neurology* 2002;59(8):1183–1186.

36. Klein C, Page CE, LeWitt P, et al. Genetic analysis of three patients with an 18p- syndrome and dystonia [In Process Citation]. *Neurology* 1999;52(3):649–651.

37. Leube B, Rudnicki D, Ratzlaff T, et al. Idiopathic torsion dystonia: assignment of a gene to chromosome 18p in a German family with adult onset, autosomal dominant inheritance and purely focal distribution. *Hum Mol Genet* 1996;5(10):1673–1677.

38. Leuzzi V, Carducci C, Carducci C, et al. Autosomal dominant GTP-CH deficiency presenting as a dopa-responsive myoclonus-dystonia syndrome. *Neurology* 2002;59(8):1241–1243.

39. Angelini L, Erba A, Mariotti C, et al. Myoclonic dystonia as unique presentation of isolated vitamin E deficiency in a young patient. *Mov Disord* 2002;17(3):612–614.

40. Mahloudji M, Pikielny RT. Hereditary essential myoclonus. *Brain* 1967;90(3):669–674.

Dystonia 4: Advances in Neurology, Vol. 94. Edited by Stanley Fahn, Mark Hallett, and Mahlon R. DeLong. Lippincott Williams & Wilkins, Philadelphia © 2004.

17

Penetrance and Expression of Dystonia Genes

*†Rachel Saunders-Pullman, *Janet Shriberg, †Vicki Shanker, and *†Susan B. Bressman

*Department of Neurology, Beth Israel Medical Center, New York, New York.
†Department of Neurology, Albert Einstein College of Medicine, Bronx, New York

Penetrance of the three known dystonia genes is incomplete: *TOR1A*/DYT1 (1) is 30% to 40% penetrant (2), *DYT5*/guanosine triphosphate (GTP)-cyclohydrolase 1 *(GCH1)* (dopa-responsive dystonia, DRD) (3) is 30% penetrant (4,5), and ε-sarcoglycan *(SGCE)/ DYT11* (myoclonus-dystonia, M-D) has reduced penetrance (6). Penetrance reflects the fraction of individuals with a genotype who have signs or symptoms of the disease. Because these genes are only partly penetrant, factors such as other genes or environmental factors must be influencing penetrance. These other factors may be exerting protective effects, decreasing penetrance. Alternatively, they may have deleterious effects and may be cofactors in the development of dystonia. All three disorders are also characterized by variable expressivity, whereby distribution and severity of dystonia may vary among affected individuals. Genetic or environmental factors are likely responsible for this variability as well.

Nondystonic features, either nondystonic motor features, or nonmotor behavioral features, may also be present in gene carriers. If these features are part of the phenotype, they affect penetrance estimates and our understanding of the degree to which other genetic or environmental factors influence penetrance. However, it is important first to establish that the feature is part of the phenotype

and not an incidental association. This chapter focuses on modifiers of gene penetrance, particularly environmental modifiers.

GENETIC MODIFIERS

The expression of dystonia genes may be modified by other genes or epigenetic modifiers. Several genes have been proposed to modify expression. A change in the D_2 receptor gene has been reported in association with M-D in one family with a *SGCE* mutation (7). Another family with M-D harboring an *SGCE* mutation also has an 18-base-pair (bp) deletion in the *DYT1* gene (8). However, the functional significance of these gene changes is unclear (9). A dopamine D_5 receptor polymorphism has been associated with expression of blepharospasm (10) and cervical dystonia (11), suggesting that the D_5 receptor may be directly pathogenic or may interact with other genes.

Epigenetic modifiers cause nonheritable changes affecting the expression of DNA without changing the DNA sequence. Epigenetic factors include imprinting gender and other environmental influences. Imprinting, where the parental origin of the allele affects the expression of the gene, appears to be a main factor in the expression of *DYT11* (6), whereby maternal imprinting decreases expression of the gene in offspring of mothers carrying the *DYT11* gene (see Chapter 16). However, this pattern of imprinting is not complete; some individuals manifest M-D despite maternal inheritance (12), and others may not manifest symptoms despite paternal inheritance. Gender is believed to play a major role in the expression of *DYT5*, as the disorder is more common in girls; however, the mechanism by which female gender predisposes, or male gender protects, is unclear [see discussion in Furukawa et al. (13)]. Genetic modifiers for *DYT1* have not yet been demonstrated, and the lack of homogeneity in expression among first-degree relatives compared to second-degree argues against a genetic modifier (S. Bressman, personal communication).

Alternatively, or in conjunction with genetic modifiers, environmental modifiers may alter the expression of *DYT1*. Childhood infection and peripheral trauma have both been posited as possible environmental triggers

(14). Because *DYT1* dystonia is an early-onset condition, we postulate that there is a critical window of vulnerability during which environmental modifiers may interact with the gene or gene products to cause dystonia to manifest. Most *DYT1* mutations are caused by the deletion of three base pairs (GAG) (1). To determine if early childhood infection is an environmental modifier associated with the expression of the GAG deletion in *DYT1*, we queried probands with *DYT1* dystonia and their family members about their history of childhood illnesses (varicella zoster, measles, and mumps). A semistructured written questionnaire was mailed out to probands and family members who were already participating in family studies and for whom gene status and a videotaped neurologic exam were completed. Those with definite dystonia and the GAG deletion were considered manifesting carriers (MCs), and without definite dystonia (including those with probable and pos-

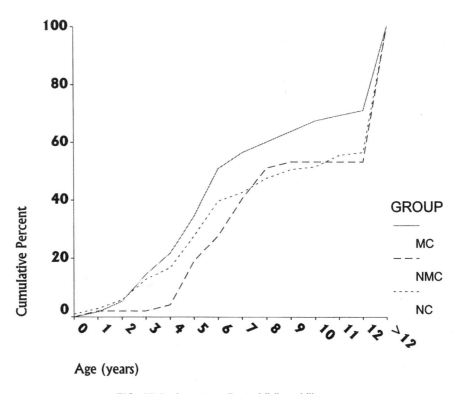

FIG. 17-1. Age at earliest childhood illness.

sible dystonia) but carrying the deletion were considered non-manifesting carriers (NMCs), and those without the deletion, noncarriers (NCs). There were 55 MCs, 47 NMCs, and 101 NCs from a total of 50 families. Families ranged from one to 13 participating family members, with the family members responding in some families where probands did not. Of the MCs, 31 were probands, mean age at onset of dystonia was 10.3 years (range 6–26 years), and 21 were relatives, mean age at onset 15 years (range 5–38 years).

The rate of any childhood illness (including those who knew the age at illness, and those who knew whether they had an illness, but did not have an age) was similar among MCs and NMCs: varicella—MCs 87%, NMCs 80%; measles—MCs 56%, NMCs 67%; mumps—MCs 39%, NMCs 49% (age at earliest childhood illness is shown in figure 17-1). When this was stratified by the illness occurring at age 6 or earlier, MCs were more likely to have had varicella (26/55 vs. 13/47, $p = .042$), measles (9/55 vs. 3/47, nonsignificant), mumps (9/55 vs. 2/47, $p = .049$) and any childhood illness (28/55 vs. 13/47, $p = 0.02$). The odds ratios are shown in Table 17-1. When we counted the MCs as having an early childhood illness *only* if the illness preceded the onset of dystonia, 25/55 MCs vs. 13/47 NMCs had varicella ($p = .064$). For all other illnesses, all MCs had onset of infection prior to the onset of dystonia (15).

Our data suggest that *DYT1* carriers who have at least one early childhood illness are more likely to develop dystonia. The relative risk is greatest for the association between mumps and manifesting dystonia; however, the confidence interval is extremely broad. The relative risk of developing dystonia after

an early (age 6 or younger) childhood illness is still more than twofold, with a narrower confidence interval. This is consistent with prior hypotheses of environmental contributions, possibly infection and trauma, to the development of dystonia (14). In a study of the *DYT1* gene in secondary dystonia, measles infection was the only etiology of secondary dystonia that was associated with the *DYT1* gene (14). Our findings are also consistent with prior case reports and retrospective studies. In their series of dystonia patients, Cooper et al. (16) noted that 30% of the individuals had viral infection within 3 months of developing symptoms. Transient lingual-mandibular dystonia has also been reported after varicella infection (17). More convincingly, a review of risk factors among spasmodic dysphonia patients found that 65% of affected patients had a history of mumps or measles, whereas only 15% of age-matched controls had these infections (18). We only found a significant difference in assessing illness occurring at age 6 or less, and did not find a difference when any childhood infection was assessed. This argues for a vulnerability window, whereby the brain is more susceptible to environmental insult at an earlier age, and parallels glutaric aciduria type 1, where gene carriers who develop early childhood infections are at risk of becoming symptomatic, but are less vulnerable after a certain age (19).

Alternately, considering the NMC gene carriers as unaffected may be too simplistic, as positron emission tomography (PET) studies demonstrate abnormal motor networks both in symptomatic and asymptomatic *DYT1* carriers. Regardless of whether they are "manifesting" or "notmanifesting" dystonia, gene carriers, *DYT1* gene carriers have relative hypermetabolism in the lentiform nucleus, supplemental motor area, and cerebellum (20). Gene carriers with overt dystonia have relative increases in the cerebellum, midbrain, and thalamus during sustained dystonic contractions (20). This suggests that the brain may be primed by the *DYT1* mutation, and one or more additional environmental in-

TABLE 17-1. *Early childhood illness among DYT1 carriers*

Childhood illness	Odds ratio	Confidence interval
Varicella	2.35	1.023–5.38
Mumps	4.40	0.901–21.51
Measles	2.87	0.729–11.30
Any of the three	2.71	1.18–6.22

sults may lead to the final step in the development of motor symptoms. Because not all manifesting carriers had a childhood illness, our study suggests that it is not a necessary factor for the development of dystonia. Because the temporal association between the early childhood illness and the onset of dystonia was usually greater than 1 year, this suggests that childhood infection may be a causal but remote early factor in the development of dystonia. The primary drawback to this study is recall bias, with the manifesting carriers having greater recall of early childhood illness. Larger samples are also needed to confirm these findings, as evidenced by the broad confidence intervals, particularly for mumps.

The mechanism for an early childhood illness precipitating dystonia is unclear. Secondary dystonia may be attributed to encephalitis (21); however, encephalitis was not reported in any of the individuals participating in the study. Indeed the effect on expression may not be the direct effect of the infection, but may be due to fever or part of the inflammatory cascade or immune response. Postinfections autoimmune phenomena are suggested in other movement disorders such as Sydenham's chorea or pediatric autoimmune neuropsychiatric disorders associated with streptococcal infections (PANDAS) (22). Because the major early childhood illness included in this study, varicella zoster, can now be prevented through vaccination, it will be important to assess whether there will be a change in the rate of manifesting dystonia.

Peripheral trauma may also be an environmental modifier. Prior studies of early-onset primary torsion dystonia have found evidence that trauma may precipitate or exacerbate dystonia (23). Although some of these cases were familial, a clear genetic etiology was not determined. In our group of *DYT1* survey respondents described above, we also queried about peripheral trauma. An individual was rated as having early peripheral trauma if there was a peripheral injury requiring and x-ray, surgery, or emergency room visit at the age of 6 or earlier. We did not find an association between peripheral trauma and mani-

festing dystonia among *DYT1* carriers (14/51 MCs had trauma and 14/43 NMCs had trauma) (15). Trauma has also been implicated in the development of other forms of dystonia, including oromandibular dystonia (24), late-onset dystonia (25), occupational (including musician's dystonia) (26), and dystonia associated with reflex sympathetic dystrophy (27). However, as our study suggests, larger systematic studies are warranted as case series may overrate the relative contribution of trauma (28).

CONCLUSION

Despite our knowledge of the *SGCE* gene in M-D, *GCH1* in DRD, and *TOR1A* in *DYT1*, our understanding of penetrance in dystonia genes remains incomplete. Expanding the phenotype to nonmotor features may improve, but does not completely explain, the penetrance patterns. Early childhood illness is an environmental modifier that is associated with manifesting dystonia among *DYT1* gene carriers. Preliminary data do not support a role for trauma in manifesting *DYT1*. As childhood infection is not necessary for the development of dystonia in all cases of *DYT1*, additional environmental and genetic factors must also underlie the incomplete penetrance patterns.

REFERENCES

1. Ozelius LJ, Hewett JW, Page CE, et al. The early-onset torsion dystonia gene (DYT1) encodes an ATP-binding protein. *Nat Genet* 1997;17:40–48.
2. Bressman SB, de Leon D, Brin MF, et al. Idiopathic dystonia among Ashkenazi Jews: evidence for autosomal dominant inheritance. *Ann Neurol* 1989;26:612–620.
3. Ichinose H, Ohye T, Takahashi E, et al. Hereditary progressive dystonia with marked diurnal fluctuation caused by mutations in the GTP cyclohydrolase 1 gene. *Nat Genet* 1994;8:239–242.
4. Nygaard TG, Wilhelmsen KC, Risch NJ, et al. Linkage mapping of dopa-responsive-dystonia (DRD) to chromosome 14q. *Nat Genet* 1993;5:386–391.
5. Nygaard TG, Trugman JM, de Yebenes JG, et al. Dopa-responsive dystonia: the spectrum of clinical manifestations in a large North American family. *Neurology* 1990;40:66–69.
6. Zimprich A, Grabowski M, Asmus F, et al. Mutations in the gene encoding epsilon-sarcoglycan cause myoclonus-dystonia syndrome. *Nat Genet* 2001;29:66–69.

7. Klein C, Brin MF, Kramer P, et al. Association of a missense change in the D2 dopamine receptor with myoclonus dystonia. *Proc Natl Acad Sci USA* 1999;96: 5171–5176.

8. Doheny D, Danisi F, Smith C, et al. Clinical findings of a myoclonus-dystonia family with two distinct mutations. *Neurology* 2002;8:1244–1246.

9. Klein C, Gurvich N, Sena-Esteves, et al. Evaluation of the role of the D2 receptor in myoclonus-dystonia. *Ann Neurol* 2000;47:369–373.

10. Misbahuddin A, Placzek Mr, Chaudhri K, et al. A polymorphism in the dopamine receptor DRD5 is associated with blepharospasm. *Neurology* 2002;58:124–126.

11. Placzek M, Misbahuddin A, Chaudhri K, et al. Cervical dystonia is associated with a polymorphism in the dopamine (D5) receptor gene. *J Neurol Neurosurg Psychiatry* 2001;71:262–264.

12. Nygaard TG, Raymond D, Chen C, et al. Localization of a gene for myoclonus-dystonia to chromosome 7q21-q31. *Ann Neurol* 1999;46:794–798.

13. Furukawa Y, Lang A, Trugman J. Gender related penetrance and de novo GTP-cyclohydrolase 1 gene mutations in dopa-responsive dystonia. *Neurology* 1998;50: 1015–1020.

14. Bressman S, deLeon D, Raymond D, et al. Secondary Dystonia and the DYT1 gene. *Neurology* 1997;48: 1571–1577.

15. Saunders-Pullman RJ, Wendt KJ, Parides MJ, et al. Environmental modifers of genetic dystonia: possible role of infection. *Neurology* 2000;54(suppl 3):A198.

16. Cooper IS, Collinan T, Riklan M. The natural history of dystonia. *Adv Neurol* 1976;14:157–169.

17. Gollomp SM, Fahn S. Transient dystonia as a complication of varicella. *J Neurol Neurosurg Psychiatry* 1987; 59:1228–1229.

18. Schweinfurth JM, Billante M, Courey MS. Risk factors and demographics in patients with spasmodic dysphonia. *Laryngoscope* 2002;112:220–223.

19. Morton DH, Bennett MJ, Sargeant LE, et al. Glutaric aciduria type 1: a common cause of episodic encephalopathy and spastic paralysis in the Amish of Lancaster County, Pennsylvania. *Am J Med Genet* 1991;41:89–95.

20. Eidelberg D, Moeller JR, Antonini A. Functional brain networks in DYT1. *Ann Neurol* 1998;44 303–312.

21. Donovan MK, Lenn NJ. Postinfectious encephalomyelitis with localized basal ganglia involvement. *Pediatr Neurol* 1989;5:311–313.

22. Swedo SE, Leonard HL, Garvey M, et al. Pediatric autoimmune neuropsychiatric disorders associated with streptococcal infections: clinical description of the first 50 cases. *Am J Psychiatry* 1998;155:264–271.

23. Fletcher NA, Harding AE, Marsden CD. The relationship between trauma and idiopathic torsion dystonia. *J Neurol Neurosurg Psychiatry* 1991;54:713–717.

24. Sankla C, Lai EC, Jancovic J. Peripherally induced oromandibular dystonia. *J Neurol Neurosurg Psychiatry*. 1998;65:722–728.

25. Jankovic J. Can peripheral trauma induce dystonia? Yes! *Mov Disord* 2001;16:7–12.

26. Frucht S, Fahn S, Ford B. Focal task-specific dystonia induced by peripheral trauma. *Mov Disord* 2000;15: 348–350.

27. Schwartzmann RJ, Kerrigan J. The movement disorder of reflex sympathetic dystrophy. *Neurology* 1990;40:57–61.

28. Weiner WJ. Can peripheral trauma induce dystonia? No! *Mov Disord* 2001;16:13.

Dystonia 4: Advances in Neurology, Vol. 94. Edited by Stanley Fahn, Mark Hallett, and Mahlon R. DeLong. Lippincott Williams & Wilkins, Philadelphia © 2004.

18

Update on Dopa-Responsive Dystonia: Locus Heterogeneity and Biochemical Features

Yoshiaki Furukawa

Movement Disorders Research Laboratory, Centre for Addiction and Mental Health-Clarke Division, Toronto, Ontario, Canada

Dopa-responsive dystonia (DRD) is a clinical syndrome characterized by childhood-onset dystonia and a dramatic and sustained response to relatively low doses of levodopa (1–3). This disorder and inherited myoclonus-dystonia are differentiated from primary dystonias and are classified under the dystonia-plus category (4,5). Patients with DRD typically present with gait disturbance due to foot dystonia, later development of some parkinsonian features, and diurnal fluctuation of symptoms (worsening of the symptoms toward the evening and their alleviation in the morning after sleep). The sustained levodopa responsiveness and no motor adverse effects of chronic levodopa therapy, such as dopa-induced dyskinesias, distinguish DRD from early-onset parkinsonism with dystonia (6).

In 1971, Segawa et al. (7) and Castaigne et al. (8) independently reported clinical details of one family each with DRD, which they called at that time "hereditary progressive basal ganglia disease with marked fluctuation" and "progressive extrapyramidal disorder," respectively. Advances in the genetics and biochemistry of DRD (3,9,10) have shown that the former had autosomal-dominant guanosine triphosphate (GTP) cyclohydrolase I (GTPCH) deficiency and the latter had autosomal-recessive tyrosine hydroxylase (TH) deficiency (11,12). The enzyme GT-PCH catalyzes the first step in the biosynthe-

sis of (6R)-L-erythro-5,6,7,8-tetrahydro-biopterin (BH4; the natural cofactor for TH, tryptophan hydroxylase, and phenylalanine hydroxylase), and TH catalyzes the rate-limiting step (the formation of dopa from tyrosine) in the biosynthesis of catecholamines (13). Dominantly inherited mutations in *GCH1*, the gene encoding GTPCH, have been identified in many patients with DRD (14). By contrast, recessively inherited *TH* mutations have been reported only in several patients with DRD (the mild form of TH deficiency) (10,12, 14–16). A recent finding of a new locus for autosomal-dominant DRD on chromosome 14q13 (*DYT14*) indicates that there are at least three causative genes for this disorder: the *GCH1* gene on chromosome 14q22.1-q22.2, the *TH* gene on 11p15.5, and an as yet undefined gene on 14q13 (9,10,17–19). Neuropathologic features (a normal population of cells with reduced melanin and no evidence of Lewy body formation in the substantia nigra pars compacta) in two DRD patients with GTPCH dysfunction were similar to those in a patient with DRD linked to the *DYT14* locus (19–21). There have been no reports of autopsied patients with TH-deficient DRD.

This chapter summarizes recent advances in DRD with a special emphasis on locus heterogeneity, genetically related disorders, and postmortem brain data, including neurochemical findings in an asymptomatic *GCH1* mutation carrier in a DRD family (22), one of the families in which Nygaard et al. (17) found the first locus for this treatable syndrome.

CLINICAL DESCRIPTION

The average age of onset of typical DRD is approximately age 6 years (range, 1–12 years) (2,23). In patients with DRD, there is no abnormality in perinatal and early postnatal periods. Motor development in infancy is usually normal. A predominance of clinically affected females is observed; the female-to-male ratio has been reported to be 2:1 to 6:1. No increased prevalence of DRD is evident in any ethnic group, and the prevalence in both England and Japan has been estimated to be 0.5 per million (1).

Initial symptoms in most patients with childhood-onset DRD are gait difficulties attributable to dystonia in the leg, typically flexion-inversion (equinovarus posture) of the foot (2,23). There is a tendency to fall and standing position often induces an increased lumbar lordosis. A relatively small number of patients have onset with arm or neck dystonia, tremor (mainly postural), or slowness of movements. A variable degree of rigidity is detected in the affected limbs. Rapid fatiguing of effort with repetitive motor tasks (e.g., foot tapping) is often observed. In addition to dystonic and parkinsonian elements, some clinical features suggestive of spasticity in the lower extremities [brisk reflexes, ankle clonus, and/or the striatal toe (this dystonic extension of the big toe may be misinterpreted as a Babinski response)] are recognized in many patients. Normal efferent cortical spinal activity in DRD using magneto-electrical stimulation of motor cortex has suggested a nonpyramidal cause of "spasticity" in this disorder (24). Diurnal fluctuation [one of the important clinical characteristics in DRD (25)] occurs in 77% of patients (23); the degree of fluctuation is variable, with some patients being normal in the morning, whereas others are only less severely affected in the morning when compared to later in the day. Some patients experience only exercise-induced exacerbation or manifestation of dystonia. There is

often an attenuation in the magnitude of diurnal fluctuation with age and disease progression. In general, the symptoms in childhood-onset patients progress gradually to generalized dystonia; typically, dystonia is more pronounced in the legs throughout the disease course. Cognitive function is normal even in advanced stages.

All patients with DRD demonstrate complete or near-complete and sustained responsiveness of symptoms to low doses of levodopa (2,23). Full motor benefit occurs within several days to a few months after beginning levodopa administration. Gradual increases of levodopa dose are recommended. Maximum benefit is usually achieved by less than 20 to 30 mg/kg/day of levodopa without a decarboxylase inhibitor (DCI) (2) or by less than 300 mg/day of levodopa with a DCI (23); some adult patients with *GCH1* mutations needed 400 mg/day of levodopa in combination with a DCI (26,27). At the initiation of levodopa treatment, some patients may develop dyskinesias. However, these dyskinesias subside following dose reduction and do not reappear with later gradual dose increments. In contrast to patients with early-onset parkinsonism, DRD patients on long-term levodopa therapy (under optimal doses of levodopa) do not develop motor response fluctuations, freezing episodes, and dopa-induced dyskinesias.

GCH1 GENE

Human GTPCH is encoded by a single copy gene, *GCH1*, which is composed of six exons spanning approximately 30 kilobases (28). There are three complementary DNA (cDNA) isoforms with different 3'-ends caused by alternative splicing and only type 1 cDNA (having the longest coding region) gives rise to the active enzyme (28–30). The atomic structure of GTPCH from *Escherichia coli* showed that this enzyme is a homodecamer formed by a face-to-face association of two pentamers (31,32). In patients with GT-PCH deficiencies [GTPCH-deficient DRD, dystonia with motor delay, and GTPCH-deficient hyperphenylalaninemia (HPA)], more than 95 independent *GCH1* mutations (missense and nonsense mutations, small deletions and insertions, and splice site mutations) have been identified (33). Approximately 70% of them are missense or nonsense mutations, and the reason why many different mutations occur throughout all of the six exons of *GCH1* remains unknown.

One polymorphism in the coding region of *GCH1* (Pro23Leu) has been reported (34). This finding is in agreement with the results of earlier studies demonstrating that (a) proline at codon 23 is not conserved across human, rat, and mouse species (29,35,36); (b) this proline is located at the GTPCH N-terminal periphery where the amino acid change probably has no consequence for oligomerization of the decameric complex enzyme (31,32,36); (c) catalytic activity of mutated recombinant GTPCH with the Pro23Leu substitution was not affected compared with that of the wild-type enzyme in a prokaryotic expression system (21); (d) kinetic parameters of purified recombinant GTPCH expressed in *Escherichia coli* were not markedly changed even after truncating its N-terminal 45 amino acid residues (37); and (e) two patients with this polymorphism on one allele and a nonsense mutation in *GCH1* on the other allele manifested the classic phenotype of DRD (without any developmental motor delay and HPA) (20,21,38).

GTPCH-Deficient Dopa-Responsive Dystonia

In the brain, BH4 is highly concentrated in the striatum, especially in the nigrostriatal dopaminergic terminals (21,22,39–41). Because intracellular BH4 content is near the Michaelis constant (K_m) of TH for the cofactor, BH4 could limit TH activity in the dopaminergic neurons (40,42,43). Therefore, both total biopterin (BP; most of brain BP exists as BH4) and total neopterin (NP) levels were measured in cerebrospinal fluid (CSF) of DRD patients before the discovery of *GCH1* mutations in this disorder and the results (re-duced BP and NP) suggested a functional abnormality of GTPCH (44–46). BP includes BH4, quinonoid dihydrobiopterin, and 7,8-dihydrobiopterin. NP consists of degradation products of dihydroneopterin triphosphate, which is synthesized from GTP by GTPCH, and thus NP is generally considered to reflect GTPCH activity. A rostrocaudal gradient for CSF BP concentrations and a significant positive correlation between BP and homovanillic acid levels in CSF suggest that CSF BP is derived from the brain (47–49). Decreased BP and NP levels in CSF were confirmed in patients with DRD caused by *GCH1* mutations (50). It has been reported that CSF pterin data can be useful for the differential diagnoses of three disorders responsive to levodopa: (a) low concentrations of both BP and NP in GTPCH-deficient DRD, (b) normal BP and NP levels in TH-deficient DRD (see below), and (c) low BP but normal NP levels in Parkinson's disease (PD) and early-onset parkinsonism, including the autosomal-recessive form caused by *parkin* mutations (3,6,14).

DRD due to *GCH1* mutations is transmitted as an autosomal-dominant trait with gender-related incomplete penetrance; the penetrance in genetically confirmed families was much higher in females (87%) than in males (38%) (51). In reports on DRD, in which a relatively large number of families was examined genetically (9,21,22,26,50–57), mutations in the coding region (including the splice sites) of *GCH1* were identified in approximately 60% of pedigrees using conventional genomic DNA sequencing of this gene (3,14). For *GCH1* "coding region mutation-negative" DRD pedigrees, including families that have an apparently sporadic patient or only a few affected siblings, possible explanations are the following: (a) a mutation in noncoding regulatory regions of *GCH1*, (b) a large deletion of one or more exons of *GCH1*, (c) an intragenic duplication or inversion of *GCH1*, (d) a recessively inherited mutation in *TH*, (e) a dominantly inherited mutation in a gene on the *DYT14* locus, and (f) a mutation in other genes on as yet unknown loci for DRD. Since neuropathologic characteristics in the patient with DRD linked to the *DYT14* locus resembled those in the DRD patients with GTPCH dysfunction (19–21), there is a possibility that the *DYT14* gene could be a regulatory gene for *GCH1* (having an influence on *GCH1* expression) or that the product of this gene might interact with GTPCH and modify the enzyme function. Point mutations in the 5'-untranslated region of *GCH1* (54,57), decreased *GCH1* messenger RNA (mRNA) expression from one allele with no *GCH1* coding region mutation (11), a large heterozygous deletion in *GCH1* (which is undetectable by usual genomic DNA sequencing of this gene) (56), and mutations in *TH* (16) have been found in *GCH1* coding region mutation-negative DRD families. After including these types of *GCH1* and *TH* abnormalities, in our series, 86% of families with DRD or dystonia with motor delay (see below) demonstrated positive results of the genetic testing (16,21,22,51,56,58; and unpublished data). Southern blotting, cDNA analysis, and quantitative duplex polymerase chain reaction (PCR) may be useful for the detection of exon deletions in *GCH1*. A wide range of symptoms and signs has been reported in genetically confirmed GTPCH-deficient DRD pedigrees: benign adult-onset parkinsonism (showing slow progression and no motor adverse effects of levodopa), DRD simulating cerebral palsy or spastic paraplegia, various types of focal dystonia, and so on (3,17, 53–55,57). In our DRD families, however, isolated scoliosis and pure writer's cramp were not always associated with *GCH1* mutations found in the probands with the classic phenotype (27,59; and unpublished data).

BH4 is the essential cofactor not only for TH but also for phenylalanine hydroxylase and tryptophan hydroxylase. However, patients with autosomal-dominant GTPCH-deficient DRD (usually heterozygotes) never develop HPA, whereas a subclinical defect in phenylalanine metabolism can often be detected by the phenylalanine loading test (60,61). Symptoms possibly relating to serotonergic hypofunction (e.g., mood changes, aggressive behavior, dysfunction of impulse control, and sleep disturbances) are not obvious in patients with typical GTPCH-deficient DRD (3). The reason for the differences in susceptibility to a BH4-deficient condition due to congenital partial GTPCH deficiency among the three aromatic amino acid hydroxylases could relate to (a) different K_m values of the hydroxylases for BH4 (3,62), (b) differences in the degree of possible regulatory effects of BH4 on stability/expression of the three hydroxylase proteins (3,14,21,22, 63–66), and (c) different *GCH1* (and GTPCH) expression levels in various tissues and in central monoamine neurons (3,67,68).

GTPCH-Deficient Hyperphenylalaninemia

Patients with autosomal-recessive GTPCH deficiency (usually homozygotes) develop BH4-dependent HPA in the first 6 months of life (28,69–71). In these patients, the neonatal phenylketonuria-screening Guthrie test can usually detect an abnormality of the phenylalanine metabolism. Two patients with GTPCH-deficient HPA, in which homozygous *GCH1* mutations were identified, had very high plasma phenylalanine levels (1,488 μM and more than 2,400 μM; normal value, less than 120 μM) (28,70). There was no detectable GTPCH activity in liver biopsy specimens in patients with GTPCH-deficient HPA (69,70). This disorder presents with severe neurologic dysfunction, including convulsions, mental retardation, swallowing difficulties, developmental motor delay, truncal hypotonia, limb hypertonia, and involuntary movements (28,69–71). In the first report of recessively inherited GTPCH deficiency by Niederwieser et al. (69), hyperreflexia with extensor plantar responses and dyskinesias probably induced by levodopa at the initiation of neurotransmitter replacement therapy (levodopa and 5-hydroxytryptophan) were also described. In contrast to GTPCH-deficient DRD patients, BH4 treatment and replacement therapy of both neurotransmitters are necessary for GTPCH-deficient HPA patients (69,71).

In coexpression studies, it has been shown that GTPCH protein with dominantly inherited *GCH1* mutations but not recessively inherited ones inactivated the wild-type enzyme, suggesting an important role of this dominant-negative effect in autosomal-dominant GTPCH-deficient DRD (72–74). In this case, the more mutant peptides, interacting with the wild-type peptides, the greater the opportunity to form nonfunctional multimers. However, Suzuki et al. (37) have suggested that the dominant negative effect is unlikely to explain low enzyme activity in phytohemagglutinin-stimulated mononuclear blood cells from GTPCH-deficient DRD patients [<20% of controls (9)] and that a reduction of the amount of GTPCH protein observed in these cells may contribute to the mechanism of dominant inheritance.

Dystonia with Motor Delay

Compound heterozygotes for significant *GCH1* mutations can develop a novel phenotype of GTPCH deficiency (dystonia with motor delay), which is clinically and biochemically intermediate between GTPCH-deficient DRD (mild) and GTPCH-deficient HPA (severe) (58). This phenotype is characterized by developmental motor delay, limb dystonia (with truncal hypotonia) that progresses to generalized dystonia, and no overt HPA in infancy.

In á four-generation family with GTPCH dysfunction, the proband developed the phenotype of dystonia with motor delay and had a maternally transmitted small deletion in *GCH1* and a paternally transmitted *GCH1* missense mutation (58). The mother as well as maternal grandmother and great-grandmother of the proband had only the heterozygous deletion and manifested the classic phenotype of DRD. Thus, the proband seems to have at least one dominant allele, whereas compound heterozygous genotypes generally involve different recessive alleles at a locus. The genetic findings in this family suggest that intrafamilial phenotypic heterogeneity in some GTPCH-deficient DRD pedigrees could be explained by an additional significant *GCH1* mutation (3). There is a possibility that the additional mutation is undetectable by the conventional genomic DNA sequence analysis of *GCH1* [e.g., a large genomic deletion in this gene (56)]. Moreover, because a relatively high spontaneous mutation rate of *GCH1* has been suggested by the discovery of different de novo mutations (51), some offspring in DRD families might have dystonia and developmental motor delay caused by compound heterozygous *GCH1* mutations; one is inherited from a parent and the other is derived from a new mutational event. Clinically, it is important to note that the proband responded remarkably to low doses of levodopa and made further improvement in motor function when BH4 was chronically added to maintenance levodopa treatment (58). This observation suggests that early combination therapy of levodopa and BH4 may be suitable for children with dystonia with motor delay due to *GCH1* mutations.

TH GENE

Human *TH* consists of 14 exons spanning approximately 8.5 kilobases (75–77). Four types of mRNA are produced through alternative splicing from a single primary transcript [now, several additional types of mRNA are known (78,79)]. The native TH enzyme is a tetramer of four identical subunits (80). As of July 2002, 13 independent *TH* mutations (ten missense mutations, two small deletions, and one branch site mutation) have been reported in patients with the mild form (TH-deficient DRD) or the severe form (infantile parkinsonism with motor delay) of TH deficiency (10,12,16,81–92). These patients are homozygous or compound heterozygous for TH mutations. Because the null mutations of *TH* are lethal as shown in *TH* (−/−) knockout mice (93), both homozygotes and compound heterozygotes appear to have some residual activity of the enzyme. There are several normal variations in this gene, and the Val112Met substitution [based on type 4 mRNA (94)] has been found frequently (95,96).

TH-Deficient Dopa-Responsive Dystonia

The clinical details of two brothers with DRD reported by Castaigne et al. (8) in 1971 are described elsewhere (12,97,98). In brief, the older brother noticed a tremor of the hands at 5 years of age and then developed gait disturbance in the following year. At age 7, he had a postural tremor in both upper extremities, equinovarus posturing of the feet when walking, and bilateral extensor plantar responses. By age 9, he could no longer walk and his whole body was fixed in a flexed position. He had rigidity of the limbs, slowness of movements, a resting tremor, and pyramidal signs. After starting levodopa administration (1 g/day, without a DCI), all of the symptoms dramatically improved. Plantar responses became flexor after beginning levodopa therapy, suggesting that the previous finding appeared to be a dystonic phenomenon (the striatal toe) rather than a Babinski response. The younger brother was normal until 2 years of age, when he manifested difficulty in walking and tremors in the upper limbs. At age 5 years, he was no longer able to walk. His left upper extremity was flexed and both lower extremities were extended and crossed. He showed flexion-inversion of the feet (pes equinovarus) and dystonic extension of the big toes. There were some parkinsonian features and bilateral extensor plantar responses. Treatment with levodopa (50 mg/kg/day, without a DCI) gave a dramatic alleviation of his symptoms. Although he developed dyskinesias after 2 months of levodopa administration, these dyskinesias subsided following dose reduction (20 mg/kg/day, without a DCI). In both brothers, a sustained response to low doses of levodopa and no motor adverse effects during chronic levodopa therapy (for more than 30 years) have been confirmed, and compound heterozygous *TH* mutations were identified (12).

According to Bartholomé and Lüdecke (15), TH-deficient DRD is characterized by leg dystonia (onset approximately 4 years of age), diurnal fluctuation of symptoms, and a good response to levodopa treatment. This group reported a homozygous *TH* mutation in two siblings with typical DRD (10,81). In two other genetically proven pedigrees with the mild form of TH deficiency, a patient in one family developed DRD simulating spastic paraplegia (16), and a patient in the other family was clinically diagnosed as hypokinetic rigid syndrome (12). The sustained levodopa responsiveness and no complications of levodopa therapy have been confirmed for 2 years in the former case and for more than 30 years in the latter case. Although further accumulation of patients with the mild form of TH-deficiency (TH-deficient DRD) is necessary to establish the clinical features of this treatable disorder, all six patients from the four families reported to date are males and have normal early development (8,10,12, 14–16,81,97,98). Thus, female predominance [which has been confirmed in GTPCH-deficient DRD (51)] may not be a clinical characteristic in TH-deficient DRD.

Infantile Parkinsonism with Motor Delay

In nine patients with the severe form of TH-deficiency from nine unrelated families, their ages at onset were less than 6 months (82–92). All of the patients had developmental motor delay, truncal hypotonia, rigidity of extremities, and hypokinesia. Ptosis and/or oculogyric crises were often observed in these patients, and three very severely affected patients demonstrated high blood prolactin concentrations (dopamine is a prolactin-inhibiting factor at the hypothalamus level) (86,88, 90,91). Diurnal fluctuation was not recognized in most of the patients with the severe form of TH-deficiency.

In a patient with infantile parkinsonism with motor delay, in which a homozygous *TH* missense mutation was identified, the mutant TH revealed only 0.3% to 16% of wild-type enzyme activity in three complementary expression systems (82,84). In contrast to this patient, in a TH-deficient DRD patient having another homozygous missense mutation of *TH*, the mutated recombinant enzyme showed approximately 15% of specific activity compared with the wild type in a coupled *in vitro* transcription-translation assay system (10, 81). A clinical comparison between two compound heterozygotes for *TH* mutations, one with the severe form of TH deficiency (83,87,89) and the other with the mild form (16), has suggested that an effect on TH activity *in vivo* of a missense mutation in the catalytic domain may be more severe than that in the tetramerization domain of this enzyme (14). Five homozygotes and one compound heterozygote with the severe form of TH deficiency, who were from four Dutch families (83,85,87,89), one Caucasian-German family (91), and one Lebanese family (92), had the same missense mutation [Arg233His, based on type 4 mRNA (94)], indicating that this *TH* mutation in the catalytic domain is a relatively common one.

DYT14 LOCUS

Very recently, Grötzsch et al. (19) have reported clinical and neuropathologic findings in a patient with autosomal-dominant DRD linked to the *DYT14* locus. In brief, this 77-year-old woman developed dystonia of the lower extremities and started walking on tiptoes by the age of 3 years. There was diurnal fluctuation of her gait disturbance. Her dystonia progressed to the upper extremities, and she was wheelchair bound by age 12 years. She had no appropriate medical assessment for her condition until age 73 years. Neurologic examination at this age revealed definite parkinsonism, including a resting tremor of the left leg, and dystonic posture of all the limbs. Levodopa administration (300 mg/day, with a DCI) dramatically alleviated the symptoms, whereas her walking remained impaired. In this patient, no mutation in either the coding region or the splice sites of *GCH1* was found. A genome-wide linkage analysis performed in her family mapped a novel causative gene for DRD to chromosome 14q13 [outside the *GCH1* gene on 14q22.1-q22.2 (9)]. A neuropathologic investigation in the substantia nigra pars compacta of the 77-year-old woman demonstrated (a) a normal number of neurons; (b) a hypomelanization of the large neurons; (c) a trend for the lateral part to be more affected by the demelanization than the medial part; and (d) no Lewy bodies and no gliosis as assessed by ubiquitin and glial fibrillary acidic protein immunostaining assays, respectively. As mentioned, these pathologic features were similar to those in the two DRD patients with GTPCH dysfunction reported previously (20,21). Neurochemical analysis was not conducted in the patient with DRD linked to the *DYT14* locus.

NEUROCHEMISTRY

In the putamen of the two autopsied DRD patients, BP levels were markedly decreased (mean, −84%) compared with age-matched normal controls (21). Both patients also had substantially reduced NP concentrations in the putamen (−62%). These brain findings are in agreement with CSF data, showing low levels of BP and NP in genetically proven patients with GTPCH-deficient DRD (50). One of the two autopsied patients (DRD patient 1) had a *GCH1* nonsense mutation (Glu65Ter) on one allele and the polymorphism in *GCH1* (Pro23Leu, see above) on the other allele (20,21) (Table 18-1). No mutation in either the coding region or the splicing junctions of *GCH1* was identified in the other autopsied patient (DRD patient 2) (21,99). Striatal subregional dopamine (DA) data pointed to an involvement of the caudal portion of the putamen, as the striatal subdivision that was most affected by DA loss (−88%) in patients 1 and 2 (20,21). By contrast, concentration of DA in this striatal subregion was normal in an autopsied patient with early-onset primary torsion dystonia having a GAG deletion in the *TOR1A* (*DYT1*) gene (100,101). The caudal putamen is known to be most affected by loss of DA in patients with PD (102,103).

In contrast to PD patients (104,105), striatal levels of dopa decarboxylase (DDC; a DA biosynthetic enzyme that does not use BH4 as a cofactor) protein, the DA transporter ([^{3}H]WIN 35428 binding), and the vesicular monoamine transporter ([^{3}H]dihydrotetrabenazine binding) were normal in patients 1

TABLE 18-1. *Clinical and genetic features of symptomatic and asymptomatic autopsied cases with GTPCH dysfunction*

Case	Sex	Age at death (years)	Age at onset (years)	Dystonia/ parkinsonism	Family history	Effect of levodopa (dose) [duration]	GCH1 mutation
DRD patient 1[a]	F	19	5	+/−	−	+ (750 mg/day) [11 yr]	Glu65Ter and a polymorphism (Pro23Leu)
DRD patient 2[b]	F	68	12	+/+	+ (DRD)	+ (100 mg/day with a DCI) [11 yr]	No mutation in the coding region (including the splice sites)
Asymptomatic carrier[c]	F	55	—	−/−	+ (DRD)	No administration of levodopa	Gly108Asp

In all three cases, neurochemical findings (decreased total biopterin and neopterin) indicated GTPCH dysfunction in the brain (14,21,22).

[a]From Rajput et al. (20) and Furukawa et al. (21).
[b]From Nygaard and Duvoisin (99) and Furukawa et al. (21).
[c]From Nygaard et al. (17) and Furukawa et al. (22).
GTPCH, guanosine triphosphate (GTP) cyclohydrolase I; *GCH1,* the gene encoding GTPCH; DRD, dopa-responsive dystonia; DCI, decarboxylase inhibitor.

and 2, indicating that striatal DA nerve terminals are preserved in GTPCH-deficient DRD (21). This postmortem brain observation is consistent with *in vivo* findings in positron emission tomography and single photon emission computed tomography studies on DRD (106,107), including the report of normal striatal fluorodopa uptake (which depends on DDC activity) in patient 2 (21,106). However, TH protein concentrations were decreased in the striatum, especially in the putamen (more than −97%), of both autopsied patients with DRD (21). These human brain data are compatible with TH protein loss but preserved DDC activity in brains of BH4-deficient mice, i.e., GTPCH-deficient *hph-1* mutants and 6-pyruvoyltetrahydropterin synthase gene (*PTS*) null mutants (63,66). Thus, the biochemical findings have suggested that striatal DA reduction in GTPCH-deficient DRD is caused not only by decreased TH activity due to low cofactor concentration but also by actual loss of TH protein without nigrostriatal DA nerve terminal loss (14,21).

Striatal TH protein reduction in GTPCH-deficient DRD may be caused by a diminished regulatory effect of BH4 on the steady-state level (stability/expression) of TH molecules (21). Gene-transfer experiments

have suggested that coexpression of GTPCH with TH stabilizes TH protein *in vivo* (64). Because TH protein levels in the substantia nigra, where striatal TH molecules are synthesized, were normal in patients 1 and 2, BH4 could control stability rather than expression of this enzyme protein (14,21). This is supported by a report demonstrating loss of TH protein but not of *TH* mRNA in brains of BH4-deficient *PTS* knockout mice (66). Alternatively, there might be an abnormality of TH protein transport from the substantia nigra to the striatum due to congenital partial GTPCH deficiency (21). A significant BP increase in the human striatum during early postnatal period (from 1 day to 12 months of age) suggests a contribution of BH4 to maturation of the nigrostriatal DA biosynthetic system (14,108).

Recently, neurochemical findings in an asymptomatic carrier of a significant mutation in *GCH1* [linked to DRD in this family (17)] have been reported (22). This asymptomatic patient had a missense mutation in *GCH1* (Gly108Asp) and died at 55 years of age (Table 18–1). In the autopsied putamen of the asymptomatic *GCH1* mutation carrier, decreases in BP and NP levels (−82% and − 57%, respectively) paralleled those in patients

1 and 2. However, TH protein and DA concentrations (-52% and -44%, respectively) in the caudal subregion of the putamen in the asymptomatic case were not as severely affected as in the symptomatic cases. Consistent with other postmortem brain data suggesting that greater than 60% to 80% of striatal DA loss is necessary for clinically overt motor symptoms to occur (103), the 44% reduction of DA in the putamen of the *GCH1* mutation carrier was not sufficient to produce any DRD symptoms. The brain biochemical findings in the asymptomatic *GCH1* mutation carrier suggest that the extent of striatal TH protein loss may be critical in determining GTPCH-deficient DRD symptomatology (22). The different degrees of striatal TH protein reduction between the asymptomatic and symptomatic DRD subjects with the same magnitude of BP and NP loss in the striatum also suggest that there are additional genetic and/or environmental factors that may modulate a regulatory effect of BH4 on the steady-state level of TH molecules.

CONCLUSION

Recent advances in the molecular genetics of DRD have demonstrated that there are at least three types of DRD: autosomal-dominant GTPCH-deficient DRD caused by mutations in the *GCH1* gene (chromosome location, 14q22.1-q22.2), autosomal-recessive TH-deficient DRD (the mild form of TH deficiency) due to mutations in the *TH* gene (11p15.5), and autosomal-dominant DRD linked to the *DYT14* locus (14q13). Neurochemical data suggest that striatal DA reduction in GTPCH-deficient DRD is caused not only by decreased TH activity resulting from a low level of BH4 (the essential cofactor for TH) but also by actual loss of TH protein without nerve terminal loss. This TH protein reduction in the striatum may be due to a diminished regulatory effect of BH4 on stability (rather than expression) of TH molecules or to a dysfunction of TH protein transport from the substantia nigra to the striatum. The extent of striatal TH protein loss could contribute to

gender-related incomplete penetrance of *GCH1* mutations in this major form of DRD. In terms of diagnosis and clinical management, all children with dystonic and/or parkinsonian symptoms of unknown etiology should be treated with low doses of levodopa (a therapeutic trial with levodopa) with the addition, if necessary, of other medications, e.g., combined administration of levodopa and BH4 for patients with dystonia with motor delay (some compound heterozygotes for *GCH1* mutations).

REFERENCES

1. Nygaard TG. Dopa-responsive dystonia: delineation of the clinical syndrome and clues to pathogenesis. *Adv Neurol* 1993;60:577–585.
2. Segawa M, Nomura Y. Hereditary progressive dystonia with marked diurnal fluctuation. In: Segawa M, ed. *Hereditary progressive dystonia with marked diurnal fluctuation.* New York: Parthenon, 1993:3–19.
3. Furukawa Y, Kish SJ. Dopa-responsive dystonia: recent advances and remaining issues to be addressed. *Mov Disord* 1999;14:709–715.
4. Fahn S, Bressman SB, Marsden CD. Classification of dystonia. *Adv Neurol* 1998;78:1–10.
5. Furukawa Y, Rajput AH. Inherited myoclonus-dystonia: how many causative genes and clinical phenotypes? *Neurology* 2002;59:1130–1131.
6. Furukawa Y, Mizuno Y, Narabayashi H. Early-onset parkinsonism with dystonia: clinical and biochemical differences from hereditary progressive dystonia or DOPA-responsive dystonia. *Adv Neurol* 1996;69: 327–337.
7. Segawa M, Ohmi K, Itoh S, et al. Childhood basal ganglia disease with remarkable response to L-DOPA: hereditary progressive basal ganglia disease with marked fluctuation. *Shinryo* 1971;24:667–672.
8. Castaigne P, Rondot P, Ribadeau-Dumas JL, et al. Affection extrapyramidale évoluant chez deux jeunes frères: effets remarquables du traitement par la L-Dopa. *Rev Neurol* 1971;124:162–166.
9. Ichinose H, Ohye T, Takahashi E, et al. Hereditary progressive dystonia with marked diurnal fluctuation caused by mutations in the GTP cyclohydrolase I gene. *Nat Genet* 1994;8:236–242.
10. Lüdecke B, Dworniczak B, Bartholomé K. A point mutation in the tyrosine hydroxylase gene associated with Segawa's syndrome. *Hum Genet* 1995;95: 123–125.
11. Inagaki H, Ohye T, Suzuki T, et al. Decrease in GTP cyclohydrolase I gene expression caused by inactivation of one allele in hereditary progressive dystonia with marked diurnal fluctuation. *Biochem Biophys Res Commun* 1999;260:747–751.
12. Swaans RJM, Rondot P, Renier WO, et al. Four novel mutations in the tyrosine hydroxylase gene in patients with infantile parkinsonism. *Ann Hum Genet* 2000;64: 25–31.

13. Furukawa Y, Shimadzu M, Hornykiewicz O, et al. Molecular and biochemical aspects of hereditary progressive and dopa-responsive dystonia. *Adv Neurol* 1998;78:267–282.

14. Furukawa Y. Genetics and biochemistry of dopa-responsive dystonia: significance of striatal tyrosine hydroxylase protein loss. *Adv Neurol* 2003;91:401–410.

15. Bartholomé K, Lüdecke B. Mutations in the tyrosine hydroxylase gene cause various forms of L-dopa-responsive dystonia. *Adv Pharmacol* 1998;42:48–49.

16. Furukawa Y, Graf WD, Wong H, et al. Dopa-responsive dystonia simulating spastic paraplegia due to tyrosine hydroxylase (TH) gene mutations. *Neurology* 2001;56:260–263.

17. Nygaard TG, Wilhelmsen KC, Risch NJ, et al. Linkage mapping of dopa-responsive dystonia (DRD) to chromosome 14q. *Nat Genet* 1993;5:386–391.

18. Tanaka H, Endo K, Tsuji S, et al. The gene for hereditary progressive dystonia with marked diurnal fluctuation maps to chromosome 14q. *Ann Neurol* 1995;37:405–408.

19. Grötzsch H, Pizzolato G-P, Ghika J, et al. Neuropathology of a case of dopa-responsive dystonia associated with a new genetic locus, *DYT 14*. *Neurology* 2002;58:1839–1842.

20. Rajput AH, Gibb WRG, Zhong XH, et al. Dopa-responsive dystonia: pathological and biochemical observations in a case. *Ann Neurol* 1994;35:396–402.

21. Furukawa Y, Nygaard TG, Gütlich M, et al. Striatal biopterin and tyrosine hydroxylase protein reduction in dopa-responsive dystonia. *Neurology* 1999;53:1032–1041.

22. Furukawa Y, Kapatos G, Haycock JW, et al. Brain biopterin and tyrosine hydroxylase in asymptomatic dopa-responsive dystonia. *Ann Neurol* 2002;51:637–641.

23. Nygaard TG, Snow BJ, Fahn S, et al. Dopa-responsive dystonia: clinical characteristics and definition. In: Segawa M, ed. *Hereditary progressive dystonia with marked diurnal fluctuation.* New York: Parthenon, 1993:21–35.

24. Müller K, Hömberg V, Lenard HG. Motor control in childhood onset dopa-responsive dystonia (Segawa syndrome). *Neuropediatrics* 1989;20:185–191.

25. Segawa M, Hosaka A, Miyagawa F, et al. Hereditary progressive dystonia with marked diurnal fluctuation. *Adv Neurol* 1976;14:215–233.

26. Steinberger D, Korinthenberg R, Topka H, et al. Dopa-responsive dystonia: mutation analysis of *GCH1* and analysis of therapeutic doses of L-dopa. *Neurology* 2000;55:1735–1737.

27. Grimes DA, Barclay CL, Duff J, et al. Phenocopies in a large GCH1 mutation positive family with dopa responsive dystonia: confusing the picture? *J Neurol Neurosurg Psychiatry* 2002;72:801–804.

28. Ichinose H, Ohye T, Matsuda Y, et al. Characterization of mouse and human GTP cyclohydrolase I genes: mutations in patients with GTP cyclohydrolase I deficiency. *J Biol Chem* 1995;270:10062–10071.

29. Togari A, Ichinose H, Matsumoto S, et al. Multiple mRNA forms of human GTP cyclohydrolase I. *Biochem Biophys Res Commun* 1992;187:359–365.

30. Gütlich M, Jaeger E, Rücknagel KP, et al. Human GTP cyclohydrolase I: only one out of three cDNA isoforms gives rise to the active enzyme. *Biochem J* 1994;302:215–221.

31. Nar H, Huber R, Meining W, et al. Atomic structure of GTP cyclohydrolase I. *Structure* 1995;3:459–466.

32. Nar H, Huber R, Auerbach G, et al. Active site topology and reaction mechanism of GTP cyclohydrolase I. *Proc Natl Acad Sci USA* 1995;92:12120–12125.

33. Furukawa Y. Dopa-responsive dystonia. In: *GeneReviews at GeneTests-GeneClinics* (database online). Seattle: University of Washington, 2002. Available at: *www.geneclinics.org.*

34. Hauf M, Cousin P, Solida A, et al. A family with segmental dystonia: evidence for polymorphism in GTP cyclohydrolase I gene (GCH I). *Mov Disord* 2000;15 (suppl 3):154–155.

35. Nomura T, Ichinose H, Sumi-Ichinose C, et al. Cloning and sequencing of cDNA encoding mouse GTP cyclohydrolase I. *Biochem Biophys Res Commun* 1993;191:523–527.

36. Maier J, Witter K, Gütlich M, et al. Homology cloning of GTP-cyclohydrolase I from various unrelated eukaryotes by reverse-transcription polymerase chain reaction using a general set of degenerate primers. *Biochem Biophys Res Commun* 1995;212:705–711.

37. Suzuki T, Ohye T, Inagaki H, et al. Characterization of wild-type and mutants of recombinant human GTP cyclohydrolase I: relationship to etiology of dopa-responsive dystonia. *J Neurochem* 1999;73:2510–2516.

38. Jarman PR, Bandmann O, Marsden CD, et al. GTP cyclohydrolase I mutations in patients with dystonia responsive to anticholinergic drugs. *J Neurol Neurosurg Psychiatry* 1997;63:304–308.

39. Levine RA, Kuhn DM, Lovenberg W. The regional distribution of hydroxylase cofactor in rat brain. *J Neurochem* 1979;32:1575–1578.

40. Levine RA, Miller LP, Lovenberg W. Tetrahydrobiopterin in striatum: localization in dopamine nerve terminals and role in catecholamine synthesis. *Science* 1981;214:919–921.

41. Sawada M, Hirata Y, Arai H, et al. Tyrosine hydroxylase, tryptophan hydroxylase, biopterin, and neopterin in the brains of normal controls and patients with senile dementia of Alzheimer type. *J Neurochem* 1987;48:760–764.

42. Kettler R, Bartholini G, Pletscher A. In vivo enhancement of tyrosine hydroxylation in rat striatum by tetrahydrobiopterin. *Nature* 1974;249:476–478.

43. Miwa S, Watanabe Y, Hayaishi O. 6R-L-erythlo-5,6,7,8-tetrahydrobiopterin as a regulator of dopamine and serotonin biosynthesis in the rat brain. *Arch Biochem Biophys* 1985;239:234–241.

44. Fink JK, Barton N, Cohen W, et al. Dystonia with marked diurnal variation associated with biopterin deficiency. *Neurology* 1988;38:707–711.

45. Furukawa Y, Nishi K, Kondo T, et al. CSF biopterin levels and clinical features of patients with juvenile parkinsonism. *Adv Neurol* 1993;60:562–567.

46. Furukawa Y, Mizuno Y, Nishi K, et al. A clue to the pathogenesis of dopa-responsive dystonia. *Ann Neurol* 1995;37:139–140.

47. Lovenberg W, Levine RA, Robinson DS, et al. Hydroxylase cofactor activity in cerebrospinal fluid of normal subjects and patients with Parkinson's disease. *Science* 1979;204:624–626.

48. Furukawa Y, Kondo T, Nishi K, et al. Total biopterin

levels in the ventricular CSF of patients with Parkinson's disease: a comparison between akineto-rigid and tremor types. *J Neurol Sci* 1991;103:232–237.

49. Furukawa Y, Nishi K, Kondo T, et al. Juvenile parkinsonism: ventricular CSF biopterin levels and clinical features. *J Neurol Sci* 1992;108:207–213.

50. Furukawa Y, Shimadzu M, Rajput AH, et al. GTP-cyclohydrolase I gene mutations in hereditary progressive and dopa-responsive dystonia. *Ann Neurol* 1996; 39:609–617.

51. Furukawa Y, Lang AE, Trugman JM, et al. Gender-related penetrance and de novo GTP-cyclohydrolase I gene mutations in dopa-responsive dystonia. *Neurology* 1998;50:1015–1020.

52. Ichinose H, Ohye T, Segawa M, et al. GTP cyclohydrolase I gene in hereditary progressive dystonia with marked diurnal fluctuation. *Neurosci Lett* 1995;196: 5–8.

53. Bandmann O, Nygaard TG, Surtees R, et al. Dopa-responsive dystonia in British patients: new mutations of the GTP-cyclohydrolase I gene and evidence for genetic heterogeneity. *Hum Mol Genet* 1996;5:403–406.

54. Bandmann O, Valente EM, Holmans P, et al. Dopa-responsive dystonia: a clinical and molecular genetic study. *Ann Neurol* 1998;44:649–656.

55. Steinberger D, Weber Y, Korinthenberg R, et al. High penetrance and pronounced variation in expressivity of *GCH1* mutations in five families with dopa-responsive dystonia. *Ann Neurol* 1998;43:634–639.

56. Furukawa Y, Guttman M, Sparagana SP, et al. Dopa-responsive dystonia due to a large deletion in the GTP cyclohydrolase I gene. *Ann Neurol* 2000;47:517–520.

57. Tassin J, Dürr A, Bonnet A-M, et al. Levodopa-responsive dystonia: GTP cyclohydrolase I or parkin mutations? *Brain* 2000;123:1112–1121.

58. Furukawa Y, Kish SJ, Bebin EM, et al. Dystonia with motor delay in compound heterozygotes for GTP-cyclohydrolase I gene mutations. *Ann Neurol* 1998;44: 10–16.

59. Furukawa Y, Kish SJ, Lang AE. Scoliosis in a dopa-responsive dystonia family with a mutation of the GTP cyclohydrolase I gene. *Neurology* 2000;54:2187.

60. Hyland K, Fryburg JS, Wilson WG, et al. Oral phenylalanine loading in dopa-responsive dystonia: a possible diagnostic test. *Neurology* 1997;48:1290–1297.

61. Saunders-Pullman RJ, Raymond D, Hyland K, et al. Markers of disease in dopa-responsive-dystonia. *Mov Disord* 1998;13(suppl 2):285.

62. Davis MD, Ribeiro P, Tipper J, et al."7-tetrahydrobiopterin," a naturally occurring analogue of tetrahydrobiopterin, is a cofactor for and a potential inhibitor of the aromatic amino acid hydroxylases. *Proc Natl Acad Sci USA* 1992;89:10109–10113.

63. Hyland K, Gunasekera RS, Engle T, et al. Tetrahydrobiopterin and biogenic amine metabolism in the *hph-1* mouse. *J Neurochem* 1996;67:752–759.

64. Leff SE, Rendahl KG, Spratt SK, et al. *In vivo* L-DOPA production by genetically modified primary rat fibroblast or 9L gliosarcoma cell grafts via coexpression of GTP cyclohydrolase I with tyrosine hydroxylase. *Exp Neurol* 1998;151:249–264.

65. Lindner M, Haas D, Zschocke J, et al. Tetrahydrobiopterin responsiveness in phenylketonuria differs between patients with the same genotype. *Mol Genet Metab* 2001;73:104–106.

66. Sumi-Ichinose C, Urano F, Kuroda R, et al. Catecholamines and serotonin are differently regulated by tetrahydrobiopterin: a study from 6-pyruvoyltetrahydropterin synthase knockout mice. *J Biol Chem* 2001; 276:41150–41160.

67. Hirano M, Imaiso Y, Ueno S. Differential splicing of the GTP cyclohydrolase I RNA in dopa-responsive dystonia. *Biochem Biophys Res Commun* 1997;234: 316–319.

68. Shimoji M, Hirayama K, Hyland K, et al. GTP cyclohydrolase I gene expression in the brains of male and female hph-1 mice. *J Neurochem* 1999;72:757–764.

69. Niederwieser A, Blau N, Wang M, et al. GTP cyclohydrolase I deficiency, a new enzyme defect causing hyperphenylalaninemia with neopterin, biopterin, dopamine, and serotonin deficiencies and muscular hypotonia. *Eur J Pediatr* 1984;141:208–214.

70. Blau N, Ichinose H, Nagatsu T, et al. A missense mutation in a patient with guanosine triphosphate cyclohydrolase I deficiency missed in the newborn screening program. *J Pediatr* 1995;126:401–405.

71. Blau N, Barnes I, Dhondt JL. International database of tetrahydrobiopterin deficiencies. *J Inherit Metab Dis* 1996;19:8–14.

72. Hirano M, Yanagihara T, Ueno S. Dominant negative effect of GTP cyclohydrolase I mutations in dopa-responsive hereditary progressive dystonia. *Ann Neurol* 1998;44:365–371.

73. Hirano M, Ueno S. Mutant GTP cyclohydrolase I in autosomal dominant dystonia and recessive hyperphenylalaninemia. *Neurology* 1999;52:182–184.

74. Hwu W-L, Chiou Y-W, Lai S-Y, et al. Dopa-responsive dystonia is induced by a dominant-negative mechanism. *Ann Neurol* 2000;48:609–613.

75. Grima B, Lamouroux A, Boni C, et al. A single human gene encoding multiple tyrosine hydroxylases with different predicted functional characteristics. *Nature* 1987;326:707–711.

76. Kaneda N, Kobayashi K, Ichinose H, et al. Isolation of a novel cDNA clone for human tyrosine hydroxylase: alternative RNA splicing produces four kinds of mRNA from a single gene. *Biochem Biophys Res Commun* 1987;146:971–975.

77. O'Malley KL, Anhalt MJ, Martin BM, et al. Isolation and characterization of the human tyrosine hydroxylase gene: identification of 5′ alternative splice sites responsible for multiple mRNAs. *Biochemistry* 1987; 26:6910–6914.

78. Dumas S, le Hir H, Bodeau-Péan S, et al. New species of human tyrosine hydroxylase mRNA are produced in variable amounts in adrenal medulla and are overexpressed in progressive supranuclear palsy. *J Neurochem* 1996;67:19–25.

79. Ohye T, Ichinose H, Yoshizawa T, et al. A new splicing variant for human tyrosine hydroxylase in the adrenal medulla. *Neurosci Lett* 2001;312:157–160.

80. Goodwill KE, Sabatier C, Marks C, et al. Crystal structure of tyrosine hydroxylase at 2.3 Å and its implications for inherited neurodegenerative diseases. *Nat Struct Biol* 1997;4:578–585.

81. Knappskog PM, Flatmark T, Mallet J, et al. Recessively inherited L-DOPA-responsive dystonia caused by a point mutation (Q381K) in the tyrosine hydroxylase gene. *Hum Mol Genet* 1995;4:1209–1212.

82. Lüdecke B, Knappskog PM, Clayton PT, et al. Reces-

sively inherited L-DOPA-responsive parkinsonism in infancy caused by a point mutation (L205P) in the tyrosine hydroxylase gene. *Hum Mol Genet* 1996;5: 1023–1028.

83. Bräutigam C, Wevers RA, Jansen RJT, et al. Biochemical hallmarks of tyrosine hydroxylase deficiency. *Clin Chem* 1998;44:1897–1904.

84. Surtees R, Clayton P. Infantile parkinsonism-dystonia: tyrosine hydroxylase deficiency. *Mov Disord* 1998;13: 350.

85. van den Heuvel LPWJ, Luiten B, Smeitink JAM, et al. A common point mutation in the tyrosine hydroxylase gene in autosomal recessive L-DOPA-responsive dystonia in the Dutch population. *Hum Genet* 1998;102: 644–646.

86. Bräutigam C, Steenbergen-Spanjers GCH, Hoffmann GF, et al. Biochemical and molecular genetic characteristics of the severe form of tyrosine hydroxylase deficiency. *Clin Chem* 1999;45:2073–2078.

87. Wevers RA, de Ruk-van Andel JF, Bräutigam C, et al. A review of biochemical and molecular genetic aspects of tyrosine hydroxylase deficiency including a novel mutation (291delC). *J Inherit Metab Dis* 1999; 22:364–373.

88. de Lonlay P, Nassogne MC, van Gennip AH, et al. Tyrosine hydroxylase deficiency unresponsive to L-dopa treatment with unusual clinical and biochemical presentation. *J Inherit Metab Dis* 2000;23:819–825.

89. de Rijk-van Andel JF, Gabreëls FJM, Geurtz B, et al. L-dopa-responsive infantile hypokinetic rigid parkinsonism due to tyrosine hydroxylase deficiency. *Neurology* 2000;55:1926–1928.

90. Dionisi-Vici C, Hoffmann GF, Leuzzi V, et al. Tyrosine hydroxylase deficiency with severe clinical course: clinical and biochemical investigations and optimization of therapy. *J Pediatr* 2000;136:560–562.

91. Janssen RJRJ, Wevers RA, Häussler M, et al. A branch site mutation leading to aberrant splicing of the human tyrosine hydroxylase gene in a child with a severe extrapyramidal movement disorder. *Ann Hum Genet* 2000;64:375–382.

92. Grattan-Smith PJ, Wevers RA, Steenbergen-Spanjers GC, et al. Tyrosine hydroxylase deficiency: clinical manifestations of catecholamine insufficiency in infancy. *Mov Disord* 2002;17:354–359.

93. Zhou Q-Y, Quaife CJ, Palmiter RD. Targeted disruption of the tyrosine hydroxylase gene reveals that catecholamines are required for mouse fetal development. *Nature* 1995;374:640–643.

94. Nagatsu T, Ichinose H. Comparative studies on the structure of human tyrosine hydroxylase with those of the enzyme of various mammals. *Comp Biochem Physiol* 1991;98C:203–210.

95. Lüdecke B, Bartholomé K. Frequent sequence variant in the human tyrosine hydroxylase gene. *Hum Genet* 1995;95:716.

96. Ishiguro H, Arinami T, Saito T, et al. Systematic search for variations in the tyrosine hydroxylase gene and their associations with schizophrenia, affective disorders, and alcoholism. *Am J Med Genet* 1998;81:388–396.

97. Rondot P, Ziegler M. Dystonia-L-dopa responsive or juvenile parkinsonism? *J Neurol Transm* 1983;suppl 19:273–281.

98. Rondot P, Aicardi J, Goutières F, et al. Dystonies dopa-sensibles. *Rev Neurol* 1992;148:680–686.

99. Nygaard TG, Duvoisin RC. Hereditary dystonia-parkinsonism syndrome of juvenile onset. *Neurology* 1986;36:1424–1428.

100. Ozelius LJ, Hewett JW, Page CE, et al. The early-onset torsion dystonia gene (*DYT1*) encodes an ATP-binding protein. *Nat Genet* 1997;17:40–48.

101. Furukawa Y, Hornykiewicz O, Fahn S, et al. Striatal dopamine in early-onset primary torsion dystonia with the *DYT1* mutation. *Neurology* 2000;54:1193–1195.

102. Kish SJ, Shannak K, Hornykiewicz O. Uneven pattern of dopamine loss in the striatum of patients with idiopathic Parkinson's disease: pathophysiologic and clinical implications. *N Engl J Med* 1988;318:876–880.

103. Hornykiewicz O. Biochemical aspects of Parkinson's disease. *Neurology* 1998;51(suppl 2):S2–S9.

104. Zhong X-H, Haycock JW, Shannak K, et al. Striatal dihydroxyphenylalanine decarboxylase and tyrosine hydroxylase protein in idiopathic Parkinson's disease and dominantly inherited olivopontocerebellar atrophy. *Mov Disord* 1995;10:10–17.

105. Wilson JM, Levey AI, Rajput A, et al. Differential changes in neurochemical markers of striatal dopamine nerve terminals in idiopathic Parkinson's disease. *Neurology* 1996;47:718–726.

106. Snow BJ, Nygaard TG, Takahashi H, et al. Positron emission tomographic studies of dopa-responsive dystonia and early-onset idiopathic parkinsonism. *Ann Neurol* 1993;34:733–738.

107. Jeon BS, Jeong J-M, Park S-S, et al. Dopamine transporter density measured by [^{123}I]β-CIT single-photon emission computed tomography is normal in dopa-responsive dystonia. *Ann Neurol* 1998;43:792–800.

108. Furukawa Y, Kish SJ. Influence of development and aging on brain biopterin: implications for dopa-responsive dystonia onset. *Neurology* 1998;51:632–634.

Dystonia 4: Advances in Neurology, Vol. 94. Edited by Stanley Fahn, Mark Hallett, and Mahlon R. DeLong. Lippincott Williams & Wilkins, Philadelphia © 2004.

19

X-Linked Recessive Dystonia Parkinsonism (XDP; Lubag; DYT3)

Andrew Singleton, Stephen Hague, and Dena Hernandez

Molecular Genetics Section, Laboratory of Neurogenetics, National Institute on Aging, National Institutes of Health, Bethesda, Maryland

CLINICAL AND PATHOLOGICAL FEATURES OF XDP

X-linked recessive dystonia parkinsonism (XDP; Lubag; DYT3) was first described in 1976 by Lee and colleagues (1) following an epidemiologic survey of Panay, an island situated in the southwest of the Philippines. XDP is estimated to affect 1/4,000 males in the Panay province of Capiz (2); however, given the phenotypic variability noted below, it is likely that this is an underestimation of the frequency in this population. XDP has also been commonly referred to as Lubag based on one of three names the disorder was given by the local Illongo. In the Illongo dialect, "Lubag" describes the twisting motion seen in some affected individuals, "wa-eg" describes the sustained postures, and "sud-sud" is an onomatopoeic term used to describe the shuffling gait that can also be commonly seen (3).

XDP often presents with a focal dystonia, commonly blepharospasm or a limb dystonia; age at onset ranges from adolescence to mid-40s, with a mean age of onset of 35 years. XDP usually progresses to a generalized form over the course of 5 to 7 years and is invariably fatal. We have recently shown that there is more variation in presentation and clinical course than previously recognized. In a series of 11 haplotype-confirmed XDP patients, we observed a number of presenting features, including essential tremor, blepharospasm, micrographia, focal limb dystonia, anterocollis, and ballism (4). Previous descriptions of XDP have noted parkinsonism in ~40% of cases (5). We have shown that parkinsonism is a more common feature of XDP than previously reported. In the series of 11 patients we reported, all 11 had definite parkinsonism during the course of the disease and five displayed parkinsonism as an early or presenting feature. Patients often have a poor response to the standard medications found useful in some dystonias and in Parkinson's disease (5), although recently a combined therapy of anticholinergics and benzodiazepines for dystonia and L-dopa for parkinsonism has been reported to confer mild relief of symptoms (4).

The pathologic basis of dystonia in general is poorly understood. There are only a small number of reports describing detailed neuropathologic analysis of dystonia cases, and those that are present often provide inconclusive or conflicting findings. There are few descriptions of the neuropathology of XDP, although there is now an XDP brain bank in the Philippines, which, it is hoped, will facilitate further neuropathologic examination (3,6,7). In 1993 Waters et al. (3) described the neuropathologic features of a 34-year-old Filipino man with XDP who displayed both dystonia and parkinsonism. The pathologic

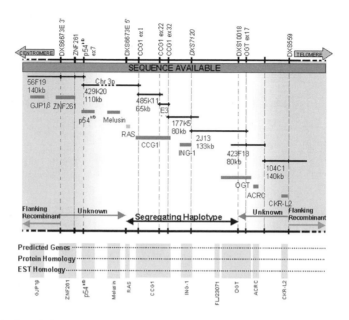

FIG. 19-1. Physical and electronic map of the X-linked recessive dystonia parkinsonism (XDP) critical region. **A:** The physically mapped clones, genes, and a number of markers. **B:** The results of the electronic data mining and analysis performed primarily using NIX (nucleotide identity X). This diagram includes the position of ESTs (expressed sequence tags), regions of homology to known proteins (all species), and predicted genes.

findings in general were unremarkable with the exception of mild Purkinje and granular cell loss in the cerebellum and subtle astrocytosis in a multifocal or mosaic pattern in the caudate and putamen. These findings were consistent with a previous report describing the neuropathology in a Filipino male with generalized dystonia (6). This particular pattern of mosaic gliosis has also been reported in a non-Filipino male with dystonia (8); however, it remains unclear whether this phenomenon is pathologically relevant to XDP. One tantalizing possibility is that this case is caused by a defect in the same gene that contains the XDP causing mutation.

We have extended the observations made in previous reports by performing detailed histopathologic analysis of a brain from an XDP patient with dystonia and prominent parkinsonism (9). We confirmed the mosaic gliosis previously noted in the striatum and described a gradient of pathology representing more marked involvement of the caudate

and putamen than the ventral and limbic striatum. Furthermore, we showed synaptic loss associated with the striatal gliosis and particularly marked synaptic loss in the globus pallidus pars interna. We suggest that the affected neurons are most likely derived from sensorimotor and association cortices. The functional significance of this pathology remains unclear; however, a current hypothesis of dystonia pathophysiology relates to γ-aminobutyric acid (GABA)ergic sensorimotor dysfunction, and hence these findings may provide some insight into the pathoetiology of XDP and other dystonias (10).

GENETICS

The restriction of known cases of XDP to descendants of Panay islanders in conjunction with the fact that no cognate disorder has been described elsewhere implies that this island may have been the geographic location of the causal germ line mutation. However, the founder mutation may have occurred prior to waves of immigration from East Malaysia and Borneo and it is feasible that this disorder may also be present in these populations (1).

XDP is inherited in an X-linked recessive fashion, the vast majority of reported cases being male. Over the past decade several groups have used a linkage approach to refine the region containing the gene defect responsible for this disease. The gene locus was originally mapped to the long arm of chromosome X, and a segregating haplotype was defined within an 1.8-megabase (Mb) YAC contig (11). Nemeth et al. (12) described a series of patients in whom flanking recombinant markers minimize the candidate region to approximately 350 kilobase (kb) at Xq13 between markers DXS559 and DXS6673E 3′. We have collected DNA samples from 50 male clinically diagnosed patients and their first-degree relatives. We have examined markers within and flanking the previously described candidate region in these cases and confirm the segregating haplotype (Table 19-1) (12). The smaller [136 base pair (bp) vs. 138 bp] allele found in five cases at marker DXS6673E 3′ may define a recombination event and thus refine the segregating region. However, it is also possible the 136-bp allele may represent an ancestral slippage event given that all of these cases possess a relatively rare (<10%) 200-bp disease segregating allele at flanking marker DXS7117. This sample series, therefore, fails to confirm the previously reported centromeric or telomeric boundaries of the disease haplotype. This may indicate that the critical interval is larger than previously suspected. A viable alternative is that a larger sample series may be required to verify these flanking recombinants; however,

the number of affected patients in our series is similar to that previously assessed ($n = 50$ vs. $n = 47$).

The advent of the human genome sequencing project has provided a formidable resource for the biologic community. Analysis of the genomic region involved in XDP, suggested to be ~350 kb in size (12), indicates the vast majority has been sequenced and ordered. Applying an electronic data-mining approach, we and others have confirmed the location of four previously mapped genes, *ZNF261, CCG1, OGT,* and $p54^{nrb}$ (11–14), and identified the position of several unmapped genes within the critical region, including melusin, *CKR-L2, ING-1,* and *ACRC* (Fig. 19-1). Our group and others have sequenced the coding region of all of these genes and failed to find any alterations that segregate with disease (12–16). In addition we have examined full-length cDNA transcripts for melusin, *CKR-L2, OGT, CCG1, ZNF261,* and $p54^{nrb}$, and failed to find any splicing differences between affected individuals and controls. To perform this analysis, we used reverse-transcriptase polymerase chain reaction (RT-PCR) amplification of messenger RNA (mRNA) derived from Epstein-Barr virus (EBV)-transformed lymphocytes from two patients and their mothers. It is possible that there may be a difference in brain-specific expression not apparent in these assays. An additional, longer 1,300-bp transcript was noted for the melusin gene. Sequencing of this product revealed the use of a previously unidentified alternative splice donor site to produce the longer transcript (unpublished observation), but no disease-causing mutations were contained within this coding region.

TABLE 19-1. *Haplotype segregating with X-linked recessive dystonia parkinsonism (XDP)*

	No.	DXS7117	DXS6673E3′	ZNF261	DXS10017	DXS10018	DXS559	DXS1124
Affected	45	**200**	**138**	**150**	**292**	**140**	**240**	**114**
	5	**200**	**136**	**150**	**292**	**140**	**240**	**114**

Note: The allele sizes shown in bold segregate with disease. The disease haplotype was found in all 50 affected patients and their mothers and in no male Filipino controls ($n = 100$).

FUTURE DIRECTIONS

Sequence analysis of all of the genes contained in the critical region (as defined by Nemeth et al.) by our group and others has failed to reveal any disease-segregating variation within the coding exons and immediate flanking regions (12,13,15,16). The most parsimonious explanation for these findings is that the genetic variation responsible for this disease is not contained within these genes, which leads us to one of three possibilities: the mutation is within a coding region not yet identified within the critical interval (either a novel exon or a novel gene); the mutation is in a regulatory region of one of the identified genes causing aberrant splicing or expression; or there is a gross structural rearrangement within the disease segregating haplotype not yet identified. In an attempt to answer these questions, we have undertaken a project aimed at cloning and sequencing the entire disease-segregating region, in a similar manner to that employed by the human genome sequencing effort. Once the mutation is identified, the problem we will face will be one of proving pathogenicity. Because all of the Filipino XDP patients carry the same disease haplotype, they will possess the same variation within that haplotype, be it benign or causal. Thus segregation of a mutation with disease in these patients implies but does not prove causation. A gross genetic change such as one causing a major alteration in the structure of a protein is a credible cause of disease; however, a mutation that confers a subtle alteration in the protein or exerts a putative effect on the splicing or expression of a gene is more difficult to prove as a cause of disease. It is vitally important to identify non-Filipino males with a disease phenotype similar to XDP. Following the identification of a mutation segregating with XDP, these patients can then be screened for a similar change in the same gene.

The disease research paradigm of gene identification followed by cellular and transgenic modeling has proven to be successful in elucidating the etiology of disease and promises to pay dividends in therapeutic design and testing. Furthermore, it seems reasonable to suggest that a similar approach applied to XDP will have implications for related disorders. Given the worldwide impact of both dystonia and parkinsonism, discovery of the causal gene defect for XDP promises to open many avenues of research in the future.

REFERENCES

1. Lee LV, Pascasio FM, Fuentes FD, et al. Torsion dystonia in Panay, Philippines. *Adv Neurol* 1976;14:137–151.
2. Kupke KG, Lee LV, Viterbo GH, et al. X-linked recessive torsion dystonia in the Philippines. *Am J Med Genet* 1990;36(2):237–242.
3. Waters CH, Faust PL, Powers J, et al. Neuropathology of Lubag (x-linked dystonia parkinsonism). *Mov Disord* 1993;8(3):387–390.
4. Evidente VGH, Advincula J, Esteban R, et al. The phenomenology of "Lubag" or X-linked dystonia-parkinsonism ('Lubag'). *Mov Disord* 2002;17:1271–1277.
5. Lee LV, Kupke KG, Caballar-Gonzaga F, et al. The phenotype of the X-linked dystonia-parkinsonism syndrome. An assessment of 42 cases in the Philippines. *Medicine (Baltimore)* 1991;70(3):179–187.
6. Altrocchi PH, Forno LS. Spontaneous oral-facial dyskinesia: neuropathology of a case. *Neurology* 1983;33 (6):802–805.
7. Lee L, Maranon E, Demaisip C, et al. The natural history of sex-linked recessive dystonia parkinsonism of Panay, Philippines (XDP). *Parkinsonism Relat Disord* 2002;9(1):29.
8. Gibb WR, Kilford L, Marsden CD. Severe generalised dystonia associated with a mosaic pattern of striatal gliosis. *Mov Disord* 1992;7(3):217–223.
9. Singleton A, Cookson N, Evidente VGH, et al. Neuropathological characteristics of a patient with X-linked recessive dystonia parkinsonism (XDP; Lubag; Dyt3). *In preparation.*
10. Levy LM, Hallett M. Impaired brain GABA in focal dystonia. *Ann Neurol* 2002;51(1):93–101.
11. Haberhausen G, Schmitt I, Kohler A, et al. Assignment of the dystonia-parkinsonism syndrome locus, DYT3, to a small region within a 1.8-Mb YAC contig of Xq13.1. *Am J Hum Genet* 1995;57(3):644–650.
12. Nemeth AH, Nolte D, Dunne E, et al. Refined linkage disequilibrium and physical mapping of the gene locus for X-linked dystonia-parkinsonism (DYT3). *Genomics* 1999;60(3):320–329.
13. Peters U, Haberhausen G, Kostrzewa M, et al. AFX1 and p54nrb: fine mapping, genomic structure, and exclusion as candidate genes of X-linked dystonia parkinsonism. *Hum Genet* 1997;100(5–6):569–572.
14. Hernandez D, Evidente VGH, Alfon JA, et al. Analysis of candidate genes within and around the critical interval for X-linked dystonia parkinsonism. *In preparation.*
15. Wilhelmsen KC, Moskowitz CB, Weeks DE, et al. Molecular genetic analysis of Lubag. *Adv Neurol* 1998;78: 341–348.
16. Nolte D, Ramser J, Niemann S, et al. ACRC codes for a novel nuclear protein with unusual acidic repeat tract and maps to DYT3 (dystonia parkinsonism) critical interval in xq13.1. *Neurogenetics* 2001;3(4):207–213.

Dystonia 4: Advances in Neurology, Vol. 94. Edited by Stanley Fahn, Mark Hallett, and Mahlon R. DeLong. Lippincott Williams & Wilkins, Philadelphia © 2004.

20

Focal Dystonia Is Associated with a Polymorphism of the Dopamine D$_5$ Receptor Gene

Anjum Misbahuddin, Mark R. Placzek, and Thomas T. Warner

Department of Clinical Neuroscience, Royal Free and University College Medical School, London, United Kingdom

Focal dystonias represent the most common form of primary torsion dystonia, with a minimum prevalence of 117 per million population in Europe (1). The most common forms are cervical dystonia (torticollis) and blepharospasm. Most cases of focal dystonia have onset in adulthood, appear to be sporadic, and have uncertain etiology.

There is mounting evidence, however, to support a role for genetic factors, and cases with clear autosomal-dominant inheritance have been described. A locus *(DYT7)* has been mapped to chromosome 18p in a German family with six members affected with torticollis and one with spasmodic dysphonia (2). Linkage studies in similar families, however, have excluded this locus (3). Recently, another family with blepharospasm inherited in an autosomal-dominant pattern has also had linkage to *DYT7* excluded (4).

Focal dystonia (usually of early onset) has been described as the sole manifestation of the *DYT1* gene, which usually causes a childhood-onset condition leading to generalized dystonia (5,6). Individuals with myoclonus-dystonia and mutations in the ε-sarcoglycan gene also often have a pure focal dystonia in addition to the myoclonus (7). Family studies also suggest a significant role for genetic factors in the etiology of focal dystonia. In one study, 25% of apparently sporadic index cases were found to have other family members with undiagnosed dystonia (8).

There is increasing evidence that a key factor in the pathogenesis of dystonic movements is abnormal dopaminergic neurotransmission. Dopamine D$_2$ receptor blocking neuroleptic drugs frequently cause dystonia (9), and a single photon emission computed tomography (SPECT) study in torticollis patients showed decreased D$_2$ receptor striatal binding (10). Experiments in primates using the nigral toxin 1-methyl-4-phenyl-1,2,3,6-tetrahydropyridine (MPTP), which selectively destroys dopamine producing neurons, produced transient dystonia (11). Dopa-responsive dystonia shows a sustained therapeutic response to low doses of levodopa and is caused by defects in either of two enzymes involved in the dopamine biosynthetic pathway—guanosine triphosphate cyclohydrolase 1 or tyrosine hydroxylase (12). *DYT1* or Oppenheim's dystonia, the most common form of primary generalized dystonia, results from a mutation in the widely expressed *DYT1* gene. *DYT1* messenger RNA (mRNA) is highly expressed in the dopaminergic neurones of the substantia nigra pars compacta (SNPC) (13). A recent study measuring levels of dopamine and its metabolites in *DYT1* postmortem brain tissue has shown evidence of an increase in dopamine turnover (14).

Disordered dopaminergic neurotransmission may not be the only abnormality needed for focal dystonia to manifest, as a rat model of blepharospasm indicates (15). In these experiments injections of 6-hydroxydopamine were used to destroy dopaminergic cells in the SNPC of the rat, and weakening of orbicularis oculi was achieved by sectioning the zygomatic branch of the facial nerve. Individually each of these lesions led to trigeminal reflex blink hyperexcitability. When both procedures were performed on the same animal, the rat developed spontaneous spasms of eyelid closure, which resembled blepharospasm in humans. This study suggested, therefore, that dopaminergic abnormalities led to an increased susceptibility of developing dystonia, but that further insults were needed before it became clinically apparent.

ALLELIC ASSOCIATION STUDIES

Allelic association studies have been performed in many multifactorial diseases in an attempt to identify predisposing genes. Case-control allelic association studies have been performed in cohorts of patients with cervical dystonia (16) and blepharospasm (17) to assess whether polymorphisms in the dopamine receptor and transporter genes may lead to an increased susceptibility to dystonia. One hundred patients with cervical dystonia and 88 patients with blepharospasm, all of whom were British Caucasians, were recruited for these studies. All patients had either cervical dystonia or blepharospasm for at least 1 year's duration and had been assessed in a movement disorder clinic. Those with secondary dystonia or a positive family history were excluded. Two sets of controls were also recruited from patients attending the hospital for nonneurologic reasons. They were matched with the patient groups for age, sex, and ethnicity.

The ten published polymorphisms studied in the D_{1-5} receptor (*DRD1–5*) and the dopamine transporter *(DAT1)* genes include both single nucleotide polymorphisms (SNPs), detected by changes in restriction fragments, and repeat polymorphisms in different areas of the genes. Details of these are given in Table 20-1. Each subject donated a blood sample from which genomic DNA was extracted by standard methods. Polymerase chain reaction (PCR) was performed with 100 ng of DNA and 20 pmol of each primer in a total volume of 25 µL. The reactions for the D_2 repeat, D_2 promoter, D_4 and D_5 polymorphisms included 10% dimethylsulfoxide (DMSO). Statistical analysis was performed using χ^2. Hardy-Weinberg equilibrium was assessed in the control population.

The details of the population groups used are given in Table 20-2.

No significant association was seen between control and patient allele frequencies for polymorphisms in the D_1 to D_4 receptor and dopamine transporter genes for either cervical dystonia or blepharospasm (data not shown). Results for the D5 microsatellite re-

TABLE 20-1. *Dopamine receptor and transporter (DAT1) polymorphisms*

Locus	Chromosomal region	Polymorphism
DAT1	5p15.3	40-base pair (bp) tandem repeat polymorphism in the 3′ untranslated region (18)
DRD1	5p31–34	Ddel RFLP in the 5′ untranslated region of the gene (19)
DRD1	5p31–34	PvuI RFLP within codon 421 (19)
DRD2	11q22–23	Microsatellite repeat in the 2nd intron (20)
DRD2	11q22–23	TaqI A RFLP 3′ flanking region of the gene (20)
DRD2	11q22–23	TaqI B RFLP within the first intron (20)
DRD2	11q22–23	BstNI RFLP from the −141 C Ins/Del within the promoter region (21)
DRD3	3q13.3	MscI RFLP within the first exon (22)
DRD4	11p	48-bp repeat polymorphism at the third exon (23)
DRD5	4p15.1–15.3	Microsatellite (CT/GT/GA)n 5′ to DRD5 (24)

RFLP, restriction fragment length polymorphism.

TABLE 20-2. *Sex and age characteristics of subject groups*

	Male:female ratio	Mean age (SD)	Mean age of onset of dystonia (SD)
Cervical dystonia	1:2.8	55.5 (12.1)	44.6 (14.2)
Controls	1:4	52.8 (17.5)	NA
Blepharospasm	1:4	63.7 (9.5)	55.8 (10.4)
Controls	1:4	60.6 (17.3)	NA

SD, standard deviation.

peat polymorphism are shown in Table 20-3. Allele 2 was significantly more common in both patient groups as compared with their control groups (cervical dystonia p = .004, blepharospasm p = .009). In addition, allele 6 of the D$_5$ repeat was significantly more common in the control group than in the cervical dystonia patient group (p = .0003). This association was not seen in the blepharospasm group.

These studies have shown that two independent cohorts of patients with focal dystonia have shown significant association with the D5 microsatellite repeat. One allele (allele 2) is overrepresented in both the cervical dystonia and blepharospasm group. It is unlikely that the microsatellite repeat itself confers any functional effect on D$_5$ receptor function, but the association may represent linkage disequilibrium with another polymorphism in the *DRD5* gene or conceivably in another gene close by, which may impart a functional variation. Thus a haplotype associated with allele 2 may lead to susceptibility to developing fo-

cal dystonia, and a haplotype associated with allele 6 of the D$_5$ repeat may confer a protective effect for cervical dystonia. *DRD5* mRNA has been identified in the SNPC (25), so a functional variant may alter dopaminergic neurotransmission.

Recently, an independent study with a group of 104 Italian cervical dystonia patients and 104 matched controls has replicated these findings by also showing that a specific allele of the same microsatellite repeat [150 base pair (bp), corresponding to allele 4] is associated with cervical dystonia (26). In addition, the 138-bp allele corresponding to allele 10 is significantly more common in the control group. The alleles in question were different from those in the previous reports (16,17), which may reflect a difference in the populations studied.

These results suggest that there may be a functional variant of the dopamine D$_5$ receptor that confers susceptibility to developing focal dystonia in later life. Based on the rat model of blepharospasm (15), it may require

TABLE 20-3. *Results of the D5 microsatellite repeat polymorphism*

D5 allele	Torticollis frequency	Control frequency	p	Blepharospasm frequency	Control frequency	p
1 (156 bp)	0	2	.154	3	2	.625
2 (154 bp)	13	2	.004	11	2	.009
3 (152 bp)	15	15	.977	9	15	.237
4 (150 bp)	31	25	.410	23	23	.902
5 (148 bp)	90	83	.536	87	84	.530
6 (146 bp)	8	29	.0003	10	18	.138
7 (144 bp)	8	6	.599	7	8	.844
8 (142 bp)	9	9	.983	6	6	.952
9 (140 bp)	9	8	.821	6	8	.631
10 (138 bp)	12	11	.849	8	7	.741
11 (136 bp)	1	7	.031	1	4	.189
12 (134 bp)	6	3	.319	3	3	.967

environmental factors later to actually trigger dystonia.

Further work will focus on identifying alternative polymorphisms within the *DRD5* gene that are more likely to produce a functional effect and on assessing whether these are associated with focal dystonias.

ACKNOWLEDGMENTS

The authors thank the Dystonia Society UK for financial support of their work.

REFERENCES

1. The Epidemiological Study of Dystonia in Europe Collaborative Group. A prevalence study of primary dystonia in eight European countries. *J Neurol* 2000;247:787–792.
2. Leube B, Rudnicki D, Ratzlaff T, et al. Idiopathic torsion dystonia: assignment of a gene to chromosome 18p in a German family with adult onset, autosomal dominant inheritance and purely focal distribution. *Hum Mol Genet* 1996;5:1673–1677.
3. Jarman PR, del Grosso N, Valente EM. et al. Primary torsion dystonia: the search for genes is not over. *J Neurol Neurosurg Psychiatry* 1999;67:395–397.
4. Defazio G, Brancati F, Valente EM. et al. Familial blepharospasm is inherited as an autosomal dominant trait and relates to a novel unassigned gene. *Mov Disord* 2003;18:207–212.
5. Bressman SB, Sabatti C, Raymond D, et al. The DYT1 phenotype and guidelines for diagnostic testing. *Neurology* 2000;54:1746–1752.
6. Gasser T, Windgassen K, Bereznai B, et al. Phenotypic expression of the DYT1 mutation: a family with writer's cramp of juvenile onset. *Ann Neurol* 1998;44:126–128.
7. Zimprich A, Grabowski M, Asmus F, et al. Mutations in the gene encoding ε-sarcoglycan cause myoclonus-dystonia syndrome. *Nat Genet* 2001;29:66–69.
8. Waddy HM, Fletcher NA, Harding AE, et al. A genetic study of idiopathic focal dystonias. *Ann Neurol* 1991;29:320–324
9. Burke R, Fahn S, Jankovic J, et al. Tardive dystonia: late onset and persistent dystonia caused by anti-psychotic drugs. *Neurology* 1982;32:1335–1346.
10. Naumann M, Pirker W, Reiners K, et al. Imaging the pre- and post-synaptic side of striatal dopaminergic synapses in idiopathic cervical dystonia: a SPECT study using [^{123}I] Epidepride and [^{123}I] beta-CIT. *Mov Disord* 1998;13:319–323.
11. Perlmutter JS, Tempel LW, Black KJ, et al. MPTP induces dystonia and parkinsonism: clues to the pathophysiology of dystonia. *Neurology* 1997;49:1432–1438.
12. Furukawa Y, Kish SJ. Dopa-responsive dystonia: recent advances and remaining issues to be addressed. *Mov Disord* 1999;14:709–715.
13. Augood SJ, Penney JB, Friberg IK, et al. Expression of the early onset torsion dystonia gene (DYT1) in the human brain. *Ann Neurol* 1998;43:669–673.
14. Augood SJ, Hollingsworth Z, Albers DS, et al. Dopamine transmission in DYT1 dystonia: a biochemical and autoradiographic study. *Neurology* 2002;59:445–448.
15. Schicatano EJ, Basso MA, Eringer C. Animal model explains the origin of the cranial dystonia benign essential blepharospasm. *J Neurophysiol* 1997;77:2842–2846.
16. Placzek MR, Misbahuddin A, Chaudhuri KR, et al. Cervical dystonia is associated with a polymorphism in the dopamine (D5) receptor gene. *J Neurol Neurosurg Psychiatry* 2001;71:262–264.
17. Misbahuddin A, Placzek MR, Chaudhuri KR, et al. A polymorphism in the dopamine receptor DRD5 is associated with Blepharospasm. *Neurology* 2002;58:124–126.
18. Le Couteur DG, Leighton PW, McCann SJ, et al. Association of a polymorphism in the dopamine-transporter gene with Parkinson's disease. *Mov Disord* 1997;12:760–763.
19. Cichon S, Nothen MM, Erdmann J, et al. Detection of four polymorphic sites in the human D1 receptor gene (DRD1). *Hum Mol Genet* 1994;3:209.
20. Hauge XY, Grandy DK, Eubanks JH, et al. Detection and characterisation of additional DNA polymorphisms in the dopamine D2 receptor. *Genomics* 1991;10:527–530.
21. Arinami T, Gao M, Hamaguchi H, et al. A functional polymorphism in the promoter region of the dopamine D2 receptor is associated with schizophrenia. *Hum Mol Genet* 1997;6:577–582
22. Lannfelt L, Sokoloff P, Martres MP, et al. Amino acid substitution in the dopamine D3 receptor as a useful polymorphism for investigating psychiatric disorders. *Psychiatr Genet* 1992;2:249–256.
23. Lichter JB, Barr C, Kennedy J, et al. A hypervariable segment in the human dopamine receptor D4 (DRD4) gene. *Hum Mol Genet* 1993;3:767–773.
24. Sherrington R, Mankoo B, Attwood J, et al. Cloning of the human dopamine D5 receptor gene and identification of a highly polymorphic microsatellite for the DRD5 locus that show tight linkage to the chromosome 4p reference marker RAF1P1. *Genomics* 1993;18:423–425.
25. Beischlag TV, Marchese A, Meador-Woodruff JH, et al. The human dopamine D5 receptor gene: cloning and characterisation of the 5'-flanking and promoter region. *Biochemistry* 1995;34:5960–5970.
26. Brancati F, Valente EM, Castori M, et al. Role of the dopamine D5 receptor (DRD5) as a susceptibility gene for cervical dystonia. *J Neurol Neurosurg Psych* 2003;74:665–666.

Dystonia 4: Advances in Neurology, Vol. 94. Edited by Stanley Fahn, Mark Hallett, and Mahlon R. DeLong. Lippincott Williams & Wilkins, Philadelphia © 2004.

21

Dystonia With and Without Deafness Is Caused by TIMM8A Mutation

Russell H. Swerdlow, Vern C. Juel, and G. Frederick Wooten

Department of Neurology, University of Virginia Health System, Charlottesville, Virginia

Mohr-Tranebjaerg syndrome (MTS) was initially described as an X-linked recessive deafness-dystonia of males. Phenotypic expression results from mutation of a gene that encodes a mitochondrial peptide import protein, the translocase of the inner mitochondrial membrane (TIMM8A) protein. It was recently shown that TIMM8A mutation also manifests as an X-dominant dystonia in females. This chapter reviews our knowledge of MTS, and discusses its broader implications for the dystonia field.

THE MOHR-TRANEBJAERG SYNDROME

Mohr and Mageroy (1) reported on a distinct form of genetic deafness in 1960. The disorder they described, later classified as DFN-1, was derived from a family in which males presented with early-life deafness in an X-linked recessive fashion. Lisbeth Tranebjaerg continued to study the original Norwegian kindred, and observed that in adolescence or young adulthood the affected males would also develop dystonia (2,3). Other phenotypically consistent families were also described (4,5). The extended phenotype subsequently became known as the Mohr-Tranebjaerg syndrome (MTS).

Although core clinical features appear universal, some degree of phenotypic heterogeneity does exist between the different MTS kindreds. For instance, deafness always develops prior to dystonia. However, the age at which deafness manifests can vary, as can the age at which dystonia does. In most kindreds, deafness develops shortly after boys attain language milestones (postlingual deafness), but onset of hearing loss can range from adolescence to before the development of any language skills. Dystonia can develop during childhood, adolescence, or young adulthood. In some kindreds, signs and symptoms are restricted to deafness and dystonia, while in others dementia, optic atrophy, cortical blindness, and behavioral/psychiatric changes are additional features that can appear years after the onset of dystonia (6). Spastic paraplegia can be seen. In some families death occurs in childhood, although affected subjects living into the seventh decade are also described. Neuropathologic descriptions are rare, but it may be the case that neuronal loss and gliosis of the caudate, putamen, and globus pallidus occur (4).

The search for the causative gene narrowed in 1995, when Xq21.3-Xq22 linkage was established (3). Mutations in a novel gene were soon identified in affected members of three different MTS kindreds (7). The investigators named this gene the dystonia/deafness peptide *(DDP)* gene. The mutations described in this report ranged from small deletions to deletion of the entire gene. Within the next several years, a limited number of other MTS kindreds were shown to have *DDP* gene mutations. In a case of molecular genetics leading to "lumping" rather than "splitting" of clinical syndromes, a related but differently named syndrome, the Jensen syndrome, was soon shown to also arise from *DDP* mutation (8,9).

The *DDP* nucleotide and amino acid sequences are shown in Fig. 21-1. In addition to the three kindreds described by Jin et al. (7) and the Jensen syndrome family (8), reports of *DDP* mutations now include a de novo transition mutation in a boy, a mutation in a Japanese kindred, and a single nucleotide deletion in a Virginia kindred (10–12). Table 21-1 catalogues the MTS mutations described to date.

1 *gcggagttcg tctctgcaag cttggtcgcc ctggg* atg gat tcc tcc tcc tct tcc tcc gcg gcg ggt ttg ggt gca gtg
                   5' UTR   M   D   S   S   S   S   S   A   A   G   L   G   A   V

81 gac cca cag ttg cag cat ttc atc gag gta gag act caa aag cag cgc ttc cag cag ctg gtg cac cag atg act
   D   P   Q   L   Q   H   F   I   E   V   E   T   Q   K   Q   R   F   Q   Q   L   V   H   Q   M   T

End of Exon 1 / Start of Exon 2

156 gaa ctt tgt tgg / gag aag tgc atg gac aag cct ggg cca aag ttg gac agt cgg gct gag gcc tgt ttt gtg aac
   E   L   C   W/   E   K   C   M   D   K   P   G   P   K   L   D   S   R   A   E   A   C   F   V   N

231 tgc gtt gag cgc ttc att gat aca agc cag ttc atc ttg aat cga ctg gaa cag acc cag aaa tcc aag cca gtt ttc
   C   V   E   R   F   I   D   T   S   Q   F   I   L   N   R   L   E   Q   T   Q   K   S   K   P   V   F

309 tca gaa agc ctt tct gac *tga tctcagcatt acctctttgg aaaaggaagg tagttcaaga aatgaagagc tgttgatggg*
   S   E   S   L   S   D stop   3' UTR

389 *atgattgaag aaacagctat gagaggattg gctcccatct tttgttactc ttgggacatc ctgtcatctg agaatgaaca aagaccaatt*

480 *ttttgtgtgt gaagcttaag ggtcatatgt ttgcttgtat tttttaatgct aatcttgtg aaaataattg acaggcgaaa gaaaactcta*

570 *tttagatgca tattactgta catgggacta tgcttttctc aaagcccccat taactgcttc ctataatttt gatagtgggga ccacatacgt*

660 *aaaaatctctc atttgtgtgg agtcatttct gatttcaggg gagatccttg tgtttatcag aaagggcag aagtaggggga agaataattt*

750 *ggtatcctta tctagtgttt gattgtcaat gctggagaaa aatatctgta agagtgttta tacagtacac ttcagttatc ttgatctccc*

840 *tttcctatat gatgatttgc ttaaatatcc atattaagta agtctcaagg tagggtaggc agcctgagag tctagaggcc tttagttata*

930 *aaggaatcta gccagtgaac ataattctta ttactagact gccacaagga agaaattaac ttaccctgta tatcagggta caaaaaattc*

1020 *agtgatgtgc ctaaataagt tataaagatt taggccaatc agaagctaac agcagtttca ggtagaggtg catgcctaat gttagttagt*

1110 *gtagattcca tttactgcat tcttctgatc actgaaataa aagctatata agattcata*

FIG. 21-1. *DDP1/TIMM8A.* Nucleotide and protein sequences. (Adapted from the National Center for Biotechnology Information and Jin H, May M, Tranebjaerg L, et al. A novel X-linked gene, DDP, shows mutations in families with deafness (DFN-1), dystonia, mental deficiency and blindness. *Nat Genet* 1996;14:177–180.)

TABLE 21-1. *DDP1/TIMM8A mutations causing Mohr-Tranebjaerg syndrome*

Total gene deletion
10-base pair (bp) deletion starting at nt 183 in exon 2
151 detT in exon 1
C233G transversion in exon 2
G105T transversion in exon 1
C273T transition in exon 2
108delG in exon 1

with accepted nomenclature, human *DDP* was also given the name *TIMM8A*. Additional investigations suggest a homologous form exists, so *TIMM8A* is sometimes referred to as *DDP1* (16). As indicated in Fig. 21-1, the *TIMM8A* gene contains two exons, which code for a 97 amino acid peptide.

AN MTS FAMILY WITH X-LINKED RECESSIVE DEAFNESS, X-LINKED DOMINANT DYSTONIA

We recently described a novel 108delG *TIMM8A* gene mutation in an MTS family (12). This mutation converts an exon 1 valine codon to a stop codon. As a consequence, translation of the 97 amino acid TIMM8A peptide terminates after just 24 amino acids. In this family this mutation is X-linked recessive for deafness, but X-linked dominant for dystonia. The family tree is shown in Fig. 21-2. The clin-

DDP1/TIMM8A

The *DDP* gene was subsequently shown to play a role in mitochondrial protein import (13,14). Mitochondrial protein import requires the coordination of two large protein families, the translocase of the inner mitochondrial membrane (TIMM) and translocase of the outer mitochondrial membrane (TOMM) protein groups (15). In yeast, the *DDP* homologue is Tim8p, and to conform

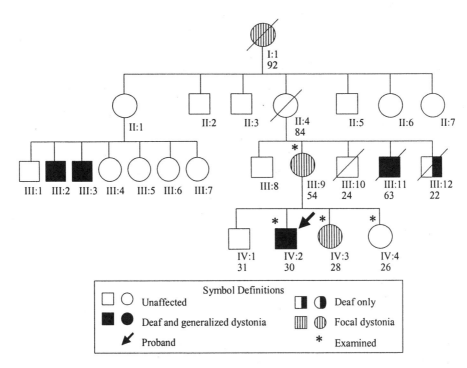

FIG. 21-2. Family tree of the Virginia Mohr-Tranebjaerg syndrome (MTS) pedigree. (Printed with permission from Wiley-Liss Inc.)

ical history of this family was previously published (12). For affected males, deafness was reportedly either present at birth or occurred within several years of birth.

The proband was noted to be deaf from very early in life, and never achieved language milestones. He did not develop dystonia until his third decade, which rapidly progressed to a generalized dystonia. He was referred to the University of Virginia Movement Disorders Clinic for the management of painful neck dystonias, which included both a head tilt and retrocollis components. Dystonic posturing of all four limbs was apparent, and dystonic movements of the lower extremities complicated his ability to ambulate. He had scoliosis, concave to the right. There was blepharospasm and facial grimacing. Rapid alternating movements were slow in both arms. He had brisk deep tendon reflexes but no pathologic reflexes. Electromyographic recordings from neck muscles using needle electrodes demonstrated coactivation of agonist-antagonist muscle pairs and an asynchronous, irregular, 4- to 6-Hz tremor involving several neck muscles. Magnetic resonance imaging of the brain was normal.

Several other male family members also developed early-onset deafness followed by dystonia later in life. One uncle of the proband was deaf but died in his early 20s, presumably before the onset of dystonia. Another deaf uncle lived until his seventh decade, developed dystonia in young adulthood, and became blind and demented during the decade prior to his death.

Interestingly, although female members of this kindred do not develop deafness or noticeable hearing loss, a number of them have developed focal dystonia syndromes. The mother of the proband has experienced oromandibular dystonias, blepharospasm, and torticollis since her third decade. In her 20s she also developed a writer's cramp, began suffering chronic neck muscle pain, and reported head shaking. Other manifestations of dystonia were absent. A sister of the proband has also suffered with writer's cramp since late in her second decade, and has a back-and-

forth head shake that results from dystonic posturing of the neck musculature. These head movements occur as "bursts," are irregular in rhythm and intensity, and the bursts differ in magnitude. Her sternocleidomastoid muscles are bilaterally hypertrophied and she occasionally shows head deviation to the right. Representations of these dystonias are shown in Fig. 21-3. Despite the more subtle clinical manifestations of dystonia in the female carriers, electromyographic recordings from neck muscles in the proband's mother and affected sister also exhibited coactivation of agonist-antagonist muscle pairs and an asynchronous, irregular, 4- to 6-Hz tremor.

The mother and symptomatic sister of the proband were genotyped for 108delG, and are carriers for the mutation (the other allele is normal). Neither of these heterozygotes complain of decreased hearing. The proband's asymptomatic sister was genotyped and has two wild-type alleles. The affected family members we have studied show variable responses to traditional treatments for dystonia, including anticholinergics, benzodiazepines, and injections of botulinum toxin.

Two distant male cousins of the proband also manifested a deafness/dystonia phenotype. Deafness manifested early in life, and dystonia developed during young adulthood. The common relative for the proband and these cousins is the proband's maternal great-grandmother, suggesting she was a carrier of the TIMM8A 108delG mutation. This great-grandmother reportedly suffered from a head shake similar to that of the proband's sister. The clinical features of this kindred are summarized in Table 21-2.

It is unclear why dystonia in this family presents in an X-dominant fashion. Several hypotheses are possible. It may result as a specific consequence of the particular abnormal protein structure. The mutation may affect patterns of X-chromosome inactivation, a concept that has some experimental support (17). Alternatively, there may be some secondary genetic feature that is unique to this family, such as the concomitant presence of mitochondrial DNA (mtDNA) mutation.

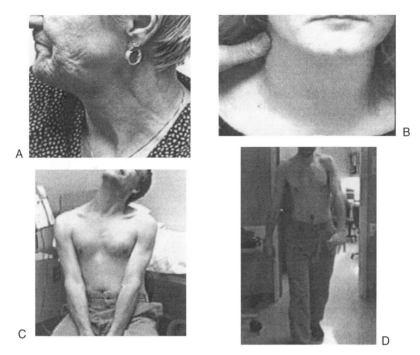

FIG. 21-3. Dystonia in the Virginia kindred Mohr-Tranebjaerg syndrome (MTS) proband, his mother, and his symptomatic sister. The mother and sister are carriers of the 108delG mutation. **A:** Head turning, oromandibular dystonia, and platysma contracture in the mother. **B:** Sternocleidomastoid hypertrophy in the sister. **C:** Proband with head tilt to the left, retrocollis with left ear down, and deviation to the right. **D:** Proband walking, with evidence of left upper extremity dystonic posturing.

TABLE 21-2. *Clinical features and age of symptom onset for affected family members*

Subject	Symptom(s)	Age of onset	Comments
I:1	Head shaking	?	—
III:2	Deafness	?	—
	Generalized dystonia	Twenties	
III:3	Deafness	?	—
	Generalized dystonia	Twenties	
III:9	Head shaking	~Age 25	—
	Torticollis	~Age 25	
	Writer's cramp	~Age 25	
III:11	Deafness	Congenital?	Died at age 63
	Generalized dystonia	Late twenties	Different father than III:9
	Blindness	Early fifties	
	Dementia	Late fifties	
III:12	Deafness	Congenital?	Died at age 22 (suicide)
			Different father than III:9
IV:2	Deafness	Congenital?	Proband
	Generalized dystonia	Age 28	
IV:3	Head shaking	Late teens	—
	Torticollis	Mid twenties	
	Writer's cramp	Mid twenties	

Studies to evaluate these possibilities are planned.

MITOCHONDRIAL MEMBRANE TRANSLOCASES AND MITOCHONDRIAL PROTEIN IMPORT

Mitochondria are dual-membrane structures. This allows one to define four anatomic regions for the organelle. From outermost to innermost, they are the (a) outer membrane, (b) intermembrane space, (c) inner membrane, and (d) matrix.

Mitochondria are protein-rich. All but 13 of the hundreds (thousands by some estimates) of mitochondrial peptides are encoded by nuclear genes and translated in the cytoplasm (15). Proteins destined for mitochondria typically contain a target sequence (18). Some can traverse mitochondrial membranes without assistance, but most require the services of an intricate import apparatus (19,20). One part consists of a multimeric complex that facilitates transport across the outer mitochondrial membrane. This is called the translocase of the outer membrane (TOM) complex. What additional import services are utilized next depends on whether the peptide is destined for insertion in the inner membrane or complete translocation into the matrix. A protein requiring inner membrane insertion is assisted by the translocase of the inner membrane 22 (TIM22) complex. Matrix-seeking proteins use a separate complex, the translocase of the inner membrane 23 (TIM23) complex.

In yeast, two proteins form a complex in the intermembrane space that assists TIM22 in the insertion of inner membrane proteins. These two proteins are Tim8p and Tim13. The Tim8p-Tim13 complex is not obligate for proper execution of TIM22-mediated inner membrane protein insertion. However, under conditions of reduced mitochondrial membrane potential ($\Delta\Psi$), Tim8p-Tim13 function becomes essential (19).

The human homologue of yeast Tim8p is TIMM8A (13,14). It appears that humans are more dependent on TIMM8A-TIM13 function than yeast is for the corresponding complex (20). In MTS, *TIMM8A* mutation causes dysfunction of TIMM8A-TIM13 (21). This impairs the ability of TIM22 to direct TIM23 proteins into the inner membrane. TIM23 dysfunction ensues, which adversely affects translocation of proteins into the mitochondrial matrix (21,22).

Surprisingly little is known about intrinsic mitochondrial function in MTS. One group did evaluate ETC (electron transport chain) complexes, mitochondrial morphology, and mitochondrial membrane potential ($\Delta\Psi$) in fibroblasts with the C66W (C233G) *TIMM8A* mutation (22). Results were reportedly unremarkable, although the specific data were not shown.

MITOCHONDRIA IN DEAFNESS AND DYSTONIA

Mitochondria contribute to particular types of both syndromic and nonsyndromic deafness. In these instances, hearing loss has a sensorineural basis (23). How mitochondrial pathophysiology drives deafness is not entirely clear. Some propose reduced adenosine triphosphate (ATP) production by mitochondria renders metabolically active hair and stria vascularis cells unable to maintain inner ear ion homeostasis (24). This presumably could impair detection and transmission of sound waves.

An epidemiologic pattern of maternally inherited hearing loss (MIHL) is recognized. Such cases are frequently associated with mtDNA mutation. Some mtDNA mutations are associated with nonsyndromic deafness, but more often they are associated with syndromic forms (24).

An mtDNA *A1555G* mutation in the 12S RNA gene can cause nonsyndromic deafness (25). In some MIHL kindreds, hearing loss deriving from this mutation occurs spontaneously. Most frequently, however, hearing loss arises only after exposure to an aminoglycoside antibiotic. Aminoglycoside-induced deafness in persons with the *A1555G* mutation is currently a quintessential example of how gene–environment interactions can effect human phenotype expression.

A role for mitochondrially relevant nuclear gene mutations in human hearing loss was previously proposed (23). Identification of *TIMM8A* mutation in MTS provides proof of principle for this concept. Various candidate nuclear genes that may determine deafness via mitochondrial dysfunction are under investigation.

Data indicate mitochondrial dysfunction occurs in dystonia (26). Complex I activity is reduced in platelets from persons with dystonia (27,28). In addition to *TIMM8A* mutation in the MTS, certain mtDNA mutations are associated with dystonia *(G3460A, G14459A)* (26,29–31). Although a pathogenic role for mitochondrial dysfunction in some forms of dystonia seems possible (since mtDNA mutation can apparently be deterministic), how pathophysiologically relevant mitochondrial dysfunction is in the majority of those with dystonia is unknown. How mitochondrial dysfunction arises in cases where no obvious mtDNA mutation is found also remains to be seen. Nevertheless, the presence of complex I dysfunction in a nontarget tissue of persons with dystonia (platelets) suggests the defect is not an inconsequential epiphenomenon of a more basic pathology. The ability of *TIMM8A* mutation to cause dystonia further emphasizes this concept.

CONCLUSION

Specific mtDNA mutations are already accepted as primary causes of both deafness and dystonia. The finding of *TIMM8A* gene mutation as the apparent cause of deafness and dystonia in MTS emphasizes the relevance of mitochondria to disorders of sensorineural hearing and movement, and especially to dystonia.

REFERENCES

1. Mohr J, Mageroy K. Sex-linked deafness of a possibly new type. *Acta Genet Statist Med* 1960;10:54–62.
2. Tranebjaerg L, Schwartz C, Huggins K, et al. X-linked recessive mental retardation with progressive sensorineural deafness, blindness, spastic paraplegia, and dystonia. *Am J Hum Genet* 1992;51:A47.
3. Tranebjaerg L, Schwartz C, Eriksen H, et al. A new X linked recessive deafness syndrome with blindness, dystonia, fractures, and mental deficiency is linked to Xq22. *J Med Genet* 1995;32:257–263.
4. Scribanu N, Kennedy C. Familial syndrome with dystonia, neural deafness, and possible intellectual impairment: clinical course and pathological findings. *Adv Neurol* 1976;14:235–243.
5. Hayes MW, Ouvrier RA, Evans W, et al. X-linked dystonia deafness syndrome. *Mov Disord* 1998;13: 303–308.
6. Tranebjaerg L, Jensen KA, van Ghelue M. X-linked recessive deafness-dystonia syndrome (Mohr-Tranebjaerg syndrome). In: Kitamura K, Steel KP, eds. *Genetics in otorhinolaryngology. Advances in Otorhinolaryngology,* vol 56. Basel: Karger, 2000:176–180.
7. Jin H, May M, Tranebjaerg L, et al. A novel X-linked gene, DDP, shows mutations in families with deafness (DFN-1), dystonia, mental deficiency and blindness. *Nat Genet* 1996;14:177–180.
8. Tranebjaerg L, Schwarz C, Huggins K, et al. Jensen syndrome is allelic to Mohr-Tranebjaerg syndrome and both are caused by stop mutations in the DDP gene. *Am J Hum Genet* 1997;51(suppl):A349.
9. Lubs H, Chiurazzi J, Arena J, et al. XLMR genes: update 1998. *Am J Med Genet* 1999;83:237–247.
10. Tranebjaerg L, Hamel BCJ, Gabreels FJM, et al. A de novo missense mutation in a critical domain of the X-linked DDP gene causes the typical deafness-dystonia-optic atrophy syndrome. *Eur J Hum Genet* 2000;8: 464–467.
11. Ujike H, Tanabe Y, Takehisa Y, et al. A family with X-linked dystonia-deafness syndrome with a novel mutation of the DDP gene. *Arch Neurol* 2001;58:1004–1007.
12. Swerdlow RH, Wooten GF. A novel deafness/dystonia peptide gene mutation that causes dystonia in female carriers of Mohr-Tranebjaerg syndrome. *Ann Neurol* 2001;50:537–540.
13. Koehler CM, Leuenberger D, Merchant S, et al. Human deafness dystonia syndrome is a mitochondrial disease. *Proc Natl Acad Sci USA* 1999;96:2141–2146.
14. Jin H, Kendall E, Freeman TC, et al. The human family of deafness/dystonia peptide (DDP) related mitochondrial import proteins. *Genomics* 1999;61:259–267.
15. Neupert W. Protein import into mitochondria. *Annu Rev Biochem* 1997;66:863–917.
16. Rothbauer U, Hofmann S, Muhlenbein N, et al. Role of the deafness dystonia peptide 1 (DDP1) in import of human Tim23 into the inner membrane of mitochondria. *J Biol Chem* 2001;276:37327–37334.
17. Plenge RM, Tranebjaerg L, Jensen KA, et al. Evidence that mutations in the X-linked DDP gene cause incompletely penetrant and variable skewed X inactivation. *Am J Hum Genet* 1999;64:759–767.
18. Pfanner N. Protein sorting: recognizing mitochondrial presequences. *Curr Biol* 2000;10:R412–415.
19. Paschen SA, Neupert W. Protein import into mitochondria. *IUBMB Life* 2001;52:101–112.
20. Bauer MF, Neupert W. Import of proteins into mitochondria: A novel pathomechanism for progressive neurodegeneration. *J Inherit Metab Dis* 2001;24:166–180.
21. Roesch K, Curran SP, Tranebjaerg L, et al. Human deafness dystonia syndrome is caused by a defect in assembly of the DDP1/TIMM8a-TIMM13 complex. *Hum Mol Genet* 2002;11:477–486.
22. Hofmann S, Rothbauer U, Muhlenbein N, et al. The

C66W mutation in the deafness dystonia peptide 1 (DDP1) affects the formation of functional DDP1.TIM13 complexes in the mitochondrial inter-membrane space. *J Biol Chem* 2002;277: 23287–23293.

23. Jacobs HT. Mitochondrial deafness. *Ann Med* 1997;29: 483–491.

24. Hutchin TP, Cortopassi GA. Mitochondrial defects and hearing loss. *Cell Mol Life Sci* 2000;57:1927–1937.

25. Prezant TR, Agapian JV, Bohlman MC, et al. Mitochondrial ribosomal RNA mutation associated with both antibiotic-induced and non-syndromic deafness. *Nat Genet* 1993;4:289–294.

26. Wallace DC, Murdock DG. Mitochondria and dystonia: The movement disorder connection? *Proc Natl Acad Sci USA* 1999;96:1817–1819.

27. Benecke R, Strumper P, Weiss H. Electron transfer com-plex I defect in idiopathic dystonia. *Ann Neurol* 1992; 32:683–686.

28. Schapira AH, Warner T, Gash MT, et al. Complex I function in familial and sporadic dystonia. *Ann Neurol* 1997;41:556–559.

29. Novotny EJ Jr, Singh G, Wallace DC, et al. Leber's disease and dystonia: a mitochondrial disease. *Neurology* 1986;36:1053–1060.

30. Jun AS, Brown MD, Wallace DC. A mitochondrial DNA mutation at nucleotide pair 14459 of the NADH dehydrogenase subunit 6 gene associated with maternally inherited Leber hereditary optic neuropathy and dystonia. *Proc Natl Acad Sci USA* 1994;91:6206–6210.

31. Thobois S, Vighetto A, Grochowicki M, et al. Leber "plus" disease: optic neuropathy, parkinsonian syndrome and supranuclear ophthalmoplegia. *Rev Neurol* 1997;153:595–598.

Dystonia 4: Advances in Neurology, Vol. 94. Edited by Stanley Fahn, Mark Hallett, and Mahlon R. DeLong. Lippincott Williams & Wilkins, Philadelphia © 2004.

22

Abnormal Brain Networks in Primary Torsion Dystonia

*Maren Carbon, †Maja Trošt, ‡Maria Felice Ghilardi, and §David Eidelberg

°*Center for Neurosciences, North Shore–Long Island Jewish Research Institute, Manhasset, New York. †Center for Neurosciences, North Shore–Long Island Jewish Research Institute, Manhasset, New York; and Department of Neurology, Division of Neurology, University Medical Centre Ljubljana, Ljubljana, Slovenia. ‡Center for Neurobiology and Behavior, Columbia College of Physicians and Surgeons, New York, New York; and INB-CNR, Milano, Italy. §Center for Neurosciences, North Shore–Long Island Jewish Research Institute, Manhasset, New York; Department of Neurology, North Shore University Hospital, Manhasset, New York; and New York University School of Medicine, New York, New York*

Primary torsion dystonia is associated with a number of genetic variants. The most frequent patient subgroup consists of the autosomal-dominant *DYT1* mutation on chromosome 9q34 that leads to a GAG deletion within the coding area for torsinA (1). This deletion, however, causes clinical manifestations of dystonia in only 30% of mutation carriers (2). The function of torsinA is currently unclear. Its classification within the AAA+ family of adenosine triphosphatases (ATPases) suggests a chaperone role in vesicle fusion, membrane trafficking, protein folding, and/or cytoskeletal dynamics (3), and its strong expression in neuronal processes may indicate a role in synaptic function (4). However, to date the pathophysiologic link between torsinA and disease manifestation remains unknown.

This chapter reviews our studies on the relationship between *DYT1* carrier status and regional brain function, focusing on clinically nonmanifesting subjects. We describe abnormalities in regional brain organization in the resting state and discuss the impact of these changes on regional activation responses during motor execution and learning. Additionally, we present preliminary data on dopamine D_2 neuroreceptor binding in gene carriers and dis-

cuss the potential relevance of these findings to the pathophysiology of the primary dystonias.

ABNORMAL RESTING STATE METABOLISM IN *DYT1* CARRIERS

Patients with primary dystonia lack specific histopathologic changes (5–7). Similarly, many functional imaging studies in dystonia patients have yielded conflicting results (8). Nonetheless, we have used a novel regional network analytical approach (9) to identify a reproducible pattern of abnormal regional glucose utilization in two independent cohorts of clinically nonmanifesting *DYT1* carriers (10,11). We found that these subjects express a specific metabolic topography characterized by increases in the posterior putamen/globus pallidus, cerebellum, and supplementary motor area (SMA) (Fig. 22-1A; see ref. 11). In an ancillary study, we demonstrated that this abnormal torsion dystonia–related pattern (TDRP) was also present in clinically affected patients, persisting even following the suppression of involuntary dystonic movements by sleep induction (10,12). Moreover, TDRP expression is not specific for the *DYT1* genotype. We have re-

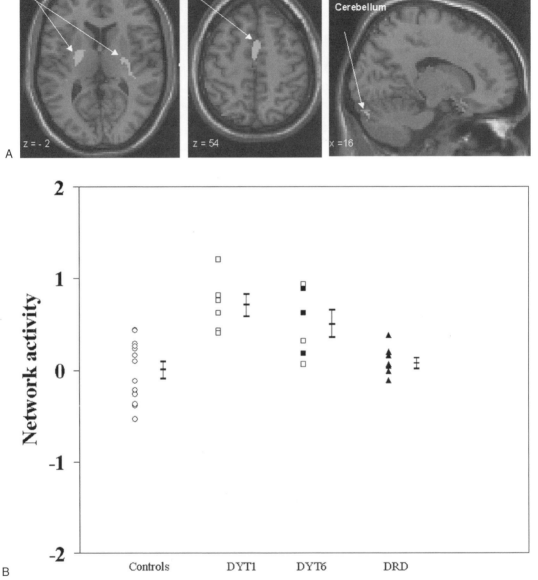

FIG. 22-1. A: Regional metabolic covariance pattern identified with fluorodeoxyglucose positron emission tomography (FDG-PET) and network analysis in nonmanifesting *DYT1* gene carriers and control subjects (see text). This torsion dystonia–related pattern (TDRP) was characterized by bilateral covarying metabolic increases in the putamen, extending into the globus pallidus (GP), the supplementary motor area (SMA), and the cerebellar hemisphere. Subject scores for this pattern discriminated the *DYT1* carriers from controls (p <.002). [The display represents voxels that contribute significantly to the network at p = .001. Voxels with positive region weights (metabolic increases) are in light grey]. **B:** Scatter diagram of TDRP subject scores computed prospectively in six new nonaffected *DYT1* gene carriers, six *DYT6* gene carriers, seven dopa-responsive dystonia (DRD) patients, and 13 control subjects. Subject scores were abnormally elevated in *DYT1* (p <.001) and *DYT6* carriers (p <.007), but not in DRD patients (p = .4). (The error bars indicate subgroup standard errors of the mean. *Circles* represent normal controls; *squares* represent subjects with genotypes associated with primary torsion dystonia; *triangles* represent DRD patients. *Open symbols* represent clinically nonmanifesting subjects; *filled symbols* represent affected dystonia patients).

cently demonstrated abnormal network activity in both manifesting and nonmanifesting carriers of the *DYT6* dystonia mutation (North American Mennonites) (Fig. 22–1B; see ref. 11). These findings suggest that TDRP expression is a feature of certain primary dystonia genotypes and is not linked to clinical phenotype. In all likelihood, this resting pattern represents a metabolic trait of dystonia. The use of positron emission tomography (PET) to quantify TDRP expression in individual family members may be valuable for gene identification in selected kindreds.

ABNORMAL BRAIN–BEHAVIOR RELATIONSHIPS IN *DYT1* CARRIERS

The presence of an abnormal resting metabolic topography in nonmanifesting gene carriers may affect the functional activity of key nodes of the motor cortico-striato-pallido-thalamo-cortical (CSPTC) loops and related cerebellar pathways (13,14). We explored the possibility that subtle behavioral changes may exist as a metabolic correlate of TDRP activity in gene-positive individuals. The basal ganglia have been shown to mediate specific aspects of motor learning, especially the process of combining individual movements into sequences (e.g., 15). We therefore selected motor sequence learning as a behavioral paradigm to study brain–performance relationships in *DYT1* carriers (16). We studied 12 nonmanifesting *DYT1* carriers and 12 healthy age-matched controls and measured psychophysical performance indices during the execution of simple movements in both timed-response and reaction time paradigms, as well as during a sequence learning task (17–19). To assess brain activation responses during task performance, we concurrently scanned seven members of each group with ^{15}O-water (H_2^{15}O) and PET.

In these tasks subjects performed paced reaching movements from a central starting point to one of eight radial targets with their dominant right hand. In the simple motor execution task (CCN), the eight targets appeared in a predictable counterclockwise order at 1 Hz. (During imaging, this task was used as a kinematically equivalent reference condition

for the motor sequence learning task). In the motor sequence learning task, the eight targets appeared in an unknown repeating order over the 90-second trial block. Subjects were instructed to learn the sequence order while reaching for the targets, to anticipate successive targets, and to reach each target in synchrony with the tone. Additionally, each subject performed a reaction time task (RAN) outside the scanner to determine the reaction time floor as a criterion for target anticipation in the sequence learning task (18,20). Lastly, subjects performed a visuospatial transformation task utilizing the same target array and rotational displacements to exclude deficits in adaptation to spatial transformation (17,21).

Movement characteristics, including spatial error, directional errors, movement time, and onset time, were quantified in all tasks (17,22). For the sequence learning task, we additionally computed the number of correct movements initiated before the floor onset time in the reaction time task. These movements reflect anticipation and successful retrieval of previously acquired targets, and represented the major descriptor of learning performance in our studies (18,20). *DYT1* carriers performed the motor execution tasks in both the timed-response and reaction time mode without significant differences from controls (Fig. 22-2A). Specifically, movement initiation and movement time during motor execution was normal in *DYT1* carriers, as were mean reaction times and floor reaction times. Thus, in contrast to clinically affected dystonia patients (23), motor preparation did not appear to be impaired in nonmanifesting *DYT1* carriers.

In contrast to the execution of simple movements, a significant defect in motor sequence learning was present in *DYT1* carriers (Fig. 22-2B). By the end of the learning task, most gene carriers correctly anticipated the appearance of three targets, compared to an average of six targets in controls ($p < .007$). By contrast, adaptation to visuospatial rotation, an implicit form of motor learning, was normal in the *DYT1* carriers. These findings demonstrate that nonmanifesting *DYT1* carriers exhibit specific defects in the explicit learning of sequential informa-

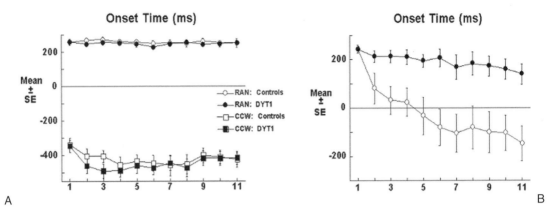

FIG. 22-2. A: Mean onset times during the execution of an internally generated timed-response motor task *(squares)* and in a kinematically identical reaction time task *(circles).* Mean onset time values (msec) in each cycle of eight movements are presented for both nonmanifesting *DYT1* carriers *(filled symbols)* and for age-matched control subjects *(open symbols).* The two groups did not differ with respect to onset time or other kinematic parameters during either task (bars indicate standard error). **B:** Mean onset times during motor sequence learning in nonmanifesting *DYT1* carriers *(filled circles)* and controls *(open circles).* Values are plotted as a function of cycles (see text). Both variables declined over time, indicating target prediction and learning (18). Learning performance in the 90-second epoch was significantly lower in the *DYT1* cohort (*p* <.001).

tion but not in movement preparation or in the learning of visuospatial transformations.

PET recordings during task performance demonstrated significant group differences in regional brain activation responses. Nonmanifesting *DYT1* carriers displayed comparative increases in SMA activation during motor execution, despite normal movement characteristics. By contrast, motor activation responses were reduced in the posterior-medial cerebellum of nonmanifesting *DYT1* carriers, perhaps as a consequence of deposition of mutant torsinA protein in this region (4,24). Given the comparatively normal motor performance of these subjects, it is possible that the changes in local activation responses represent an effective means of compensating for impaired resting metabolic dysfunction within key nodes of the major motor pathways.

While neural resources within the motor CSPTC loops may compensate for baseline metabolic dysfunction in *DYT1* carriers performing simple movements, this may not be the case for sequences of movements. During sequence learning, *DYT1* carriers showed significantly greater activation than controls in the right pre-SMA and posterior parietal cortex,

the right anterior cerebellum, and the left prefrontal cortex. Nonetheless, this overactivation did not result in normal learning performance. These PET findings are limited to mean differences between the two groups and do not relate these changes to the behavioral abnormalities that were detected in the *DYT1* carriers.

To examine the nature of these brain–behavior relationships, we first determined whether a previously validated learning network in normal subjects accurately predicted performance in *DYT1* carriers. In earlier sequence learning studies (18), we found that a specific covariance pattern, characterized mainly by caudate, prefrontal, and posterior parietal activation, accurately correlated with the learning achieved during imaging in both healthy volunteers and in patients with Parkinson's disease (PD). While reproducible in these populations (19), this learning network failed to predict performance in the *DYT1* carrier group. To determine whether a different network mediated sequence learning in these subjects, we performed an exploratory analysis restricted only to the *DYT1* carriers (25) and detected a novel pattern that correlated with learning in this cohort (Fig. 22-3). Indeed, this candidate topography incorpo-

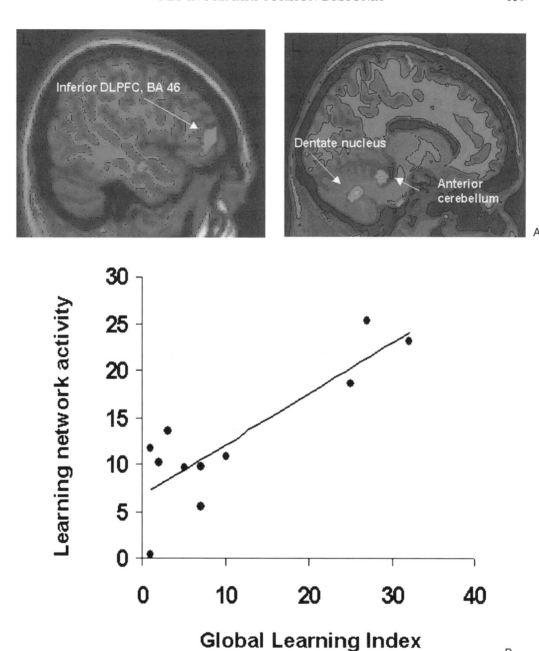

FIG. 22-3. Voxel-based network analysis of $H_2{}^{15}O$/positron emission tomography (PET) data from seven nonmanifesting *DYT1* carriers scanned during motor sequence learning: retrieval pattern. **A:** This network topography was characterized by covarying learning-related activations *(arrows)* in the cerebellum and dentate nucleus *(left)*, and in the inferior dorsolateral prefrontal cortex (DLPFC) *(right)*. [Positive region weights *(light grey)* were thresholded at $Z = +2$ to display clusters contributing significantly ($p < .01$) to the network (see text)]. **B:** Subject scores for this topography, representing network activity in individual gene carriers, correlated with the learning that was achieved concurrently during the scanning epoch ($R^2 = 0.72$, $p < .001$).

rated several regions not used by control subjects, such as the cerebellar cortex and dentate nucleus, as well as the ventral prefrontal cortex. Interestingly, the caudate nucleus contributed significantly to the learning network in normals (18,19), but not to that identified in *DYT1* carriers.

These findings suggest that sequence learning in *DYT1* carriers is not mediated by the activation network utilized by normal cohorts or by patients with later-onset conditions such as parkinsonism. The presence of a different learning network in nonmanifesting gene carriers raises the possibility of functional reorganization of frontostriatal pathways in these subjects, perhaps on a genetic/developmental basis. Indeed, a shift from striatal to cerebellar processing may be a feature of the *DYT1* carrier state. The status of network–performance relationships in clinically affected *DYT1* patients and potential changes in these relationships with treatment (26) is a topic of ongoing investigation.

DOPAMINE RECEPTOR BINDING

Decreased D_2 receptor availability has been suggested as a possible mechanism of striatal dysfunction in primary dystonia (27). In our cohort of nonmanifesting *DYT1* gene carriers, ^{11}C-raclopride binding was significantly reduced in both the putamen and caudate (18% and 12% of control values, respectively). These reductions are somewhat lower than the 29% mean reduction in D_2 receptor binding measured in focal dystonia (27). Although preliminary, these data suggest that a subthreshold reduction in D_2 receptor availability may be needed for the development of clinical manifestations of *DYT1* carriers. Furthermore, there may be a link between dopaminergic neurotransmission in the caudate nucleus to deficits in sequence learning in the nonmanifesting *DYT1* carriers. In ancillary studies, we have detected correlations between dorsolateral prefrontal cortex (DLPFC) activation and caudate dopaminergic functioning in normal volunteers, early-stage PD patients (26), and in preclinical carriers of the

Huntington disease mutation. It is not known whether comparable relationships exist in primary dystonia.

The identification of abnormal brain networks in dystonia has several practical implications. As mentioned above, the resting TDRP metabolic network can potentially be used as a marker in linkage studies to identify potential gene carriers among family members of dystonia patients. Additionally, disease-related networks can prove useful for assessing mechanisms of therapeutic interventions, as has been demonstrated in PD (28,29). A combined network–performance approach may be especially relevant in characterizing the effects of treatment on higher order motor functioning (14,19).

ACKNOWLEDGMENTS

This work was supported by the National Institutes of Health (NIH) grant RO1 NS 37564 and the Dystonia Medical Research Foundation. Dr. Ghilardi and Dr. Eidelberg were supported by NIH grants KO8 NS 01961 and NIH K24 NS 02101, respectively. The authors wish to thank Dr. Thomas Chaly for radiochemistry support, and Christine Edwards and Sherwin Su for editorial assistance. Special thanks to Dr. Silvestri for the analysis of behavioral data. We acknowledge the valuable technical support provided by Dr. Abdel Belakhleff and Claude Margouleff.

REFERENCES

1. Ozelius LJ, Hewett JW, Page CE, et al. The early-onset torsion dystonia gene (*DYT1*) encodes an ATP-binding protein. *Nat Genet* 1997;17(1):40–48.
2. Bressman SB, deLeon D, Kramer PL, et al. Dystonia in Ashkenazic Jews: clinical characterization of a founder mutation. *Ann Neurol* 1994;36(5):771–777.
3. Breakefield XO, Kamm C, Hanson PI. TorsinA: movement at many levels. *Neuron* 2001;31(1):9–12.
4. Konakova M, Huynh DP, Yong W, et al. Cellular distribution of torsin A and torsin B in normal human brain. *Arch Neurol* 2001;58(6):921–927.
5. Zeman W. Pathology of the torsion dystonias (dystonia musculorum deformans). *Neurology* 1970;20(11):79–88.
6. Zweig RM, Hedreen JC, Jankel WR, et al. Pathology in brainstem regions of individuals with primary dystonia. *Neurology* 1988;38(5):702–706.
7. Walker R, Brin M, Sandu D, et al. TorsinA immunore-

activity in brains of patients with *DYT1* and non-*DYT1* dystonia. *Neurology* 2002;58(1):120–124.

8. Ceballos-Baumann AO, Brooks DJ. Activation positron emission tomography scanning in dystonia. *Adv Neurol* 1998;78:135–152.

9. Eidelberg D, Moeller JR, Ishikawa T, et al. The metabolic topography of idiopathic torsion dystonia. *Brain* 1995;118(pt 6):1473–1484.

10. Eidelberg D, Moeller JR, Antonini A, et al. Functional brain networks in *DYT1* dystonia. *Ann Neurol* 1998;44(3):303–312.

11. Trŏst M, Carbon M, Edwards C, et al. Primary dystonia: is abnormal functional brain architecture linked to genotype? *Ann Neurol* 2002;52(6):853–856.

12. Hutchinson M, Nakamura T, Moeller JR, et al. The metabolic topography of essential blepharospasm: a focal dystonia with general implications. *Neurology* 2000;55(5):673–677.

13. Wichmann T, DeLong MR. Functional and pathophysiological models of the basal ganglia. *Curr Opin Neurobiol* 1996;6(6):751–758.

14. Carbon M, Eidelberg D. Modulation of regional brain function by deep brain stimulation: studies with positron emission tomography. *Curr Opin Neurol* 2002;15(4):451–455.

15. Soliveri P, Brown RG, Jahanshahi M, et al. Learning manual pursuit tracking skills in patients with Parkinson's disease. *Brain* 1997;120(8):1325–1337.

16. Ghilardi MF, Ghez C, Eidelberg D. Visuospatial learning may be impaired in non-manifesting carriers of the *DYT1* mutation. *Neurology* 1999;52(6):A516.

17. Ghilardi MF, Ghez CP, Moeller JR, et al. Patterns of regional brain activation associated with different aspects of motor learning. *Brain Res* 2000;871(1):127–145.

18. Nakamura T, Ghilardi MF, Mentis M, et al. Functional networks in motor sequence learning: abnormal topographies in Parkinson's disease. *Hum Brain Mapp* 2001;12(1):42–60.

19. Carbon M, Ghilardi MF, Feigin A, et al. Learning networks in health and Parkinson's disease: reproducibility and treatment effects. *Hum Brain Mapp* 2003;19(3):197–211.

20. Fukuda M, Ghilardi MF, Carbon M, et al. Pallidal stimulation for parkinsonism: improved brain activation during sequence learning. *Ann Neurol* 2002;52(2):144–152.

21. Krakauer JW, Ghilardi MF, Ghez C. Independent learning of internal models for kinematic and dynamic control of reaching. *Nat Neurosci* 1999;2(11):1026–1031.

22. Fukuda M, Ghilardi MF, Mentis MJ, et al. Functional correlates of pallidal stimulation for Parkinson's disease. *Ann Neurol* 2001;124(8):1601–1609.

23. Jahanshahi M, Rowe J, Fuller R. Impairment of movement initiation and execution but not preparation in idiopathic dystonia. *Exp Brain Res* 2001;140(4):460–468.

24. Augood SJ, Martin DM, Ozelius LJ, et al. Distribution of the mRNAs encoding torsinA and torsinB in the normal adult human brain. *Ann Neurol* 2000;46(5):761–769.

25. Carbon M, Ghilardi MF, Dhawan V, et al. Brain networks subserving motor sequence learning in *DYT1* gene carriers. *Neurology* 2002;58(7):A203.

26. Carbon M, Ghilardi MF, Ma Y, et al. Target acquisition in motor sequence learning correlates with caudate dopamine transporter density in early Parkinson's disease. *Mov Disord* 2002;17(5):S181.

27. Perlmutter JS, Stambuk MK, Markham J, et al. Decreased (18F) spiperone binding in putamen in idiopathic focal dystonia. *J Neurosci* 1997;17(2):843–850.

28. Fukuda M, Mentis MJ, Ma Y, et al. Networks mediating the clinical effects of pallidal brain stimulation for Parkinson's disease: a PET study of resting-state glucose metabolism. *Brain* 2001;124(8):1601–1609.

29. Feigin A, Ghilardi MF, Fukuda M, et al. Effects of levodopa on motor activation responses in Parkinson's disease. *Neurology* 2002;59:220–226.

Dystonia 4: Advances in Neurology, Vol. 94. Edited by Stanley Fahn, Mark Hallett, and Mahlon R. DeLong. Lippincott Williams & Wilkins, Philadelphia © 2004.

23

Dysfunction of Dopaminergic Pathways in Dystonia

*Joel S. Perlmutter and †Jonathan W. Mink

*Departments of Neurology, Radiology, and Anatomy and Neurobiology, Washington University School of Medicine, St. Louis, Missouri. †Departments of Neurology, Neurobiology, and Pediatrics, University of Rochester School of Medicine; and Department of Child Neurology, Golisano Children's Hospital, Rochester, New York

Multiple investigations, including neuroimaging studies, indicate that dysfunction of dopaminergic pathways contributes to the pathophysiology of dystonia. Early structural imaging studies helped identify the lenticular nuclei and other brain regions as sites of pathology in secondary dystonias. Later, imaging studies with positron emission tomography (PET) and functional magnetic resonance imaging demonstrated dysfunction in the putamen and cortical-basal ganglia circuits including specific abnormalities of dopaminergic pathways. These findings fit well with recent observations of reduced cortical inhibition in people with dystonia.

ANATOMY AND STRUCTURAL IMAGING

Many investigators have used computed tomography (CT) or magnetic resonance imaging (MRI) to correlate the site of an identifiable brain lesion with the development of secondary dystonia. Since most of the sites involve the basal ganglia or its connections, we will briefly review the anatomy of the basal ganglia (Fig. 23-1). The basal ganglia have two major pathways leading from the putamen to the globus pallidus internal (GPi) segment, the major output nucleus of the basal ganglia for limb movement: (a) a "direct" inhibitory pathway from the putamen to the GPi; and (b) an "indirect" net excitatory pathway consisting of an inhibitory projection from the striatum to the globus pallidus external segment (GPe), an inhibitory projection from the GPe to the subthalamic nucleus (STN), and an excitatory projection from the subthalamic nucleus to the GPi. The indirect and the direct pathways converge on the GPi, which then sends its inhibitory output to the motor thalamus, which projects to cortical motor areas. One may view the function of the indirect pathway as broadly inhibiting unwanted movement during an intentional movement and the direct pathway as focally permitting the selected movement (1). Multiple additional connections among basal ganglia nuclei may modify the activity of these two pathways. Perhaps the most important modifying circuit is the dopaminergic input to the striatum from the substantia nigra pars compact. The dopamine input differentially modulates the direct and indirect pathways from the putamen to the GPi. Postsynaptic dopamine D_2-like receptors predominantly localize to and inhibit the striatopallidal neurons of the indirect pathway projecting to the GPe, whereas

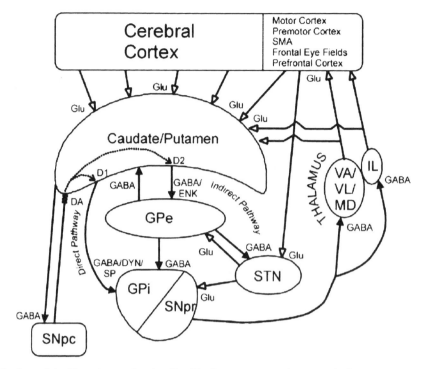

FIG. 23-1. A model of basal ganglia circuitry. Excitatory connections are indicated by *open arrows*, inhibitory connections by *filled arrows*, and the modulatory dopamine projection by a *three-headed arrow*. DA, dopamine (with D_1 and D_2 receptor family subtypes); Dyn, dynorphin; Enk, enkephalin; GABA, γ-aminobutyric acid; Glu, glutamate; GPe, globus pallidus external segment; GPi, globus pallidus internal segment IL, intralaminar thalamic nuclei; MD, mediodorsal thalamic nucleus; SNpc, substantia nigra pars compacta; SNpr, substantia nigra pars reticulata; SP, substance P; STN, subthalamic nucleus; VA, ventral anterior thalamic nucleus; VL, ventral lateral thalamic nucleus.

postsynaptic dopamine D_1-like receptors predominately localize to and facilitate the neurons of the direct pathway that project from the striatum to the GPi (2–6). D_1 and D_2 receptors are co-localized on some individual striatal neurons (7), but complete separation is not required for preferential control via specific dopamine receptors of direct and indirect pathways (8–10).

Structural abnormalities have been found in the basal ganglia contralateral to the symptomatic side in hemidystonic patients (11–13). The putamen has been the most commonly described site of such lesions in secondary dystonias (14–22), but lesions in-

volving other components of the basal ganglia thalamocortical motor circuit have been found including the thalamus, caudate (23), internal pallidum (24), and midbrain (25), as well as the posterior fossa in a few people with cervical dystonia (26). Although primary dystonias do not appear to be associated with easily visible structural defects in basal ganglia, high field strength MRI has demonstrated prolonged T2 times in the lentiform nucleus in patients with cervical dystonia (27), and volumetric analyses revealed about a 10% increased volume of putamen in those affected by primary cranial or hand dystonia (28).

FUNCTIONAL IMAGING

Positron emission tomographic (PET) measurements of regional cerebral blood flow or metabolism either at rest or during activation have provided key insights into the pathophysiology of dystonia. Resting-state studies have identified abnormal function of the putamen in patients with primary and secondary forms of dystonia, as well as alterations in function at other sites in cortical basal ganglia motor circuits (29–33). Activation studies have identified dysfunction in sensory motor processing in primary dystonias (including cranial, hand, and unilateral dystonias) and alterations in brain activity during motor tasks (34–36). Interestingly, abnormal cortical sensory responses to vibration in dopa-responsive dystonia may normalize after administration of levodopa, suggesting that sensory motor processing at the cortical level is influenced by dopaminergic pathways, most likely through basal ganglia cortical circuits (37). Other investigations using PET have found that primary and some secondary forms of dystonia may be associated with reduced activity of presynaptic dopaminergic nigrostriatal neurons (25,38–40). Studies of [^{18}F]fluorodopa (FD) uptake measured with PET has demonstrated decreased putaminal FD uptake in primary dystonias, but normal uptake in dopa-responsive dystonia despite deficient tyrosine hydroxylase activity (41,42).

PET measurements of radiolabeled dopaminergic ligands have provided additional insights into the function of dopaminergic pathways in dystonia. Nonhuman primates treated with intracarotid 1-methyl-4-phenyl-1,2,3,6-tetrahydropyridine (MPTP), which selectively destroys dopaminergic neurons, develop transient hemidystonia prior to hemiparkinsonism with flexed posture, bradykinesia, and postural tremor that persists up to 1½ years (43). Dystonia corresponded temporally with a decreased striatal dopamine content (97% to 98%) and a transient decrease (about 30%) in D_2-like receptor number in the putamen (44). The transient dystonia followed by persistent parkinsonism is analogous to lower limb dystonia as the first, frequently transient, symptom of Parkinson's disease in humans (45).

The relevance of these findings to primary dystonias comes from comparison with PET studies in humans. PET measurement of the *in vivo* binding of the dopaminergic radioligand [^{18}F]spiperone in the putamen in 21 patients with cranial and hand dystonia revealed a significant 29% mean decrease in a binding index called the combined forward rate constant (the product of the association rate constant and the maximum number of available specific binding sites) in dystonics compared to normals (46). These findings are consistent with decreased D_2-like binding in putamen and were the first demonstration of a receptor abnormality in primary dystonia (46). This closely matches the findings in nonhuman primates with transient dystonia and provides further evidence for the relevance of these findings to the pathophysiology of dystonia (47). It is important to note that [^{18}F]spiperone is relatively nonspecific; about 70% binding to D_2-like receptors and 30% to S_2-type receptors in primate putamen (48), but this method has been carefully validated for *in vivo* measurements (48–50). Others have found reduced uptake of the more specific D_2-like radioligand [^{123}I]epidepride using single photon emission computed tomography in ten patients with cervical dystonia (51). In contrast, [^{11}C]raclopride, another D_2-like radioligand, had increased binding in patients with dopa-responsive dystonia compared to normals in two different studies (52,53). However, endogenous dopamine competes for [^{11}C]raclopride binding sites; therefore, these findings do not distinguish an increase in dopamine receptors from a reduction in striatal dopamine (which is expected in dopa-responsive dystonia). No studies have directly quantified D_1 binding in primary dystonia, since suitable PET radioligands have not been available.

CORROBORATING EVIDENCE OF DOPAMINERGIC DYSFUNCTION

Other evidence confirms that dystonia may be associated with decreased striatal dopamine activity. The syndrome of dopa-responsive dystonia has remarkable symptomatic response to levodopa. An autosomal-dominant form of this disease is associated with deficiency of guanosine triphosphate (GTP) cyclohydrolase, which leads to reduction of tyrosine hydroxylase activity, the rate-limiting enzyme for dopamine production (54); the autosomal-recessive form is caused by a direct defect in tyrosine hydroxylase (55). Either defect produces striatal dopamine deficiency, despite no loss of nigrostriatal neurons. Additionally, drugs that block dopamine receptors can produce acute dystonic reactions (56–58). A recent postmortem study of several people with *DYT1* dystonia suggests that D_1 and D_2 receptors may be reduced in the striatum (59). Furthermore, the expression of messenger RNA that encodes torsinA, which is the protein product of the *DYT1* gene, is particularly concentrated in the dopamine neurons of the pars compacta in the substantia nigra (60). However, it is clear that the relationship between reduced striatal dopamine dysfunction and development of symptoms is either more selective or more complicated than in Parkinson's disease, since patients with Parkinson's disease usually have a dramatic clinical response to levodopa, whereas most patients with primary dystonias do not.

An interesting rodent model of cranial dystonia suggests that mild striatal dopamine deficiency may be a permissive factor that permits subsequent modest injury to the lid-closing orbicularis muscle to produce bilateral forceful blinking of the eyelids that resembles blepharospasm (61). These observations may connect the findings of reduced D_2 binding in the putamen, which may reduce dopaminergic control of the indirect pathway. This may also explain the relatively low penetrance of the *DYT1* gene defect in generalized dystonia since only about 30% of those with the gene defect develop clinical manifestations. A "two-hit" pathophysiologic mechanism may be necessary to develop symptoms, and the dopaminergic deficit may be the permissive condition allowing a second injury to cause dystonia. Such a permissive state may be identifiable as the movement-related pattern identified by fluorodeoxyglucose (FDG) PET in patients with the *DYT1* gene defect, whether or not they have developed clinical dystonia (31), or as the bilateral abnormalities of blood flow responses in patients with unilateral dystonic manifestations (35,62). One may postulate that an injury or defect in sensory processing could be the second "hit" in patients with dystonia, and several studies suggest that there may be sensory processing abnormalities in a variety of different types of dystonia (34,35,41,62–66).

CONCLUSION

Substantial evidence implicates dysfunction of dopaminergic pathways in the pathophysiology of dystonia. PET measures of dopaminergic receptor binding in patients with dystonia and in an animal model with transient dystonia suggest that this involvement may preferentially affect D_2-mediated pathways, which implicates the indirect pathway of the basal ganglia motor circuit. As noted above, one primary function of indirect pathway may be to broadly inhibit unwanted movement during an intended movement (1) (Fig. 23-2). Conceivably, signal processing through the indirect pathway could be influenced at many different points. Regardless of the site of primary pathology, we hypothesize that dysfunction of the indirect pathway could lead to the loss of lateral inhibition both within the basal ganglia and at the level of the cerebral cortex, producing abnormal central sensory processing (Fig. 23-3). The normalization by levodopa of the vibration-induced blood flow response in dopa-responsive dystonia, is suggestive, but

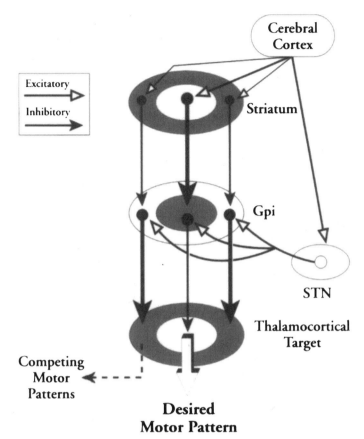

FIG. 23-2. Functional organization of the basal ganglia output. When a voluntary movement is initiated by cortical mechanisms, a corollary signal is sent to subthalamic nucleus (STN), exciting it. The STN projects in a widespread pattern and excites the globus pallidus internal segment (GPi)/substantia nigra pars reticulata (SNpr). The increased GPi/SNpr activity causes inhibition of thalamocortical motor mechanisms. In parallel to the pathway through the STN, signals are sent from all areas of the cerebral cortex to the striatum. The striatum projects in a focused pattern and inhibits the GPi. The resulting focally decreased activity in GPi/SNpr selectively disinhibits thalamocortical motor mechanisms involved in the desired movement. The net result of basal ganglia activity during a voluntary movement is broad inhibition of competing motor patterns and focused facilitation of the selected voluntary movement. Excitatory projections are indicated with *open arrows*; inhibitory projections are indicated with *filled arrows*. Relative magnitude of activity is represented by line thickness.

not proof, of this notion. Additional studies measuring the function of the direct pathway through the basal ganglia will help clarify its role. Finally, development and application of new neuroimaging tools will likely help address some of these unsettled issues and provide new insights into the pathophysiology of dystonia.

ACKNOWLEDGMENTS

This work is supported by the Greater St. Louis Chapter of the American Parkinson Disease Association (APDA), National Institutes of Health grants NS41248, NS41509, NS31001, and NS49821, the APDA Advanced Center for PD Research at Washing-

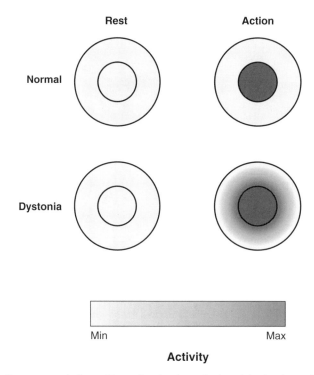

FIG. 23-3. Schematic representation of hypothesized cortical activity in dystonia. The center of the annulus represents activity of cortical mechanisms involved in a desired movement. The surrounding ring represents the activity of mechanisms involved in unwanted competing movements. In normals, action is associated with a discrete activation of the desired movement with suppression of unwanted movements. In dystonia, the surrounding inhibition is reduced. This abnormality may cause unwanted muscle contractions and movements.

ton University, the Ruth Kopolow Fund, and the Sam and Barbara Murphy Fund.

REFERENCES

1. Mink JW. The basal ganglia: focused selection and inhibition of competing motor programs. *Prog Neurobiol* 1996;50:381–425.
2. Albin, RL, Young AB, Penney JB. The functional anatomy of basal ganglia disorders. *Trends Neurosci* 1989;12:366–375.
3. Alexander GE, Crutcher MD. Functional architecture of basal ganglia circuits: neural substrates of parallel processing. *Trends Neurosci* 1990;13:266–271.
4. Gerfen CR, Engber TM, Mahan LC, et al. D1 and D2 dopamine receptor-regulated gene expression of striatonigral and striatopallidal neurons. *Science* 1990;250: 1429–1432.
5. Gerfen CR. The neostriatal mosaic: multiple levels of compartmental organization. *Trends Neurosci* 1992;15: 133–139.
6. Keefe KA, Gerfen CR. D1-D2 dopamine receptor synergy in striatum: effects of intrastriatal infusions of dopamine agonists and antagonists on immediate early gene expression. *Neuroscience* 1995;66:903–913.
7. Surmeier D, Song W, Yan Z. Coordinated expression of dopamine receptors in neostriatal medium spiny neurons. *J Neurosci* 1996;16:6579–6591.
8. Gerfen CR, McGintry JF, Young WS. Dopamine differentially regulates dynorphin, substance P and enkephalin expression in striatal neurons: in situ hybridization histochemical analysis. *J Neurosci* 1991;11:1016–1031.
9. Black KJ, Gado MH, Perlmutter JS. PET measurement of dopamine D2 receptor-mediated changes in striatopallidal function. *J Neurosci* 1997;17:3168–3177.
10. Black, KJ, Hershey T, Gado M, et al. A dopamine D1 agonist activates temporal lobe structures in primates. *J Neurophysiol* 2000;84:549–557.
11. Demierre B, Rondot P. Dystonia caused by putaminocapsulo-caudate vascular lesions. *J Neurol Neurosurg Psychiatry* 1983;46:404–409.
12. Grimes J, Hassan M, Quarrington A, et al. Delayed-onset post-hemiplegic dystonia: CT demonstration of basal ganglia pathology. *Neurology* 1982;32:1033–1035.
13. Pettigrew L, Jankovic J. Hemidystonia: a report of 22 patients and a review of the literature. *J Neurol Neurosurg Psychiatry* 1985;48:650–657.
14. Bhatia K, Marsden CD. The behavioural and motor con-

sequences of focal lesions of the basal ganglia in man. *Brain* 1994;117:859–876.

15. Fross RD, Martin WR, Li D, et al. Lesions of the putamen: their relevance to dystonia. *Neurology* 1987;37: 1125–1129.

16. Giroud M, Lemesle M, Madinier G, et al. Unilateral lenticular infarcts: radiological and clinical syndromes, aetiology, and prognosis. *J Neurol Neurosurg Psychiatry* 1997;63:611–615.

17. Kawano H, Takeuchi Y, Misawa A, et al. Putaminal necrosis presenting with hemidystonia. *Pediatr Neurol* 2000;22:222–224.

18. Krauss J, Mohadjer M, Braus D, et al. Dystonia following head trauma: a report of nine patients and review of the literature. *Mov Disord* 1992;7:263–272.

19. Lee M, Rinne J. Dystonia after head trauma. *Neurology* 1994;44:1374–1378.

20. Lyoo CH, Oh SH, Joo JY, et al. Hemidystonia and hemichoreoathetosis as an initial manifestation of moyamoya disease. *Arch Neurol* 2000;57:1510–1512.

21. Obeso J, Gimenez-Roldan S. Clinicopathological correlation in symptomatic dystonia. *Adv Neurol* 1988;50: 113–122.

22. Rutledge J, Hilal S, Silver A, et al. Magnetic resonance imaging of dystonic states. *Adv Neurol* 1988;50:265–275.

23. Lehericy S, Vidailhet M, Dormont D, et al. Striatopallidal and thalamic dystonia. A magnetic resonance imaging anatomoclinical study. *Arch Neurol* 1996;53:241–250.

24. Munchau A, Mathen D, Cox T, et al. Unilateral lesions of the globus pallidus: report of four patients presenting with focal or segmental dystonia. *J Neurol Neurosurg Psychiatry* 2000;69:494–498.

25. Vidailhet M, Dupel C, Lehericy S, et al. Dopaminergic dysfunction in midbrain dystonia: anatomoclinical study using 3-dimensional magnetic resonance imaging and fluorodopa F 18 positron emission tomography. *Arch Neurol* 1999;56:982–989.

26. Gupta AK, Roy DR, Conlan ES, et al. Torticollis secondary to posterior fossa tumors. *J Pediatr Orthop* 1996;16:505–507.

27. Schneider S, Feifel E, Ott D, et al. Prolonged MRI T_2 times of the lentiform nucleus in idiopathic spasmodic torticollis. *Neurology* 1994;44:846–850.

28. Black KJ, Ongur D, Perlmutter JS. Putamen volume in idiopathic focal dystonia. *Neurology* 1998;51:819–824.

29. Perlmutter JS, Raichle ME. Pure hemidystonia with basal ganglion abnormalities on positron emission tomography. *Ann Neurol* 1984;15:228–233.

30. Stoessl AJ, Martin WR, Clark C, et al. PET studies of cerebral glucose metabolism in idiopathic torticollis. *Neurology* 1986;36:653–657.

31. Eidelberg D, Moeller JR, Antonini A, et al. Functional brain networks in DYT1 dystonia. *Ann Neurol* 1998;44: 303–312.

32. Eidelberg D, Moeller JR, Ishikawa T, et al. The metabolic topography of idiopathic torsion dystonia. *Brain* 1995;118:1473–1484.

33. Hutchinson M, Nakamura T, Moeller JR, et al. The metabolic topography of essential blepharospasm: a focal dystonia with general implications. *Neurology* 2000; 55:673–677.

34. Feiwell RJ, Black KJ, McGee-Minnich LA, et al. Diminished regional blood flow response to vibration in patients with blepharospasm. *Neurology* 1999;52:291–297.

35. Tempel LW, Perlmutter JS. Abnormal cortical responses to vibration in patients with writer's cramp. *Neurology* 1993;43:2252–2257.

36. Playford ED, Passingham RE, Marsden CD, et al. Increased activation of frontal areas during arm movement in idiopathic torsion dystonia. *Mov Disord* 1998;13:309–318.

37. Perlmutter JS, Mink JW. The pathophysiology of dystonia: clues from neuroimaging. *Medlink Neurol* 2001. www.medlink.com

38. Playford E, Fletcher N, Sawle G, et al. Striatal [^{18}F]dopa uptake in familial idiopathic dystonia. *Brain* 1993;116: 1191–1199.

39. Leenders KL, Frackowiak RS, Quinn N, et al. Ipsilateral blepharospasm and contralateral hemidystonia and parkinsonism in a patient with a unilateral rostral brainstem-thalamic lesion: structural and functional abnormalities studied with CT, MRI, and PET scanning. *Mov Disord* 1986;1:51–58.

40. Brashear A, Mulholland GK, Zheng QH, et al. PET imaging of the pre-synaptic dopamine uptake sites in rapid-onset dystonia-parkinsonism (RDP). *Mov Disord* 1999;14:132–137.

41. Byl NN, McKenzie A, Nagarajan SS. Differences in somatosensory hand organization in a healthy flutist and a flutist with focal hand dystonia: a case report. *J Hand Ther* 2000;13:302–309.

42. Jeon BS, Jeong JM, Park SS, et al. Dopamine transporter density measured by [123I]beta-CIT single-photon emission computed tomography is normal in doparesponsive dystonia. *Ann Neurol* 1998;43:792–800.

43. Perlmutter JS, Tempel LW, Black KJ, et al. MPTP induces dystonia and parkinsonism: clues to the pathophysiology of dystonia. *Neurology* 1997;49:1432–1438.

44. Todd RD, Carl J, Harmon S, et al. Dynamic changes in striatal dopamine D2 and D3 receptor protein and mRNA in response to MPTP denervation in baboons. *J Neurosci* 1996;16:7776–7782.

45. Lucking CB, Durr A, Bonifati V, et al. Association between early-onset Parkinson's disease and mutations in the parkin gene. French Parkinson's Disease Genetics Study Group. *N Engl J Med* 2000;342:1560–1567.

46. Perlmutter JS, Stambuk MK, Markham J, et al. Decreased [18F]spiperone binding in putamen in idiopathic focal dystonia. *J Neurosci* 1997;17:834–842.

47. Perlmutter JS, Tempel LW, Black KJ, et al. MPTP induces dystonia & parkinsonism: clues to the pathophysiology of dystonia. *Neurology* 1997;49:1432–1438.

48. Perlmutter JS, Moerlein SM, Huang DR, et al. Nonsteady-state measurement of in vivo radioligand binding with positron emission tomography: specificity analysis and comparison with in vitro binding. *J Neurosci* 1991;11:1381–1389.

49. Perlmutter JS, Larson KB, Raichle ME, et al. Strategies for the in vivo measurement of receptor binding using positron emission tomography. *J Cereb Blood Flow Metabol* 1986;6:154–169.

50. Perlmutter JS, Kilbourn MR, Welch MJ, et al. Nonsteady-state measurement of in vivo receptor binding with positron emission tomography: "dose-response" analysis. *J Neurosci* 1989;9:2344–2352.

51. Naumann M, Pirker W, Reiners K, et al. Imaging the pre- and postsynaptic side of striatal dopaminergic synapses in idiopathic cervical dystonia: a SPECT study using [123I] epidepride and [123I] beta-CIT. *Mov Disord* 1998;13:319–323.

52. Kunig G, Leenders KL, Antonini A, et al. D2 receptor

binding in dopa-responsive dystonia. *Ann Neurol* 1998; 44:758–762.

53. Kishore A, Nygaard TG, de la Fuente-Fernandez R, et al. Striatal D2 receptors in symptomatic and asymptomatic carriers of dopa-responsive dystonia measured with [11C]-raclopride and positron-emission tomography. *Neurology* 1998;50:1028–1032.

54. Nygaard T. Dopa-responsive dystonia. *Curr Opin Neurol* 1995;8:310–313.

55. Knappskog PM, Flatmark T, Mallet J, et al. Recessively inherited L-DOPA-responsive dystonia caused by a point mutation (Q381K) in the tyrosine hydroxylase gene. *Hum Mol Genet* 1995;4:1209–1212.

56. Garver D, Davis J, Dekirmenjian H, et al. Dystonic reactions following neuroleptics: time course and proposed mechanisms. *Psychopharmacology* 1976;47:199–201.

57. Kolbe H, Clow A, Jenner P, et al. Neuroleptic-induced acute dystonic reactions may be due to enhanced dopamine release on to supersensitive postsynaptic receptors. *Neurology* 1981;31:434–439.

58. Rupniak N, Jenner P, Marsden CD. Acute dystonia induced by neuroleptic drugs. *Psychopharmacol* 1986;88: 403–419.

59. Augood SJ, Hollingsworth Z, Albers DS, et al. Dopamine

transmission in DYT1 dystonia: a biochemical and autoradiographical study. *Neurology* 2002;59:445–448.

60. Augood SJ, Martin DM, Ozelius LJ, et al. Distribution of the mRNAs encoding torsinA and torsinB in the normal adult human brain. *Ann Neurol* 1999;46:761–769.

61. Schicatano EJ, Basso MA, Evinger C. Animal model explains the origins of the cranial dystonia benign essential blepharospasm. *J Neurophysiol* 1997;77:2842–2846.

62. Tempel LW, Perlmutter JS. Abnormal vibration-induced cerebral blood flow response in dystonia. *Brain* 1990; 113:691–707.

63. Reilly JA, Hallett M, Cohen LG, et al. The N30 component of somatosensory evoked potentials in patients with dystonia. *Electroencephalogr Clin Neurophysiol* 1992;84:243–247.

64. Elbert T, Candia V, Altenmuller E, et al. Alteration of digital representations in somatosensory cortex in focal hand dystonia. *Neuroreport* 1998;9:3571–3575.

65. Sanger TD, Tarsy D, Pascual-Leone A. Abnormalities of spatial and temporal sensory discrimination in writer's cramp. *Mov Disord* 2001;16:94–99.

66. Bara-Jimenez W, Shelton P, Hallett M. Spatial discrimination is abnormal in focal hand dystonia. *Neurology* 2000;55:1869–1873.

Dystonia 4: Advances in Neurology, Vol. 94. Edited by Stanley Fahn, Mark Hallett, and Mahlon R. DeLong. Lippincott Williams & Wilkins, Philadelphia © 2004.

24

Clinical Presentation and Progression of Sporadic and Familial Primary Torsion Dystonia in Italy

*Anna Rita Bentivoglio, *Antonio E. Elia, †Graziella Filippini, ‡Enza Maria Valente, *Alfonso Fasano, and §Alberto Albanese

*Istituto di Neurologia, Universita Cattolica del Sacro Cuore, Rome, Italy.
†Istituto Nazionale Neurologico Carlo Besta, Milan, Italy. ‡Istituto CSS Mendel, Rome, Italy.
§Istituto di Neurologia, Universita Cattolica del Sacro Cuore, Rome, Italy; and Istituto Nazionale Neurologico Carlo Besta, Milan, Italy.

Dystonia is a syndrome of sustained muscle contractions, causing twisting and repetitive movements or abnormal posture. The disease is usually classified based on etiology as idiopathic (primary) or symptomatic (secondary). Primary torsion dystonia (PTD) encompasses sporadic and familial cases. Four different PTD loci and nine loci for other inherited dystonias have been identified so far. Dystonia is a clinically and genetically heterogeneous disease that is difficult to schematize based on simple phenotype-genotype correlation.

The natural history of PTD is characterized by focal onset and frequent spread to other body parts with a variable time course. In many cases, dystonia remains focal or spreads only to the adjacent musculature. Sufficient data are not available on the progression of dystonia, particularly in the European population. Moreover, few studies have focused on the clinical features of familial dystonia in large series. This chapter reviews a series of 460 PTD patients referred to the Movement Disorders Clinic of the Gemelli Hospital in Rome; we analyze the onset and progression of sporadic dystonia and describe the clinical features of familial cases.

SUBJECTS AND METHODS

The Movement Disorders Clinic was started in 1986 at the Gemelli Hospital in Rome. During an interval of 15 years, 4,581 in- or outpatients were recorded in a movement disorders registry. Patients in the registry received a clinical diagnosis of dystonia based on the observation of dystonic postures and dystonic movements occurring in combination, either at rest or following a voluntary motor task (1). The observation of sensory tricks provided an additional diagnostic criterion for a definite clinical diagnosis. Isolated head or limb tremors were not considered reliable criteria for the diagnosis. The registry included cases of PTD, of dystonia plus syndromes (2) and of secondary dystonia (e.g., due to cerebral palsy, stroke, neoplasm, drug induced, or psychogenic). The etiologic classification was based on clinical and laboratory workout including neuroimaging (3). The patients were evaluated at least twice a year by a staff neurologist, who reviewed the diagnosis and the treatment plan.

The following clinical data were retrieved from the registry: gender, ethnic origin, age, disease duration, distribution of dystonia at onset and at the time of the last visit, disease site, and family history of movement disorders. Continuous data were expressed as mean (± standard deviation, SD) and were compared by Student's t-test. Categorical data were compared by means of chi square (χ^2) test. The analysis of variance (repeated measures) was performed (4) to estimate the mean number of sites progressively involved during the follow-up in sporadic and in familial cases.

To examine the clinical features of familial dystonia, we considered the patients who reported at least one family member with dystonia. All index cases were asked for participation of their relatives in the study. Only one index subject was considered for each family. In 39 index cases, the diagnosis of familial dystonia was confirmed personally as we examined family members. Thirty-three index patients were not further investigated.

RESULTS

The Gemelli dystonia registry encompassed 593 patients (356 women and 237 men) with primary or secondary dystonia who were followed in the period 1986–2001. The patients originated mostly from Central and Southern Italy (Lazio, Campania, Apulia, and Abruzzo regions). One hundred thirty-three patients were affected by secondary dystonia, 460 (296 women and 164 men) had PTD.

The mean age at onset in PTD cases (48.3 ± 17.7 years) was higher than that of secondary cases (30.1 ± 23.0; $p < .001$). Perinatal cerebral injury was the commonest cause of secondary dystonia (33.3%), and treatment with neuroleptics was the second most common cause (28.0%); in 5.3% of cases a psychiatric condition not related to neuroleptic intake was associated with dystonia (obsessive-compulsive disorder, psychosis). Head trauma, brain neoplasm, thalamotomy, stroke, parkinsonism, or Fahr's disease were the causes of the remaining secondary cases.

A detailed history revealed that 380 cases were affected by sporadic PTD, whereas 80 patients reported at least one relative affected with dystonia.

The 380 sporadic PTD patients had a mean age at disease onset of 49.1 ± 17.2 years. At the last available clinical examination, 234 patients presented a focal dystonia (124 cranial, 43 cervical, 21 laryngeal, 43 upper limb, and three lower limb). Segmental cases were 124, encompassing 52 patients affected by cranial-cervical dystonia, 23 by cranial-cervical and upper limb dystonia, 24 by Meige's syndrome, 17 by neck and upper limb, six by neck and trunk, two by neck and laryngeal dystonia. Multifocal dystonia occurred in seven patients and generalized dystonia in 15. There was a male-to-female ratio of 1:1.85, mainly caused by a preponderance of women with blepharospasm or cranial-cervical dystonia (M:F ratio of 1:2.6 and 1:3.7, respectively).

Of the 460 patients with PTD, 80 (17.6%) reported a family history of dystonia; eight had relatives included in the registry, and therefore, the frequency of familial cases was 15.9%. In 39 cases, familial dystonia was ascertained by direct examination of the affected relatives or indirect evidence based on medical records confirming the diagnosis. These families were studied in detail. Among the families studied, 15 presented a prevalent phenotype of focal dystonia, 16 had a segmental phenotype, and eight a generalized phenotype.

Sporadic PTD

Disease Onset

At onset, all PTD patients presented with focal symptoms, and a large variability of body districts involved. Most cases (55.3%) had cranial onset, with blepharospasm in almost all, and oromandibular dystonia in just eight. Cervical dystonia was observed in 77 patients (20.3%); 29 patients (7.6%) had spasmodic dysphonia at onset; 64 patients (16.8%) had limb onset involving one upper limb in most cases (64, 14.2%) and a lower limb in the remaining 10 (2.6%). The mean age at onset was 49.1 ± 17.2 years; age at onset varied apparently in correlation with the site of onset—

ascended from lower to upper body either in women or in men. Patients with lower limb dystonia had the youngest age at disease onset (p <.001, when compared to the other subgroups), whereas the mean age of patients with cranial onset was the highest (p <.001). Cranial, cervical, laryngeal, and lower limb onset were observed more frequently in women than in men (M to F ratio 1:2.7, 1:1.8, 1:2.6, 1:4.0, respectively). Interestingly, onset in the upper limb was more frequent in men than in women (M to F ratio 2.8:1) and the age at disease onset was higher in men (p <.05).

Progression

In most patients (234, 61.5%) dystonia did not progress after a mean disease duration of 7.2 ± 6.4 years, but remained confined to the site of onset. In 124 patients (32.6%, mean disease duration: 10.1 ± 9.4 years) dystonia progressed to a segmental distribution; in 22 patients (5.6%, mean disease duration: 14.2 ± 15.8 years) dystonia progressed to a multifocal or generalized distribution (Table 24-1).

Patients with generalized dystonia had a lower age at disease onset than patients with focal, segmental, or multifocal distributions (17.9 ± 16.7, compared to 50.2 ± 17.3 years for segmental, 48.4 ± 17.7 for multifocal, and 50.4 ± 15.2 for focal cases; p <.001 in each case); there were no differences in age at disease onset among patients with focal, segmental, and multifocal dystonia.

When patients were compared on the basis of the body area affected at onset, it was observed that clinical progression occurred in a higher percentage of patients with lower limb onset (75%), than of those with cervical (48.0%), cranial (40.4%), laryngeal (27.6%), or upper limb onset (20.3%). No gender-related difference occurred in the progression of dystonia.

The progression rate varied in relation to the site affected at disease onset. In the majority of patients with cranial onset in whom spread of dystonia occurred, the disease progressed to cranial-cervical involvement or to Meige's syndrome, with very few cases of generalization. Cervical (and laryngeal) dystonia progressed to cranial-cervical or cervical-brachial segmental dystonia; generalization occurred in 9% of patients with cervical onset and in no patient with laryngeal onset. In 11 out of 54 patients with upper limb onset, dystonia progressed to other sites, mostly to a

TABLE 24-1. *Presentation of dystonia at the last examination in sporadic cases*

Features of dystonia	Number	M/F	Age at onset	Disease duration
Focal PTD				
Cranial	124	35/89	57.4 ± 9.4	6.6 ± 5.6
Blepharospasm	122	34/88	57.3 ± 9.4	6.7 ± 5.6
Low face	2	1/1	47.5 ± 24.7	1.0 ± 0.0
Cervical	43	17/26	42.0 ± 14.5	9.5 ± 8.0
Laryngeal	21	7/14	55.0 ± 17.4	5.9 ± 6.1
Upper limb	43	34/9	38.0 ± 15.9	7.7 ± 6.6
Lower limb	3	1/2	33.3 ± 22.0	3.3 ± 4.2
Total of focal forms	234	94/140	50.4 ± 15.2	7.2 ± 6.4
Segmental PTDs				
Meige's syndrome	24	8/16	57.9 ± 9.2	8.8 ± 7.3
Cranial-cervical	52	11/41	53.1 ± 15.3	9.2 ± 8.8
Neck and upper limb	17	8/9	37.9 ± 21.5	15.8 ± 11.6
Neck and trunk	6	1/5	40.8 ± 18.5	5.3 ± 2.8
Neck and laryngeal	2	0/2	51.0 ± 12.7	6.0 ± 0.0
Cranial-cervical and upper limb	23	4/19	47.3 ± 19.9	11.2 ± 11.3
Total of segmental forms	124	32/92	50.2 ± 17.3	10.1 ± 9.4
Multifocal dystonia	7	1/6	48.4 ± 17.7	5.7 ± 4.7
Generalized dystonia	15	6/9	17.9 ± 16.7	18.3 ± 17.7
Total	380	133/247	49.1 ± 17.2	8.6 ± 8.5

PTD, primary torsion dystonia

cervical or cranial-cervical involvement. Seven out of 10 patients with onset in the lower limb had a clinical progression, which led to a generalized form in all.

Duration of clinical history was directly related to the spread of symptoms (p <.001), thus revealing that dystonia is a progressive disease. The most relevant clinical progression occurred during the first 5 years; after that period the disease was more stable (Fig. 24-1).

Primary Torsion Dystonia Families

The frequency of familial inheritance in the registry was estimated to be 15.9%. This was calculated by considering that eight patients, out of 80 who had at least one relative with dystonia, were already on record. Thirty-nine PTD families were studied; in 15 the prevalent phenotype was focal, in 16 segmental, and in eight generalized. Age at onset was adult (>21 years) in 34 families; onset was early (≤21 years) in three families; in two families age at onset was variable.

In nine families the prevalent phenotype was cranial-cervical dystonia with occasional generalization, two families had cranial-cervical dystonia with upper limb involvement, and three had a cranial-cervical form. Cervical dystonia was the prevalent phenotype in seven families (with occasional lower limb involvement in four of them). Cranial dystonia (blepharospasm, with or without lower cranial involvement) was the most common presentation in five families; focal laryngeal dystonia occurred in three families, and isolated writer's cramp in two. Generalized dystonia occurred in eight families (in two of them with rapid movements resembling myoclonic dystonia); two non-Jewish families and one Sephardi Jewish family had the *DYT1* mutation; some family members of the non-Jewish

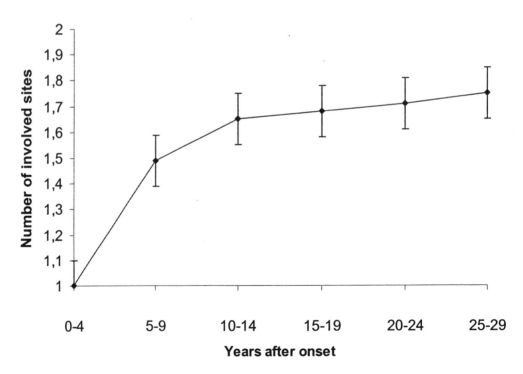

FIG. 24-1. Clinical progression of dystonia in a population of 380 patients with sporadic primary torsion dystonia (PTD), who were followed up after disease onset. Number of involved sites is shown as average ± standard error of the mean.

families presented with atypical clinical features. We did not observe any familial case of focal oromandibular dystonia or isolated lower limb dystonia.

Genetic Data

We screened 163 subjects for the GAG deletion on the DYT1 gene; 13 of them (8%) carried the mutation (Table 24-2). Three of them were affected by sporadic PTD and ten were members of three families. Three patients (two familial PTD and one sporadic), out of 140 with adult onset, carried the *DYT1* GAG deletion. Overall, we identified 11 *DYT1* cases of PTD and two unaffected carriers. *DYT1* patients had a mean age at onset of 23.3 ± 19.7 years, and mean disease duration of 17.4 ± 17.4 years. Men-to-women ratio was of 1.2:1. All cases presented with limb onset; in five cases onset was in a lower limb.

Among familial *DYT1* cases there was an unaffected gene carrier who presented a clinically definite form of psychogenic dystonia (5). She was the mother of a 21-year-old man affected by classic generalized *DYT1* PTD. Two other women in the same family presented with early-onset upper limb dystonia and mild progression: in one case dystonia progressed to a segmental distribution involving the upper body; in the other, dystonia remained confined to the upper limb. A typical form of *DYT1* PTD affected four patients with early onset in a lower limb and rapid generalization.

Four *DYT1* carriers with generalized dystonia had limb onset and spread to cervical muscles (in one case there was also laryngeal and oromandibular involvement). The mean age at disease onset was 10.0 ± 5.4 years. One *DYT1* carrier presented dystonia of the right shoulder at age 42; progression included scoliosis and action-induced tremor of the right hand. Two years later she presented tremor in the left hand, 20 years after the onset she also presented head tremor.

In four families that were large enough for linkage studies, linkage to the *DYT6* and *DYT7* loci was excluded.

The set of families with cervical dystonia and occasional generalization included a large family with 11 affected members linked to a novel PTD locus *(DYT13)* located on chromosome 1p36.13-36.32 (6). The prevalent phenotype revealed focal or segmental dystonia with prominent involvement of the cranial-cervical region and the upper limbs (7). The age at onset in the affected subjects was variable, ranging from 5 to 45 years. No anticipation (of age at onset and severity) was documented among generations. Onset occurred either in the cranial-cervical region (in six patients) or in the upper limb (in two patients), and was apparently segmental (both upper

TABLE 24-2. *Genetic classification of primary torsion dystonia (PTD) patients and families (not considering dystonia plus syndromes)*

Genetic characterization	No. of patients (no. of families)	Clinical features	Age at onset
DYT1+	10 (3)	Limb onset and rapid generalization	Juvenile
DYT1−	4 (2)	Blepharospasm	Adult
	2 (1)	Cranial-cervical	Juvenile
	6 (3)	Cranial-cervical	Adult
	2 (1)	Cranial-cervical or upper limb	Adult
	3 (1)	Cranial-cervical or generalized	Juvenile
	15 (4)	Cranial-cervical or generalized	Adult
	2 (1)	Cervical	Juvenile
	3 (1)	Cervical or generalized	Adult
	4 (2)	Upper limb	Adult
	2 (1)	Generalized	Juvenile
	4 (1)	Myoclonic	Juvenile
DYT13+	11 (1)	Cervical or generalized	Variable

limbs) in one. Progression was mild and the disease course was relatively benign in all the affected individuals. All the patients with long disease duration had a spread of symptoms to other body regions; in two patients the disease progressed to generalization, but their functional impairment remained mild. The estimated penetrance of the *DYT13* gene in this family was 58%.

DISCUSSION

The present series includes 460 PTD patients referred to the Gemelli Movement Disorders Clinic during a 15-year interval (1986–2001). Population data are influenced by several conditions: the center is a referral clinic for adult cases from central and southern Italy; children are not referred routinely, and this may bias the estimated prevalence of both early-onset PTD and secondary dystonias (particularly those secondary to birth injury). In the present series, early-onset cases accounted for 10.2% of the total and secondary dystonias for 22.4%. This is at odds with earlier series collected in other movement disorders centers where patients with early onset were approximately 20% of the total (8,9). This may indicate between-center differences in the catchment areas or in the availability of pediatric neurologists. Another difference is in the population collected by different centers; North American series encompass many Ashkenazi Jewish patients, who are poorly represented in European registries. Genetic heterogeneity between this and other series provides an intriguing glimpse on differences in populations.

Most patients with sporadic PTD in the present series (61.6%) had a final phenotype of focal dystonia, 32.6% had a segmental form, 1.8% were multifocal, and 3.9% had generalization. This is in agreement with data indicating that most patients with adult-onset PTD have focal dystonia, whereas segmental or multifocal dystonia represent altogether 22% of cases (10). According to the prevalence data estimated by an earlier study, patients with focal dystonia are ten times more

numerous than those with generalized forms (11). Considering focal PTD, most patients in this series were affected by blepharospasm or by cervical dystonia. This is consistent with the results of several studies indicating that blepharospasm is more frequent in southern Italy (12) than in the United States, Japan, or northern Europe, where cervical dystonia is the most common focal dystonia (11,13,14). Interestingly, an epidemiologic study performed in Segovia, Spain, found that blepharospasm was the commonest focal dystonia, thus providing a parallel between the two Mediterranean countries (15). Nevertheless, the relative frequency of blepharospasm and of cervical dystonia may be overestimated in the Gemelli series because patients affected by these focal forms were referred specifically for botulinum toxin treatment. This is probably a common bias in all clinical series collected during the last 15 years that attempt to deduce prevalence of dystonia on the basis of patient series collected at movement disorders clinics.

The present study confirms that generalized dystonia presents at an earlier age at onset than focal or segmental forms (16) and that the age at onset is inversely related to the diffusion of dystonia (9). In the present series, the mean age at onset was 17.9 ± 16.7 years for generalized dystonia, 50.2 ± 17.3 for segmental, and 50.4 ± 15.2 for focal dystonia. The present series also indicates sex-related differences in age at disease onset: in patients with cranial, cervical, or laryngeal dystonia age at onset was higher in women than in men, while in patients with upper limb dystonia age at onset was higher in men. This observation is in keeping with earlier reports (13,17,18) and points to a role of sex hormones in the pathophysiology of dystonia (19,20).

Significant differences were observed when patients with focal onset were categorized by their age at onset, in keeping with the observation that the mean age at onset increases as the site of onset ascends in the body (9). In patients with cranial dystonia, a progression to other body areas occurred in

40.4% of cases; this figure is similar to that reported in another series of Italian patients affected by blepharospasm (21). In the North American population, however, it has been observed that a spread of symptoms occurred in 73% of 107 patients with cranial onset (9). In the present series, cervical and laryngeal dystonia have a higher rate of progression to other body areas (cervical dystonia: 48.0%; laryngeal dystonia: 27.6%). Previous studies have found that spread of disease occurs in only 22% of non-Jewish patients with adult onset (9), in 31.9% of cervical dystonia cases (22), and only in 14% of laryngeal PTD cases (9). As far as upper limb dystonia is concerned, the rate of progression observed in the Gemelli registry (20.4%) is lower than that of previous studies reporting figures of 41% for adult-onset cases, 72% for early-onset cases (9), and 60% for *DYT1* negative Ashkenazi Jewish patients (23). This discrepancy may be due to the higher age at onset of patients in the present series that encompasses many patients with writer's cramp or occupational dystonia, who do not have progression to generalization.

The frequency of cases with family history of dystonia among our PTD population was estimated to be 15.9%, in keeping with previous studies, which estimated familial occurrence between 18% (24) and 23% (25) of patients. The latter study reported that the incidence of dystonia among first-degree relatives of patients with torticollis and blepharospasm is higher than expected on the basis of population data. Furthermore, familiarity has been considered a risk factor for PTD in an epidemiologic study performed in Italy (26).

The analysis of familial cases of the Gemelli registry showed that among 140 PTD patients with adult onset who were screened for the *DYT1* mutation, three had the *DYT1* GAG deletion. In two patients with familial dystonia, the age at onset was 50; in the sporadic patient, age at onset was 42. This observation provides caveats on the possibility of exporting to the European population the testing proposed for North American patients

seeking genetic testing for the *DYT1* mutation (27). Further comparisons should probably account for differences in genetic backgrounds between North America and Europe.

REFERENCES

1. Fahn S, Eldridge R. Definition of dystonia and classification of the dystonic states. *Adv Neurol* 1976;14:1–5.
2. Fahn S, Bressman S, Marsden CD. Classification of dystonia. *Adv Neurol* 1998;78:1–10.
3. Bressman SB. Dystonia. *Curr Opin Neurol* 1998;11: 363–372.
4. Diggle PJ, Liang KY, Zegler SL. *The analysis of longitudinal data.* New York: Oxford University Press, 1994.
5. Bentivoglio AR, Loi M, Valente EM, et al. Phenotypic variability of DYT1-PTD: does the clinical spectrum include psychogenic dystonia? *Mov Disord* 2002;17: 1058–1063.
6. Valente EM, Bentivoglio AR, Cassetta E, et al. DYT13, a novel primary torsion dystonia locus, maps to chromosome 1p36.13-36.32 in an Italian family with cranial-cervical or upper limb onset. *Ann Neurol* 2001;49: 362–366.
7. Bentivoglio AR, Del Grosso N, Albanese A, et al. Non-DYT1 dystonia in a large Italian family. *J Neurol Neurosurg Psychiatry* 1997;62:357–360.
8. Bressman SB, Fahn S. Childhood dystonia. In: Watts RL, Koller WC, eds. *Movement disorders.* New York: McGraw-Hill, 1997:419–429.
9. Greene P, Kang UJ, Fahn S. Spread of symptoms in idiopathic torsion dystonia. *Mov Disord* 1995;10: 143–152.
10. The Epidemiological Study of Dystonia in Europe (ESDE) Collaborative Group. A prevalence study of primary dystonia in eight European countries. *J Neurol* 2000;247:787–792.
11. Nutt JG, Muenter MD, Aronson A, et al. Epidemiology of focal and generalized dystonia in Rochester, Minnesota. *Mov Disord* 1988;3:188–194.
12. Defazio G, Livrea P. Epidemiology of primary blepharospasm. *Mov Disord* 2002;17:7–12.
13. Duffey POF, Butler AG, Hawthorme MR, et al. The epidemiology of the primary dystonias in the north of England. *Adv Neurol* 1998;78:121–125.
14. Nakashima K, Kusumi M, Inoue Y, et al. Prevalence of focal dystonias in the Western area of Tottori prefecture in Japan. *Mov Disord* 1995;10:440–443.
15. Sempere AP, Duarte J, Coria F, et al. Prevalence of idiopathic focal dystonia in the province of Segovia, Spain. *J Neurol* 1994;241:S124.
16. Fahn S. Concept and classification of dystonia. *Adv Neurol* 1988;50:1–8.
17. Epidemiological Study of Dystonia in Europe (ESDE) Collaborative Group. Sex-related influences on the frequency and age of onset of primary dystonia. *Neurology* 1999;53:1871–1873.
18. Soland VL, Bhatia KP, Marsden CD. Sex prevalence of focal dystonias. *J Neurol Neurosurg Psychiatry* 1996; 60:204–205.
19. Kompoliti K. Estrogen and movement disorders. *Clin Neuropharmacol* 1999;22(318):326.
20. Loscher W, Blanke T, Richter A, et al. Gonadal sex hor-

mones and dystonia: experimental studies in genetically dystonic hamsters. *Mov Disord* 1995;10:92–102.

21. Defazio G, Berardelli A, Abbruzzese G, et al. Risk factors for spread of primary adult onset blepharospasm: a multicentre investigation of the Italian movement disorders study group. *J Neurol Neurosurg Psychiatry* 1999; 67:613–619.

22. Jahanshahi M, Marion MH, Marsden CD. Natural history of adult-onset idiopathic torticollis. *Arch Neurol* 1990;47:548–552.

23. Bressman SB, de Leon D, Kramer PL, et al. Dystonia in Ashkenazi Jews: clinical characterization of a founder mutation. *Ann Neurol* 1994;36:771–777.

24. Leube B, Kessler KR, Goecke T, et al. Frequency of familial inheritance among 488 index patients with idiopathic focal dystonia and clinical variability in a large family. *Mov Disord* 1997;12:1000–1006.

25. Stojanovic M, Cvetkovic D, Kostic VS. A genetic study of idiopathic focal dystonias. *J Neurol* 1995;242: 508–511.

26. Defazio G, Berardelli A, Abbruzzese G, et al. Possible risk factors for primary adult onset dystonia: a case-control investigation by the Italian Movement Disorders Study Group. *J Neurol Neurosurg Psychiatry* 1998;64: 25–32.

27. Bressman SB, Sabatti C, Raymond D, et al. The DYT1 phenotype and guidelines for diagnostic testing. *Neurology* 2000;54:1746–1752.

Dystonia 4: Advances in Neurology, Vol. 94. Edited by Stanley Fahn, Mark Hallett, and Mahlon R. DeLong. Lippincott Williams & Wilkins, Philadelphia © 2004.

25

Cognition and Affect in Patients with Cervical Dystonia With and Without Tremor

*Drake D. Duane and †Kendall J. Vermilion

°*Arizona Dystonia Institute, Scottsdale, Arizona and Arizona State University, Tempe, Arizona.*
†*Wayne State University, College of Medicine, Detroit, Michigan*

One might reasonably ask why should cognition and affect be investigated in any neurologic disorder, especially one as uncommon as focal cervical dystonia. Furthermore, why investigate the co-occurrence of tremor as a potential variable? To clarify, behavior is recognized to have three major components: *cognition,* the information management aspect of behavior; *emotional state,* relating to feelings and motivation; and *executive function,* which controls how behavior may be expressed (1). These three components likely have underlying neuroanatomic and neurochemical correlates.

There are four classes of cognitive function:

1. Receptive functions, which involve abilities to select, acquire, classify, and integrate information.
2. Memory and learning, which relate to information storage and retrieval.
3. Thinking, which relates to the mental organization and reorganization of information.
4. Expressive functions, which are the means through which information is communicated or acted upon (1).

Although injury may induce changes in cognition or affect as well as in executive function, there are patterns of these behaviors that are constitutional and lifelong, maturing with the individual. Since these components

are brain-based, when the nervous system becomes disordered, the dysfunction may be reflected in disorder in some aspect of behavior, whether cognitive, affective, or executive in nature.

The examination of cognitive function as in the motor system examination in clinical neurology reflects brain function, so that in a disorder in which localization of the source(s) of the motor dysfunction are in dispute, avenues that may reflect the source site or related sites of dysfunction may be helpful in revealing the underlying mechanism and its location.

Since therapies including medication, surgery, and perhaps botulinum toxin may affect cognition through chemical derangement or structural destruction, baseline and posttherapeutic cognitive evaluation may determine what and how much change has occurred in thinking or behavior, which may influence the degree of enthusiasm for some forms of treatment.

Attempting to assess cognition is a challenge, because it is not always clear what constitutes deviation from the norm on a cognitive task and whether that deviation localizes precisely in that subject's nervous system. Additional confounds include mood and pain, both of which may adversely influence cognition and therefore need to be monitored; the patient's social milieu; and the effects of age, gender, and other sources of disability, such as health problems unrelated to dystonia and their therapy, for example, hypertension (2).

The affective state refers to the extent to which one's temperament or personality has become depressed, anxious, worrying, ruminative, or delusional, as opposed to the healthy state of emotional adjustment. Mood states putatively have both anatomic and neurochemical correlates, for example the observation that left temporal lobe seizure disorders have a higher risk of concomitant depression (3). The catecholamine theory of depression (4) has resulted in catecholamine-modifying drug therapies, such as fluoxetine, the selective serotonin reuptake inhibitor facilitating serotonin metabolism; the tricyclics, which facilitate norepinephrine metabolism; or bupropion, which affects both dopamine and norepinephrine metabolism. Consequently, the rates of disorders of affect might reflect underlying anatomic and/or neurochemical characteristics of the primary disorder of brain function, which has potential heuristic and therapeutic value.

A limiting factor in the assessment of affect is that the mood state of the subject may be a reflection of pain, disability, or the treatment employed, as well as the social milieu and age, thereby not representing a direct concomitant of the disorder under investigation or of the central nervous system. Consequently, these issues need to be assessed and factored just as they should be in the investigation of cognition. Whether assessing affect or cognition, sufficient numbers of subjects, and where possible age- and gender-matched controls, enhance the capacity to test hypotheses regarding the role of cognitive and affective dysfunction in focal dystonia.

With respect to the investigation of subgroups of dystonic subjects, there are a variety of potentially meaningful subcategories including age of onset; distribution of dystonic symptoms, i.e., so-called cervical dystonia plus (CD+) versus isolated cervical dystonia (CD); a verified family history of movement disorder; and ascertaining whether the disorder is primary or essential versus secondary to some acquired disorder of the nervous system. Nonetheless, acquired mechanisms may offer models for better understanding idiopathic dystonia. Tremor holds appeal for us, even though what constitutes primary or secondary tremor in focal dystonia has been in dispute. The observation of the high rate of occurrence of tremor in relatives of CD patients (5), its common occurrence in those with CD when rigorously defined and not necessarily in the region of the dystonic involvement, i.e., hand tremor in those with CD (6–9), as well as the antecedent history of tremor in up to 10% of those with CD (10) raise the possibility that there is a relationship between what usually has been referred to as *essential* tremor and focal dystonia. Characterizing the differences between patients who manifest tremor and those who do not may assist in the explication of the relationship between these two conditions. The differential rate of occurrence of tremor in the general population versus idiopathic focal CD presents a potential confound unless reasonable numbers of subjects are available for the comparison.

For the purposes of this discussion, tremor refers to a fixed-rate rhythmic oscillation of head, voice, and/or hands. The upper limb component is expressed with postural adjustment, and the rhythmicity and rate have been confirmed by objective measurements, such as, in our studies, an oscilloscopic voice analysis, accelerometer, or Motus tremometer recording. If there is an observed difference between the populations of patients with CD and tremor (CD/T) versus CD without tremor (CD/no T), then there may be either two distinct entities or one entity in which there is a comorbid factor producing tremor. Consequently, studies of cognition and affect may help discern whether there are similarities or differences between patients with focal dystonia, patients with essential tremor (ET), and patients who appear to have both phenomena.

Since 1990, our pattern of patient assessment has included a widening array of psychological and affective measures to address the relationship among CD/T, CD/no T, and ET. In the following studies, the population sizes differ, reflecting the stage of the evolution of these studies. Similarly, there may be variation in the assessment instruments used as the protocol has matured. All the studies carry a similar reservation in that they involve a referral population from a wide distribution within North America assessed in an outpatient university affiliated facility, but all patients have been examined in a similar manner, and in most instances patients have been followed for at least a few years by the same examiner and seen on more than one occasion.

STUDY I: BASELINE COGNITION AND THE EFFECT OF ANTICHOLINERGIC MEDICATIONS

In the fall of 1991 at the Movement Disorders Section meeting preceding the American Neurological Association meeting in Seattle, we presented data on 123 patients with CD, 74 of whom were evaluated while on no medications, and 49 of whom were evaluated while taking agents with anticholinergic properties (11). The two groups were similar with regard to gender split, favoring females versus males; the patients in both groups were in their early 50s at the time of the study; and the patients in both groups had similar durations of torticollis symptoms and similar severity using a 0 through 3 scale with a 0.5-gradation step. Fifteen of these patients were evaluated both on and off medications. All patients had at least two cognitive studies. The first was a measure of visual sustained attention or vigilance developed initially for assessing cognition in the use of antiepileptic drugs, the so-called 3-Letter Cancellation Task (LCT) (1). The second was the Rey version of the Auditory Verbal Learning Test (AVLT), in which two components—the learning curve and the recall or verbal memory component—were analyzed (1). Of the 49 patients on anticholinergic medications, 37 were on typical anticholinergic drugs used for dystonia, which, in order of the frequency of use, were ethopropazine, procyclidine, and trihexyphenidyl. An additional 18 patients were assessed while using antidepressant medications, namely, amitriptyline, imipramine, and maprotiline. Mean dosages in both categories of anticholinergic medications were low, 170 mg for ethopropazine, 12.5 mg for procyclidine, and 8 mg for trihexyphenidyl, and, in the second group, 85 mg for amitriptyline, 50 mg for imipramine, and 100 mg for maprotiline.

Because of the potential impact of anxiety and depression on cognition, the Minnesota Multiphasic Personality Inventory (MMPI) was completed by the patients and processed at the Mayo Clinic, Rochester, Minnesota, where one of the authors had previously been a staff member (12). Results were based on a research scale called the Purdue Anxiety Index, the Primary Depression Scale, and two research depression scales known as the Objective Depression Scale and Johnson 9. T scores at or above 68 were construed as significant for anxiety or depression.

Analysis of the 18 patients observed both on and off anticholinergic medications showed that only one patient had an improvement in LCT performance while on anticholinergic medications; 33% of the patients were worse in LCT performance, 20% were worse on verbal learning, and 73% had impairment in verbal memory on versus off medication. This suggests that anticholinergic medications increase the risk of verbal memory impairment.

In contrasting the means for the groups on versus off medication ($n = 74$ versus $n = 49$), impaired LCT performance was prevalent in both groups, in 30 of the 74 patients taking no medication (41%), and in 24 of the 49 on medication (49%). In each group the prevalence of anxiety, depression, or both was reasonably high—43% of those taking no medication and 42% of those taking anticholinergic drugs. Patients who were not using medication only occasionally demonstrated impairment in auditory verbal learning, as seen in 11 of 74 patients (15%), whereas 16 of the 49 (33%) on medications had impaired verbal learning. Four of the 11 patients (36%) off medications with impaired verbal learning had concomitant anxiety, depression, or both, whereas two of the 16

(13%) on medications with impaired verbal learning had concomitant anxiety, depression, or both. Verbal memory was impaired in 8 of the 74 (11%) not on medication, whereas 18 of the 49 (37%) on anticholinergic medication had impaired verbal recall. The difference between the two groups regarding verbal memory was significant (p <.005). Off medications, three of the eight patients with impaired AVLT performance had anxiety, depression, or both, whereas three of 18 (17%) with impaired recall on medication had evidence of anxiety, depression, or both.

From these data, it appears that the psychological states of depression or anxiety alone did not account for cognitive impairment, and that, in general, patients off medications with untreated CD had the greatest difficulty in cognition on a task of attention, whereas only if they were on anticholinergic medication was there a high frequency of verbal memory impairment. Of additional interest is the observation that some patients with profound adverse effects on short-term verbal recall were relatively young, in their mid-30s, and on doses of procyclidine as low as 5 mg per day. That observation raised the possibility that perhaps there was something unique about these patients, if not the entire population of those with CD, in which unusual sensitivity to anticholinergic drugs was manifest.

Among the limitations in interpreting these data is that there was no control group of asymptomatic patients of similar age treated with these drugs to see if there was an induced problem in verbal recall, nor was there a control pain population to ascertain the prevalence of cognitive impairment versus those with dystonia. A similar negative impact on verbal learning and recall in patients with dystonia treated by anticholinergic medications had been reported earlier that same year by Taylor and colleagues (13).

In contrast with subsequent studies we have performed, this investigation did not segregate patients on the basis of the presence or absence of tremor. What was observed, however, was that the probabilities of having difficulty in verbal learning and recall were greatest in those subjects with a phasic form of CD or in which there was an extension of the dystonic manifestation outside of the neck, whether into the upper extremity or lower cranial area or both (CD+).

A slight correlation between the emotional state and cognition was observed on the task of visual vigilance (LCT). Of the 29 patients who had impaired performance on this task, but on no medication, ten, more than a third, had concomitant evidence of anxiety as measured by the MMPI.

STUDY 2: AFFECT IN CERVICAL DYSTONIA VERSUS SPINE PAIN CONTROLS

At the Second International Congress of Movement Disorders in Munich, Germany, in June 1992, we presented data on the occurrence of emotional symptoms of depression, anxiety, and the relationship between antecedent stress and the onset of CD by contrasting the history and examinations of 201 CD patients with those of 135 spine pain control subjects who had been evaluated at the Arizona Dystonia Institute, all evaluated by the same examiner (14).

The gender ratio was similar in this study between the two groups, favoring females over males, with a mean age in the early 50s. One hundred ninety-one of the subjects with CD had completed the MMPI, the Beck Depression Inventory (15), and/or the Spielberger Anxiety Scale (16), whereas 96 of the 135 pain controls had similar assessment. All subjects provided a personal and family history and pain severity data. Duration of symptoms was twice as long in the CD subjects at 9½ years versus a little more than 4½ years in the spine pain control subjects. Both groups, surprisingly, had an antecedent to the onset of their spine pain or CD, a 20% risk in the case of CD and an 18% risk in those with spine pain, of prior psychiatric diagnosis and treatment. In the year prior to the first symptom of CD or of the spine pain syndrome, 50% of the patients with CD had had major emotional stressor(s) versus 32% of those in the spine pain group (p = .01). A psychiatric diagnosis and treatment after the onset of symptoms in these two groups was 13% in those with CD and 3% in those with spine pain (p <.001).

Of the 180 CD patients who completed the MMPI, 18% had evidence of depression, with T scores in excess of 68 on the primary D scale, whereas 33% had evidence of anxiety as shown on the Purdue Anxiety Index, with T scores above 68. In contrast, in the spine pain control group, 63 of whom had completed the MMPI, 13% had evidence of depression (p <.05). There was a statistically insignificant difference in anxiety, 37% in the control group.

Our subsequent clinical studies have suggested the use of the Toronto Western Spasmodic Torticollis Rating Scale (TWSTRS) (17), because the presence of depression, as defined by the MMPI, is associated with higher scores for disability and objective severity scores for the dystonia. The mechanism of production of this aggravation of the latter score particularly is unclear, unless mechanisms of compensation utilized by the emotionally intact patient are more effective in suppressing the contraction of the dystonic muscles, or unless it is the case that depression activates dystonic pathophysiology.

STUDY 3: URINARY 24-HOUR MHPG LEVELS IN CERVICAL DYSTONIA

In the fall of 1994, at the Movement Disorders Section meeting preceding the American Neurological Association meeting in San Francisco, we presented a paper on the ranges of levels of 24-hour urinary 3-meth-hydroxy-phenylglycol (MHPG) in patients with CD versus a control group (18). The measurements were performed on 198 CD patients and contrasted with the results from 94 control subjects. One hundred forty-eight of the CD patients were female versus 47 of the control subjects. Controls were subjects used by the Mayo Clinic, Rochester, Minnesota, to establish normative MHPG levels. Samples were collected over 24 hours, and analyses were performed at the Mayo Clinic, whose staff coauthored the study.

Our CD group had a mean age of 54 years versus 41 years for the control group. Neither the control patients nor the CD patients were using medication during the collection of urine.

Limitations of the study included the lack of clarity as to the extent to which peripheral sources of MHPG rather than central sources of this norepinephrine degradation product affect the urinary measurements. In psychiatry, low urinary MHPG levels have been associated with treatment success when the concomitant mood disorder is treated with the tricyclic agent imipramine (19). A possible value of studying MHPG is that it might explain why depression is common in patients with CD or it might provide a means by which depression, when present, may be treated. However, it is possible that levels of anxiety might contribute to elevated norepinephrine levels. The primary central nervous system (CNS) site for norepinephrine is the locus ceruleus within the brainstem. The brainstem is a recognized potential source for dystonic symptoms, especially cranial, but cervical as well (20). Since CD is not a uniform disorder, in that some patients have concomitant tremor and some have spread of dystonic symptoms to other body parts, perhaps measurements such as MHPG levels would correlate with one or more subtype characteristic.

The analysis of variance (ANOVA) showed insignificant differences between male controls and male CD patients, focal CD and segmental dystonia, dark-colored and light-colored eyes [i.e., blue, green, gray or hazel, which are overrepresented in patients with CD (11)], as well as insignificant differences with regard to age of CD onset, prior drug exposure, presence of tremor, and MMPI evidence of depression or anxiety. What did significantly correlate with low urinary MHPG levels (p ≤.05) were all males versus all females, controls versus CD patients, female controls versus female CD patients, CD patients without antecedent trauma versus those with antecedent trauma, and CD patients with no family history of tremor versus those with family history of tremor. In each of these comparison pairs, the second had a lower level of MHPG. This evidence of lowered urinary MHPG levels in patients versus controls suggests a lowered central norepinephrine level of activity, which might result in the use of noradrenergic therapies such as imipramine. Our clinical experience includes some anecdotal occurrences of reduction in CD symptoms to the level of remission with tricyclic agent therapy, such as with imipramine or its breakdown product desipramine.

STUDY 4: AFFECT AND COGNITION IN ESSENTIAL TREMOR

To investigate the possible relationship between tremor presumably of the essential type (ET) and dystonia (CD) we embarked in 2001 on a retrospective analysis of 55 ET patients evaluated at the Arizona Dystonia Institute, many of whom were assessed with a cognitive battery expanded in comparison to the limited one in use in our CD study of 1991 (21). In addition, mood measures included the MMPI, the Spielberger Anxiety Index (Spiel-Anx), and the Hamilton Depression Rating Scale (Ham-D) (22). The results of this investigation were presented at the International Symposium on Mental and Behavioral Dysfunction in Movement Disorders in Montreal in the fall of 2001. Sixty-two percent of the patients were female, their mean age of onset was 46 years, and the mean age at evaluation was 57 years. Tremor location was head only in 14%, hands only in 69%, and both head and hands in 16%. The mean educational level of the group was 14 years. Overall, the tremor was mild as judged by a mean Tremor Rating Scale of 12 ± 4 (23). At the time of the cognitive assessment no medications were in use.

The family history of this group for nonparkinsonian tremor was 49%; for three fourths of the patients the tremor was described as being in the hands only, dystonia in 2%, scoliosis in 5.5%, and Parkinson's disease in 2%. Family psychiatric history, using criteria of the *Diagnostic and Statistical Manual of Mental Disorders*, 4th edition (DSM-IV) (24), showed anxiety in 7%, depression in 31%, obsessive-compulsive disorder in 9%, and alcohol abuse in 18%.

The patients' personal evidence of psychiatric dysfunction as measured by the psychological studies mentioned previously and by using T scores on the MMPI of 68 or higher, Ham-D scores of 15 or higher, and Spiel-Anx scores of 40 or higher yielded the following: anxiety alone in 13%, depression alone in 7%, anxiety and depression in 42%, and obsessive-compulsive disorder in 15%. In other words, 55% demonstrated anxiety and 49% depression.

The cognitive test battery employed included the Rey AVLT, Rey Osterrieth Complex Figure (ROCF), LCT, Digit Span (DS), Wisconsin Card Sorting Test (WCST) and in some instances the Test of Variables of Attention (TOVA) and/or the Conners Continuous Performance Test (CPT) (1).

In the analysis, we differentiated patients on the basis of whether they exceeded the age-normed performance above the 15th percentile of control subjects listed for these instruments. The percentage of patients demonstrating impairment of a specific cognitive function as measured by the instrument was as follows: visual-motor skill (ROCF) 2/40 (5%), digital memory (DS) 6/31 (19%), auditory verbal memory (AVLT) 9/46 (20%), auditory verbal learning (AVLT) 11/46 (24%), visual spatial memory (ROCF) 11/40 (28%), executive function (WCST) 5/18 (28%), visual attention (LCT) 25/45 (56%), and visual attention as assessed by TOVA or CPT 12/17 (71%).

Presented at the same meeting and published just prior to it, Lombardi et al. (25) described cognitive deficits in 18 ET patients in Utah, ten of whom were male, all of whom had only upper limb tremor, whose average age was 66 years, who had been symptomatic for an average of 36 years, and who had, on average, 14 years of education. Their tremor rating scale scores were 19 ± 8, and eight of the 18 patients were taking either primidone or propranolol. These findings were contrasted with those of 18 parkinsonian patients.

The assessment of these 18 patients included measures of depression, the WCST, DS, the California Verbal Learning Test, a test of verbal fluency, and the Boston Naming Test. We have since contrasted our data with those of 79 patients who have CD and tremor, just as Lombardi et al. had contrasted their data with a population of similar size of Parkinson's patients.

The results in the two studies differed, with a much higher proportion of patients who had difficulty with verbal learning and memory in the Utah population. Three of four patients in our investigation had no impairment of either verbal learning or memory. Only 19% of our patients underperformed on DS. Only 28% of our patients underperformed on the WCST. Both patient populations did well on visual spatial skills and both had a high rate of depression, 49% in our population. We included visual attention tasks that were not part of the Utah protocol. In our study, visual attention impairment was observed in the majority of patients studied, whether it was the LCT, TOVA, or CPT. The next study section in this chapter addresses the comparison between CD/T and ET.

In a letter to the editor of *Neurology,* we discussed the differences between the two study groups: the Utah group included patients on medications, was older, and had greater severity of tremor, as the patients were being considered for surgery (26).

The question of the effects of surgery for tremor on cognition or affect is not germane to our discussion. However, there are several studies that suggest that uncomplicated surgical treatment is cognitively well tolerated (27).

STUDY 5: COGNITION AND AFFECT IN CERVICAL DYSTONIA WITH TREMOR

From our database of CD patients, we analyzed 79 subjects with CD/T (28). All patients completed the MMPI, many completed the Ham-D and Spiel-Anx, and some completed the Yale-Brown Obsessive-Compulsive Rating Scales (29). Virtually all patients had completed the AVLT, LCT, and ROCF, many completed the DS, and some completed the WCST, TOVA, or CPT. Sixty-nine (87%) were female, mean age for the group was 59 years at the time of study, mean age at CD onset was 47 years and the same for tremor; however, in one fourth of the patients tremor preceded dystonia and in one fourth dystonia preceded tremor. Tremor was defined and evaluated as described previously. Tremor location was head only in 68%, hands only in 5%, and both head and hands in 27%. Therefore, head tremor occurred in 75 of 79 patients.

A family history of involuntary movement disorder occurred as follows: non-parkinsonian tremor in 48% (18% head, 22% hands, 10% both head and hands), dystonia in 17%, scoliosis in 14%, and Parkinson's disease in 8%. As has been our custom for a number of years, to aid patients in distinguishing between essential forms of tremor and parkinsonian tremor, we demonstrated examples of these and the additional manifestations of parkinsonian states, to assist in clarification of the affected family member who had to have been observed by the patient.

A family history of psychiatric disorder was as follows: anxiety 13%, depression 22%, obsessive-compulsive disorder 6%, psychosis 5%, and alcohol abuse 37%. In the patients themselves using the criteria defined previously, anxiety was present in 52%, depression in 72%, and obsessive-compulsive disorder in 9%. These are even higher than the rates we observed in our 1992 study and significantly greater than the rates for the spine pain control group in that study.

Just as we have done with respect to essential tremor patients, we defined impaired neuropsychological performance as the bottom 15% on age-normed performance. By analyzing the components of the neuropsychological battery, we determined the findings with regard to impairment to be as follows: visual-motor skill (ROCF) 1/68 (1%), auditory verbal memory (AVLT) 6/72 (8%), digital memory (DS) 4/41 (10%), auditory verbal learning curve (AVLT) 9/72 (13%), visual spatial memory (ROCF) 11/68 (16%), executive function (WCST) 12/21 (57%), visual attention (LCT) 46/72 (64%), and visual attention (TOVA/CPT) 13/14 (93%).

Our interpretation of the data was that visual attention is a prominent deficit in a relatively young patient group on no medications, in which both tremor and dystonia are manifest. Furthermore, there is a high frequency of family history of tremor as well as dystonia and scoliosis, but not especially of parkinsonism. Although psychiatric family history was prevalent, it did not seem prevalent enough to explain the frequency of psychiatric manifestations in these patients. A weakness of the study is that there is no parallel cognitive study as was the case with the affective measures in our spine pain control subjects in 1992. Finally, the risk for depression or anxiety, but especially the former, is significantly higher in patients who have their tremor manifestation primarily in the head versus the hands and who have concomitant dystonia of at least the neck. Whether this represents the effects of pain, disfigurement in a readily observable body location, or an intrinsic difference between the disorders has not been determined.

STUDY 6: AFFECT AND COGNITION IN CERVICAL DYSTONIA WITHOUT TREMOR

From the same database from which we had derived our CD/T subjects, we analyzed 165 CD/No T patients, 117 of whom (71%) were female, and 29% of whom had at least one additional dystonic site (CD+) but not generalized dystonia (30). For this group the mean age at the evaluation was 52 years, with a mean duration of symptoms of 8 years, i.e., onset at around age 44. All had completed the MMPI; many had completed the Ham-D and/or Spiel-Anx; most had completed the AVLT, LCT, and ROCF; more than half had completed the DS; and about a fifth had completed the WCST. Eighteen had completed the TOVA or CPT.

The family history of psychiatric disorder showed anxiety in 9%, depression in 35%, obsessive-compulsive disorder in 10%, alcohol

abuse in 33%, and psychosis in 5%. On the MMPI and related instruments, anxiety was observed in 50% and depression in 62%.

Family history of movement disorder included nonparkinsonian tremor 32% (in half it was only the head, in a quarter only the hands, and in a quarter both head and hands), dystonia 10%, scoliosis 17%, and parkinsonism 10%.

The cognitive assessments revealed impairment in the following pattern: impaired verbal learning (AVLT) 19/138 (14%), impaired verbal memory (AVLT) 15/138 (11%), impaired auditory digital memory (DS) 11/89 (12%), impaired visual vigilance (LCT) 87/135 (64%), impaired visual spatial memory (ROCF) 19/126 (15%), impaired visual attention (TOVA/CPT) 7/18 (39%), and impaired executive function (WCST) 25/35 (71%).

CONCLUSION: ESSENTIAL TREMOR VERSUS CERVICAL DYSTONIA WITH TREMOR VERSUS CERVICAL DYSTONIA WITHOUT TREMOR

Table 25-1 summarizes the findings of the last three studies pertaining to ET, CD/T, and CD/no T. Although the population sizes are not equal, it is not inappropriate to compare and contrast the findings in these three groups as the sample size is reasonable. All three groups are of similar age. There are more females than males in all three groups, with the highest ratio of females to males in the CD/T group. Further analysis might be required of the ET group females to see if their characteristics are more similar to those in the CD/T group.

All three groups have a high frequency of occurrence of family history of movement disorder, especially with respect to tremor. They are virtually equivalent in the ET and CD/T group, both with a higher rate of occurrence than in these CD/no T. Dystonia is much more common in the two CD groups, with or without tremor, as contrasted with the ET group. The rate of scoliosis is statistically higher in the CD/T and CD/No T group versus the ET group. Parkinsonism is a bit more common in CD/T and CD/No T and equiva-

TABLE 25-1. *Essential tremor (ET) versus cervical dystonia with tremor (CT/T) versus cervical dystonia with no tremor (CD/No T)*

	ET	CD/T	CD/No T	p
Psychiatric disorder				
n	55	79	165	
F/M	34/21	69/10	117/48	
Mean age at study (yr)	57	59	53	
Family history psychiatric disorder[a]				
Anxiety	4 (7%)	10 (13%)	15 (9%)	NS
Depression	17 (31%)	11 (14%)	58 (35%)	<.05[b]
Alcohol abuse	10 (18%)	27 (37%)	55 (33%)	<.01[c]
Personal evidence psychiatric disorder[d]				
Anxiety	30 (55%)	41 (52%)	84 (51%)	NS
Depression[e]	27 (49%)	66 (84%)	103 (62%)	<.01[c]
Family history movement disorders				
n	55	79	165	
Tremor Total	27 (49%)	38 (48%)	60 (36%)	NS
Head only	4 (15%)	13 (34%)	29 (48%)	
Hands only	20 (74%)	17 (45%)	15 (25%)	.05[f1]
Both head and hands	3 (11%)	8 (21%)	16 (27%)	
Dystonia	1 (2%)	13 (16%)	16 (10%)	<.01
Scoliosis	3 (5%)	11 (14%)	27 (16%)	.09
Parkinson's disease	1 (2%)	6 (8%)	17 (10%)	NS
Patient tremor location				
Head only	8 (14%)	54 (68%)	—	
Hands only	38 (69%)	4 (5%)	—	<.01[f2]
Both head and hands	9 (16%)	21 (27%)	—	
Cognitive impairment[g]				
Female/male	34/21	69/10	117/48	
Mean age at study (yr)	57	59	53	
Mean years of education	14	14	14	
Cognitive function (test)				
Impaired performance				
Verbal learning (AVLT)	11/46 (24%)	9/72 (13%)	19/138 (14%)	NS
Verbal memory (AVLT)	9/46 (20%)	6/72 (8%)	15/138 (11%)	.07
Visual attention (LCT)	25/45 (56%)	46/72 (64%)	87/135 (64%)	NS
Digital memory (DS)	6/31 (19%)	4/41 (10%)	11/89 (12%)	NS
Visual motor/memory (ROCF)	11/40 (28%)	11/68 (16%)	19/126 (15%)	NS
Executive function (WCST)	5/18 (28%)	12/21 (57%)	25/35 (71%)	.07[h], <.05[i]

[a]*Diagnostic and Statistical Manual of Mental Disorders,* 4th ed. (DSM-IV) criterion referenced first-degree relatives.

[b]*p* <.05 CD/T vs. ET, CD/No T.

[c]*p* <.01 CD/T, CD/No T vs. ET.

[d]Minnesota Multiphasic Personality Inventory (MMPI) T score >68.

[e]In-spine pain controls (*n* = 63), anxiety 37% (NS), depression 13%; *p* ≤.05 for all three groups (14).

[f1]Head vs. hand tremor in CD/T, vs. ET.

[f2]No tremor.

[g]Bottom 15% for age-matched norms.

[h]ET vs. CD/T.

[i]ET vs. CD/No T.

AVLT, Rey Auditory Verbal Learning Test; LCT, 3 Letter Cancellation Test; DS, Digit Span Test; ROCF, Rey-Osterrieth Complex Figure; WCST, Wisconsin Card Sorting Test.

lent between these two; it is higher in both groups than in the ET population.

With respect to family history of psychiatric disorder, it is roughly equivalent for all three populations with regard to reported family history of anxiety. Depression was least common among the CD/T population and roughly equivalent in the ET and CD/No T populations. The rates are relatively high in these groups versus the control studies of 14% that we had reported in a poster at the American Psychiatric Association annual meeting in 1993 (31). A statistically significant higher rate of occurrence of family history of alcohol abuse is noted in both CD groups, with or without tremor, when contrasted with the ET population.

All three populations have personal evidence of anxiety at levels that are even higher than we previously observed in 1992 in our CD population that was not subgrouped, and much higher when contrasted with the control group of that study. Depression is prevalent also in all three populations, but is statistically significantly increased in the CD/T versus both CD/No T and ET and slightly higher in the CD/No T group versus the ET group.

In those patients demonstrating tremor in this study, there was a bias of patients with hand tremor in the ET population and head tremor in the CD/T population. An interesting examination would be to evaluate only patients with head tremor or head and hand tremor to see if there are more parallels between that subgroup of ET patients and the CD/T population.

With respect to cognition, both CD/T and CD/No T have a lower rate of occurrence of verbal learning and verbal memory difficulty ($p = .07$ and $p = .11$, respectively), and a much higher rate of occurrence of executive dysfunction as measured by the WCST ($p = .07$). All three populations have difficulty in visual attention as measured by the LCT. However, the small population in each that has undergone TOVA and/or CPT does not reach statistical significance ($p = .12$). All three populations have low rates of occurrence of visual perception, visual-motor, or visual memory problems. Thus, like the study of Lombardi et al. (25), semantic memory is a far more common deficit in the ET population. In our study, age is not a factor, as both groups are of comparable middle age.

In contrast to the study of Jahanshahi et al. (32), this much larger study in focal dystonia does not appear to support the absence of executive dysfunction but rather suggests that in the majority of patients with focal dystonia with or without tremor and in contrast to those with ET, there is impaired basal ganglion to frontal neocortical function. These data also lend support to an al-

ternative mechanism of cerebellar dysfunction in essential tremor in contrast to that in focal dystonia.

ACKNOWLEDGMENT

This study was supported in part by the Foundation for Clinical Neuroscience.

REFERENCES

1. Lezak MD. *Neuropsychological assessment,* 3rd ed. New York: Oxford University Press, 1995.
2. Rao SM. Neuropsychological assessment. In: Fogel BS, Schiffer RB, Rao SM, eds. *Neuropsychiatry.* Baltimore: Williams & Wilkins, 1996:29–45.
3. Bear D, Fedio P. Quantitative analysis of interictal behavior in temporal lobe epilepsy. *Arch Neurol* 1977;34: 454–467.
4. Schildkraut JJ, Kety SS. Biogenic amines and emotion. *Science* 1967;156:21–30.
5. Duane DD, Clark M, LaPointe LL, et al. Tremor characteristics and family history of patients with essential tremor versus cervical dystonia associated with tremor. *Can J Neurolog Sci* 1993;20(40):S237.
6. Jankovic J, Leder S, Warner D, et al. Cervical dystonia: clinical findings and associated movement disorders. *Neurology* 1991;41:1088–1091.
7. Jedynak CP, Bonnet AM, Agid Y. Tremor and idiopathic dystonia. *Mov Disord* 1991;6:230–236.
8. Duane DD, Clark M, Gottlob L, et al. The influence of family history of tremor on cervical dystonia. *Mov Disord* 1993;8:313–314.
9. Deuschl G, Heinen F, Guchlbauer B, et al. Hand tremor in patients with spasmodic torticollis. *Mov Disord* 1997; 12:547–552.
10. Duane DD, Case JL, LaPointe LL. Cognition in treated and untreated spasmodic torticollis. *Mov Disord* 1991; 6:274.
11. Duane DD. Spasmodic torticollis: clinical and biologic features and their implications for focal dystonia. *Adv Neurol* 1988;50:473–792.
12. Hathaway SR, McKinley JC. *The Minnesota Multiphasic Personality Inventory.* Minneapolis: University of Minnesota Press, 1943, 1970.
13. Taylor AE, Lang AE, Saint-Cyr JA, et al. Cognitive processes in idiopathic dystonia treated with high-dose anticholinergic therapy: implications for treatment strategies. *Clin Neuropharmacol* 1991;14: 62–77.
14. Duane DD, Berman MB. Depression and anxiety in cervical dystonia patients versus spine pain controls. *Mov Disord* 1992;7:124.
15. Beck AT, Ward CH, Mendelson M, et al. An inventory for measuring depression. *Arch Gen Psychiatry* 1961; 41:561–571.
16. Spielberger CD, Gorsuch RL, Lushene RE. *STAI Manual for the State-Trait Anxiety Inventory.* Palo Alto, CA: Consulting Psychologists Press, 1970.
17. Consky ES, Lang AE, Clinical assessments of patients with cervical dystonia. In: Jankovic J, Hallett M, eds.

Therapy with botulinum toxin. New York: Marcel Dekker, 1994:211–237.

18. Duane DD, Gottlob L, Brennan ME, et al. Urinary MHPG levels in cervical dystonia: a possible aid to subtyping. *Mov Disord* 1994;9:487.

19. Maas JW, ed. *MHPG: basic mechanisms and psychopathology.* New York: Academic Press, 1983.

20. Jankovic J, Patel SC. Blepharospasm associated with brainstem lesions. *Neurology* 1983;33:1237–1240.

21. Duane DD, Vermilion K, Stone A. Cognition and affect in idiopathic-essential tremor. *Mov Disord* 2001;16:(suppl 1):S30.

22. Hamilton M. A rating scale for depression. *J Neurol Neurosurg Psychiatry* 1960;23:56–62.

23. Fahn S, Tolosa E, Marin C. Clinical rating scale for tremor. In: Jankovic J, Tolosa E, eds. *Parkinson's disease and movement disorders,* 2nd ed. Baltimore: Williams & Wilkins, 1993:271–280.

24. American Psychiatric Association. *Diagnostic and statistical manual of mental disorders,* 4th ed. Washington, DC: American Psychiatric Association, 1994.

25. Lombardi WJ, Woolson BA, Roberts JW, et al. Cognitive deficits in patients with essential tremor. *Neurology* 2001;57:785–790.

26. Duane DD, Vermilion K. Cognitive deficits in patients with essential tremor. *Neurology* 2002;58:1706.

27. Troster AI, Fields JA, Pahwa R, et al. Neuropsychological and qualitative life outcome after thalamic stimulation for essential tremor. *Neurology* 1999;53:1774–1780.

28. Vermilion K, Johnson J, Duane D. Cognition and affect in patients with cervical dystonia and tremor. *Mov Disord* 2002;17:1138.

29. Goodman WK, Price LH, Rasmussen SA, et al. The Yale-Brown Obsessive-Compulsive Scale. I. Development, use, and reliability. *Arch Gen Psychiatry* 1989;46:1006–1011.

30. Vermilon K, Peterson J, Duane D. Cognition and affect in patients with cervical dystonia without tremor. *Mov Disord* 2002;17(suppl 5):S281.

31. Duane DD, Brennan ME, Wallrichs S, et al. Familial occurrence of ADHD, reading disorder, mood disorder, sleep disorder in ADHD with and without reading disorder. *American Psychiatric Association New Research Program and Abstracts* 1993;NR563:201.

32. Jahanshahi M, Rowe J, Fuller R. Cognitive executive function in idiopathic dystonia. *Mov Disord* 2002;17:1120.

Dystonia 4: Advances in Neurology, Vol. 94. Edited by Stanley Fahn, Mark Hallett, and Mahlon R. DeLong. Lippincott Williams & Wilkins, Philadelphia © 2004.

26

Clinical Features of the *Geste Antagoniste* in Cervical Dystonia

*Saša R. Filipović, †Marjan Jahanshahi, ‡Ramachandran Viswanathan, §Peter Heywood, ‖Daniel Rogers, and ‡Kailash P. Bhatia

Burden Neurological Institute, and Departments of Neurology and Neuropsychiatry, Frenchay Hospital, Bristol, United Kingdom. †Sobell Department of Motor Neurosciences and Movement Disorders, Institute of Neurology, Queen Square, London, United Kingdom. ‡Institute of Neurology, and National Hospital for Neurology and Neurosurgery, Queen Square, London, United Kingdom. §Department of Neurology, Frenchay Hospital, Bristol, United Kingdom. ‖Department of Neuropsychiatry, Frenchay Hospital, Bristol, United Kingdom

Patients with dystonia, particularly those with focal dystonias, are often able to reduce or even eliminate their abnormal postures, movements, or associated feelings of pain and tenderness by using certain maneuvers that involve tactile or proprioceptive stimulation. This distinctive phenomenon, usually referred to as *geste antagoniste* (GA) or "sensory trick," has been well established as a clinical feature of dystonia, and particularly of cervical dystonia (CD) (1–3). The physiologic mechanisms behind this phenomenon are unknown, and the GA has only rarely been the subject of clinical, physiologic, or epidemiologic studies.

In fact, most epidemiologic studies of CD registered the frequency of occurrence of GA, sometimes assessing a few of its other characteristics, but as a rule fell short of evaluating this phenomenon in detail. Only a few published studies have systematically evaluated the phenomenon of GA in dystonia (4–7). However, these studies have primarily tried to measure the physiologic effects of GA (4–6) or to objectively quantify its effects (7). Consequently, they have predominantly targeted groups of patients with well-expressed GA effects, and comparisons with patients devoid of this phenomenon are usually lacking. In addition, the population of patients studied has generally been limited in size and in geographic location.

To assess the phenomenon of GA in more detail, we developed a questionnaire and administered it to a series of consecutive patients with idiopathic CD attending two large botulinum toxin (BT) injection clinics with geographically distinct catchment areas. This chapter addresses the following issues: (a) whether there are any clinical features that distinguish patients with and without GA, (b) the natural history of GA, (c) the magnitude and other characteristics of GA effects, and (d) whether there are any clinical features that influence the magnitude of the GA effect.

METHOD

Subjects

The population base for the study was formed from the patients attending one of two participating BT injection outpatient clinics. The clinics were at the National Hospital for Neurology and Neurosurgery in London (led by K.P.B.) and the Frenchay Hospital in Bristol (led by D.R. and P.H.). Both clinics were to a large extent dedicated to patients with CD.

Only patients presenting with idiopathic CD, either isolated or as a part of segmental dystonia, of a severity to require regular BT injections, were included in the study. Patients were given a questionnaire (see Appendix) and were asked to complete it at home and to mail it back in the self-addressed and stamped envelope provided. The voluntary and anonymous nature of the questionnaire was clearly stressed.

The Questionnaire

The questionnaire consisted of 27 questions that were thematically divided into three parts. The first part addressed basic demographic (age, gender) and clinical characteristics (duration, type of head/neck deviation, presence of head tremor). In addition, patients were asked to gauge how much control they had over their head and neck position on a scale from 0 (no control at all) to 10 (complete control). Patients were also asked whether they had been receiving BT injections, and if they did, to gauge the effect of injections on their CD over time. Finally, the concept of GA was explained and patients were asked whether they had ever been able to reduce the severity of their CD by touching certain parts of their face or neck. If the answer to this was no, they were asked to check whether they nevertheless had GA by systematically touching defined regions of the head and neck. If the answer was still no, then the questionnaire was considered completed. However, if the patients responded affirmatively to the GA question at any stage, they were asked to continue further.

The second part of the questionnaire targeted the global features of the clinical effect of GA, i.e., when it was first noticed, whether it was still present and if not when it had stopped, and its relationship with the effect of BT injections. Also, the variability of GA occurrence and effectiveness, as well as the perceived magnitude of the GA's effect, when it had been most effective, were determined. Patients were first asked to assess the GA's ability to improve their CD in general. They were

then asked about effectiveness of the GA in (a) correcting the position of the head, neck, or shoulder ("position"); (b) restoring neck and shoulder movements ("movements"); and (c) in relieving the feelings of tension, tenderness, or aching in the neck and/or shoulder ("pain").

The third part of the questionnaire dealt with detailed phenomenology of the GA maneuver (e.g., target sites on the head and neck, their laterality, the exclusiveness of the parts of the hand able to elicit GA effect). These data form an essentially distinct thematic subset, and space limitations prevent us from presenting them here.

Statistics

The age, age at CD onset, and duration of CD were the only continuous variables, and they were analyzed using a parametric method, i.e., Student's t-test. All other variables were either interval or categorical and they were analyzed using nonparametric methods; the method that has been used in each instance is cited (8). Since this was an exploratory study, no correction for number of comparisons was used and the level of significance was set at $p < .05$.

RESULTS

A total of 150 questionnaires were given to patients; 108 were returned (57 from London patients and 51 from Bristol patients), and of these, six had a significant proportion of data missing or were inadequately completed. Therefore, our analysis was based on 102 adequately completed or almost completed (i.e., more than 80% of questions answered)[1] questionnaires. The mean age of this group was 56 years [standard deviation (SD) 12.2, range 30–82], the mean age at the onset of CD was 43 years (SD 13.8, range 5–76), and mean CD duration was 13 years (SD 8.3, range 1–50); 65.4% of the patients in this group were

---

[1] When answers to some questions were missing, the actual number of patients who provided the answers to the question is indicated in the text (*n*).

women. The most frequent feature of CD was rotacollis (89%), defined to the patients as turning of the head to one side, followed by laterocollis (44%), defined as leaning of the head toward the shoulder; retrocollis (19%) and anterocollis (7%), defined as bending of the neck backward and forward, respectively, were the least frequent. The isolated presence of only one of these features was reported by 47% of patients, while in the remaining 53% they were combined (complex CD). The rotacollis was the most frequent feature of simple CD (87.5%), and an almost ubiquitous feature of complex CD (96%). Head tremor was present in 59% of the patients. All but two of the patients had received BT injections at least once prior to answering the questionnaire.

Sixty-five patients (64%) reported that they had a GA (GA+). In comparison to the subgroup of patients without a GA (GA−), the GA+ subgroup was marginally younger and had a marginally longer duration of CD at the time of completing the questionnaire, while there was no difference in gender distribution between the groups (Table 26-1). However, the GA+ subgroup had a significantly earlier onset of CD than the GA− subgroup (Table 26-1).[2] This was mainly due to the fact that almost all of the GA− patients had CD onset after the age of 32; there was only one GA− patient with CD onset at the age of 19. However, in 18 (28%) of the CD+ patients, the CD started before or at the age of 32. Moreover, when only patients with CD onset after the age of 32 were compared, neither the age at CD onset nor the actual age and duration of CD differed between GA+ and GA− subgroups (student test (77) <1.5, p >.15 for all comparisons).

Rotacollis was significantly more frequent in GA+ than in GA− patients, while there was no difference in the frequency of occurrence of laterocollis, retrocollis, anterocollis, head tremor, or complex CD between two subgroups (Table 26-1). Also, there was no difference in the perceived severity of CD, indexed as the feeling of control over one's neck/head position, or in the perceived effect of BT injections between the two subgroups (Table 26-1).

---

[2]Although mathematically related, the age, the age at onset, and the duration of the disease all have sound theoretical reasons to be able to independently influence the target variable (i.e., patients reporting of presence or absence of GA).

TABLE 26-1. *Comparison of the demographic and clinical characteristics of the two subgroups of cervical dystonia (CD) patients*

	No GA (GA−)	GA present (GA+)	Statistics
Age (years)*	59.2 (10.1)	54.3 (13.1)	$t(100) = 1.99$, $p = .05$[1]
Age at onset of the CD (years)*	48.8 (11.7)	40.0 (14.2)	$t(96) = 3.13$, $p = .002$[1]
Duration of the CD (years)*	11.0 (5.9)	14.5 (9.3)	$t(96) = 2.02$, $p = .05$[1]
Gender (female/male ratio)	1.65	1.96	$Chi^2(1) = 0.17$, NS[2]
Clinical characteristics			
Rotacollis (%)	77.8	95.4	$Chi^2(1) = 5.70$, $p = .017$[3]
Laterocollis (%)	50.0	41.5	$Chi^2(1) = 0.67$, NS[2]
Retrocollis/anterocollis (%)	19.4/11.1	18.5/4.6	$Chi^2(2) = 1.60$, NS[2]
Complex CD (%)			
Head tremor (%)	63.9	56.3	$Chi^2(1) = 0.56$, NS[2]
Feeling of control (10-point scale)*	5.0 (2.7)	5.4 (2.3)	$Z = 0.65$, NS[4]
Botulinum toxin effect			
1. Excellent from the beginning and still the same (%)	31.3	31.1	
2. Excellent from the beginning but diminished with time (%)	25.0	29.5	
3. Moderate from the beginning (%)	31.3	24.6	
4. Variable (%)	12.5	14.8	$Chi^2(3) = 0.58$, NS[2]

*Values presented as mean (standard deviation).
GA, geste antagoniste.
[1]Student's t-test; [2]Chi² test; [3]Chi² test with Yates correction; [4]Mann-Whitney U Test.

Of GA+ patients, 60% discovered the presence of a GA at the time of CD onset, while 37% became aware of their GA some time after the onset of CD (median 5 years, range 1–34). Two patients (3%) discovered their GA while completing the questionnaire. In the great majority (92%) of the patients (*n* = 63), the GA was still effective, while only five patients (8%) noticed that their GA stopped being effective. However, the beneficial effect

of BT injections made 30% of GA+ patients (*n* = 60) use their GA rarely if ever, while 53% were still using it and considered its effect unchanged. Only 13% of GA+ patients had found that the GA effect had become weaker or disappeared after they started BT injections (Fig. 26-1A). The good BT effect was predominant (88.9%) among the rare GA users, while among persistent GA users good and not-so-good (unpredictable or unsatisfac-

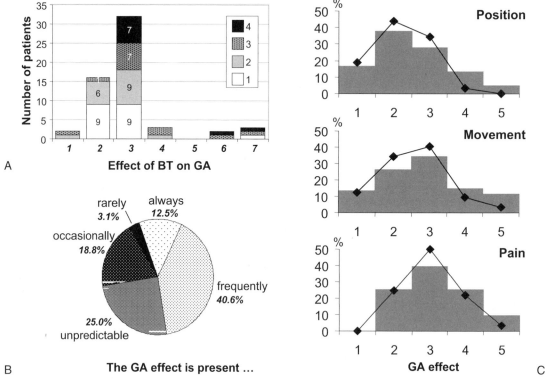

Fig. 26-1. Some characteristics of the *geste antagoniste* (GA). **A:** Interaction between patients' perceived effect of botulinum toxin (BT) injections on cervical dystonia (CD) (*shading:* 1 = excellent from the beginning and still the same, 2 = excellent from the beginning but diminished with time, 3 = moderate from the beginning, and 4 = variable) and the effect of BT on GA (x-axes: 1 = not using/not need GA since started BT, 2 = hardly using GA because BT is so good, 3 = still using GA and it works as usual, 4 = still using GA but works less than before, 5 = still using GA and works better than before, 6 = still using GA but works much more unpredictably than before, 7 = since BT started, GA not working anymore); y-axes, percentage of total number of GA+ patients. **B:** How often the GA is effective (frequently = more than 75% of the time, unpredictable = about 50% of the time, occasionally = less than 50% of the time, rarely = less than 25% of the time). **C:** The magnitude of the GA effect on the three main aspects of CD [x-axes: 1 = complete improvement (100%), 2 = significant improvement (75%), 3 = moderate improvement ("to some extent," ~50%), 4 = small improvement (25%), 5 = no impact; y-axes: percentage of patients]; histogram represents the results from all patients with GA, line represents the results from 32 patients who had "effect of BT on GA" = 3 (see Fig. 26–1A).

tory) BT effects were equally distributed (56% and 44%, respectively) (Fig. 26-1A); a significant difference in distribution (Yates corrected $Chi^2 = 4.24$, $p = .039$).

More than 50% of the patients ($n = 64$) indicated that their GA was effective, either "always" or "frequently" (i.e., "more than 75% of the time") (Fig. 26-1B). When present, the effect of the GA was judged as "always the same" by 40% of the patients ($n = 60$), while it was judged as "variable" by the remaining 60% of patients. The majority (71%) of the patients ($n = 63$) were of the opinion that during the period when it was the most effective, the GA was able to improve their CD in general by at least 50% (30% even considered that the improvement associated with the GA was 75% or better). In contrast, 14% of the patients found that the GA effect was only "minimal" (i.e., "less than 25% better"). A greater than 50% improvement associated with the GA was reported by 82% of the patients ($n = 61$) regarding correcting "position," by 74% ($n = 61$) regarding improvement of "movements," and by 65% ($n = 63$) regarding feelings of "pain."

The pattern of effectiveness of the GA (Fig. 26-1C) significantly differed across the effects on position, movements, and pain [Friedman analysis of variance (ANOVA) $Chi^2 = 23.21$ ($n = 61$, degrees of freedom [df] = 2), $p < .00001$]: the GA effect was significantly better for position than for movements or pain [Wilcoxon Matched Pairs Test, $Z = 3.114$ ($n = 61$), $p = .0018$; and $Z = 3.831$ ($n = 61$), $p = .00013$, respectively]. Additionally, the GA effect was significantly better for movements than for pain [Wilcoxon Matched Pairs Test, $Z = 2.129$ ($n = 61$), $p = .033$]. To exclude a possible bias from the patients who were rarely using their GA (and therefore probably not very accurate in quantification of its effects), a subgroup of GA+ patients who declared that they were still using their GA and that it was working as usual (unchanged) was separately analyzed (Fig. 26-1C). However, the overall pattern of GA effects remained the same and the aforementioned differences became even sharper [Friedman ANOVA $Chi^2 = 19.88$ ($n = 32$, df = 2), $p < .00005$).

The general improvement of CD symptoms brought about by the GA was not correlated with the patients' age or their age at CD onset (Gamma correlation[3]: Gamma = 0.127, $Z = 1.265$, $p = .21$; and Gamma = -0.076, $Z = -0.756$, $p = .45$, respectively). In contrast, a longer CD duration was significantly associated with a worse GA effect in general (Gamma = 0.232, $Z = 2.287$, $p = .022$). However, when specific aspects of the GA effect were examined, a longer CD duration was significantly associated with a worse GA effect on movements only (Gamma = 0.222, $Z = 2.195$, $p = .028$).

The general improvement of CD symptoms associated with the GA was not influenced by the direction of head deviation (i.e., rotacollis, laterocollis, and antero/retrocollis), the complexity (i.e., simple vs. complex CD), or by the presence of head tremor. This was also true for all three features of the GA-induced improvement (position, movements, and pain) when analyzed separately. The only exception was that the presence of head tremor was associated with a significantly lower rating of the GA effect regarding improvement in position and movements (Mann-Whitney U test ($n = 61$): $Z = -2.213$, $p = .027$; and $Z = -2.283$, $p = .022$, respectively). The effect of BT injections was not associated with any aspect of the improvement brought about by the GA. However, the perceived severity of CD as indexed by the patients' ratings of the feeling of control over their head and neck movements was significantly associated with GA-induced improvement of the CD in general (Gamma = -0.270, $Z = -2.533$, $p = .011$), and particularly with the improvement of "pain" (Gamma = -0.263, $Z = -2.407$, $p = .016$).

DISCUSSION

Validity of the Data and Representatives of the Sample

One of the limitations of this study is the self-reported nature of the data collected. To

---

[3]The Gamma statistic is a nonparametric measure of correlation between two variables that is particularly suited when the data contain many tied (i.e., of equal value) observations (8).

preserve anonymity, there was no independent and objective confirmation of the data provided by the patients. Although this may mean that description and quantification of clinical phenomena were not always accurate, the strong subjective nature of the GA-induced improvement makes self-report an important method of assessment. From the patient's point of view, the quality and the magnitude of the perceived disease-induced disability and its improvement by GA are more important parameters than any objective measures of disease severity.

A second limitation of this study is a relatively selective patient sample. The population of patients evaluated in this study was restricted to the patients attending specialized BT injection clinics and therefore excluded were subjects with very mild CD, patients with very complicated CD not helped by BT injections, as well as patients who stopped responding to BT. Nevertheless, the essential clinical characteristics, such as mean age at CD onset, gender ratio, the frequencies of occurrence of rotacollis, laterocollis, retrocollis, and anterocollis, as well as of head tremor, were consistent with previously reported as typical for CD (3,9,10). Only the proportion of complex CD cases was slightly below what has usually been reported (i.e., 66% to 80%) (3,10). This was probably due to the self-reported nature of the data and the patient's incomplete awareness of all aspects of disturbed head, neck, and shoulder positions in CD.

Comparisons of GA+ and GA– Patients

Almost two thirds of all CD patients reported the presence of a GA. This is similar to, although more on the conservative side than, the values usually reported (7,9,11). By comparing patients with and without GA, we were unable to determine any feature of the CD clinical presentation that would be meaningfully associated with GA presence. The only exception was the almost ubiquitous presence of GA in patients with earlier

onset of CD (i.e., even before the age of 32). This has not been reported before and warrants further study. The apparent higher occurrence of rotacollis in the subgroup of GA+ patients could have been a chance finding due to the relatively high presence of rotacollis in the studied group of patients in general.

The Natural History of GA

The GA seems to be a commonly associated feature of the clinical presentation of CD. In most patients it was apparent from the onset of CD symptoms or within the first 5 years. This is in line with findings of most epidemiologic studies that CD usually progresses within the first 5 years and then reaches a plateau or sometimes even regresses (3,9,10). In addition, it seems that if GA is present, it is usually persistent throughout the course of CD. The findings of Müller et al. (7), which is the only study to have evaluated the natural history of GA in CD, agree with this. However, the use of GA may be reduced or discontinued due to good effects of BT in reducing CD symptoms, which was the case in 30% of the patents in this study. This purely behavioral/psychological interaction between the use of GA and BT effect has not been previously considered, but it may be responsible for the higher rates of patients who stopped using GA that are reported in some studies (11). Nevertheless, slightly more than a half of GA+ patients were still using GA and considered the GA effect to be unchanged. As would be expected, the BT effect was considered less than satisfactory by almost half of the patients in this subgroup. Since they did not obtain sufficient relief from BT injections, these patients persisted in using GA. Only a minority of patients had noticed a decrease or even a disappearance of the GA effect after starting BT injections. However, it is not clear whether this was truly an effect of the BT injections or merely a manifestation of the spontaneous reduction of the GA effect.

The Magnitude of the GA Effect

Even if not always reliable regarding its occurrence and magnitude of its effect, when effective, GA tends to bring considerable relief (i.e., reduction of symptoms by 50% or more) to a majority of patients. The GA effect is maximal for improvement of head, neck, and shoulder position. This was followed by an effect on neck movements. The effect was the least, though still very good, on pain and tenderness in the neck and shoulders. Müller et al. (7) reported a slightly higher percentage of patients with a clinically significant effect of the GA (82%), but they defined their threshold for "good" effect as a 30% reduction in head deviation, which was lower than in our study, and they used a more objective rating by an investigator, which was more likely to detect even small changes that may escape patients' self-awareness. However, when patients were asked to rate the GA effect themselves, 74% declared it as good or excellent, which was almost identical with the percent in our study.

The magnitude of the GA effect is comparable to the usually reported results from BT injections (3,10,12). However, the pattern of benefits seems to differ slightly between BT and GA. In several studies, BT has been found to be slightly more effective on pain than on movements and position of the head, neck, and shoulders (13,14). Exactly the opposite was the case for GA in this study. This is an interesting finding that may be related to the opposite modes of action of the two—the peripheral blockage of the effectors in the case of BT and a probable central reorganization of sensorimotor programs in the case of the GA (15).

Clinical Features that Influence the Magnitude of GA Effect

No clinical characteristic has been found to influence the magnitude of the benefit brought about by the GA. Interestingly, this is different from the effect of BT that tends to be better in simple CD cases, and particularly in rotacollis (12,16). Only the presence of head tremor appeared to interfere with the beneficial effect of the GA on position and movements of the head, neck, and shoulders. Whether this is due to a certain pathophysiologic specifics of head tremor in CD is an interesting question for further study. Although GA remained present throughout the course of CD in the great majority of patients, the beneficial effect of GA tended to decline with the duration of CD. This trend has been already noted by clinicians (3), but has never been statistically confirmed. Interestingly, the beneficial effect of GA was significantly associated with the patients' perception of the severity of CD: the greater the relief of CD in general, and particularly the greater the relief of pain, associated with the use of GA, the better the patients perceived their ability to control their head and neck movements. However, it remains unclear whether GA had a better effect in milder cases of CD or if the patients have a tendency to perceive the severity of their CD as milder if an effective GA is present. Further studies with additional objective quantification of CD severity and GA effectiveness are needed to clarify this issue.

CONCLUSION

This study increases our understanding of the phenomenon of GA in CD due to its large population base and a number of issues evaluated that were not addressed in previous studies. Although no particular clinical characteristics of CD predictive of GA presence were identified, a high prevalence of GA in CD together with its remarkable efficacy as well as a significant association with the patients' perception of the severity of CD, warrants further investigation of its clinical phenomenology, natural history, and physiology. Better appreciation of the phenomenon of GA as well as the mechanisms of the sensorimotor interactions underlying it may provide clues for an understanding of the neurobiology of dystonias in general and open new avenues for their treatment.

REFERENCES

1. Podivinsky F. Torticollis. In: Vinken PJ, Bruyn GW, eds. *Diseases of the basal ganglia. Handbook of clinical neurology,* vol 6. Amsterdam: Elsevier, 1969:567–603.
2. Fahn S. Concept and classification of dystonia. In: Fahn S, Marsden CD, Calne DB, eds. *Dystonia 2. Advances in neurology,* vol 50. New York: Raven Press, 1988:1–8.
3. Dauer WT, Burke RE, Greene P, Fahn S. Current concepts on the clinical features, aetiology, and management of idiopathic cervical dystonia. *Brain* 1998;121:547–560.
4. Leis AA, Dimitrijevic MR, Delapasse JS, et al. Modification of cervical dystonia by selective sensory stimulation. *J Neurol Sci* 1992;110:79–89.
5. Wissel J, Müller J, Ebersbach G, et al. Trick manoeuvres in cervical dystonia: investigation of movement- and touch-related changes in polymyographic activity. *Mov Disord* 1999;14:994–999.
6. Naumann M, Magyar-Lehmann S, Reiners K, et al. Sensory tricks in cervical dystonia: perceptual dysbalance of parietal cortex modulates frontal motor programming. *Ann Neurol* 2000;47:322–328.
7. Müller J, Wissel J, Masuhr F, et al. Clinical characteristics of the geste antagoniste in cervical dystonia. *J Neurol* 2001;248:478–482.
8. Siegel S, Castellan NJ. *Nonparametric statistics for the behavioral sciences.* New York: McGraw-Hill, 1988.
9. Tsui JKC. Cervical dystonia. In: Tsui JKC, Calne DB, eds. *Handbook of dystonia.* New York: Marcel Dekker, 1995:115–127.
10. Velickovic M, Benabou R, Brin MF. Cervical dystonia pathophysiology and treatment options. *Drugs* 2001;61:1921–1943.
11. Jahanshahi M. Factors that ameliorate or aggravate spasmodic torticollis. *J Neurol Neurosurg Psychiatry* 2000;68:227–229.
12. Comella C. Cervical dystonia: treatment with botulinum toxin serotype A as BOTOX or Dysport. In: Brin MF, Jankovic J, Hallett M, eds. *Scientific and therapeutic aspects of botulinum toxin.* Philadelphia: Lippincott Williams & Wilkins, 2002:359–364.
13. Lees AJ, Turjanski N, Rivest J, et al. Treatment of cervical dystonia hand spasms and laryngeal dystonia with botulinum toxin. *J Neurol* 1992;239:1–4.
14. Brans JW, de Boer IP, Aramideh M, et al. Botulinum toxin in cervical dystonia: low dosage with electromyographic guidance. *J Neurol* 1995;242:529–534.
15. Hallett M. Is dystonia a sensory disorder? *Ann Neurol* 1995;38:139–140.
16. Tsui JKC. Applications of botulinum toxin: cervical and limb dystonia. In: Tsui JKC, Calne DB, eds. *Handbook of dystonia.* New York: Marcel Dekker, 1995:115–127.

APPENDIX–QUESTIONNAIRE: SENSORY TRICKS IN TORTICOLLIS

The aim of this questionnaire is to find out about the use of sensory tricks by people who have torticollis. "Sensory trick" refers to the fact that some people with torticollis are able to reduce the severity of their torticollis by touching certain parts of their face. This information about sensory tricks may help us understand the physiologic basis of torticollis better. When completing the questionnaire, please remember that there are no right or wrong answers. We are simply interested in your own experiences of torticollis. The information you provide will be kept strictly confidential and will be used for research purposes only. Please try to answer the questions as accurately as possible. If you are unable to answer a question, then place a question mark ("?") in front of it.

Many thanks for your help.

1. How long have you had torticollis?
_____ (Please give the most accurate estimate possible.)

2. In which direction(s) does your head "want" to go? (Please check all that apply to you.)
☐ Turn to the left or turn to the right
☐ Lean/tilt toward the left shoulder or lean/tilt toward the right shoulder
☐ Bend backward or bend forward

3. Does your head shake?
☐ YES / ☐ NO

4. Please indicate how much control you feel you have over your head position by circling an appropriate number on the scale below:
No control at all   Complete control
    0 1 2 3 4 5 6 7 8 9 10

5. Do you receive botulinum toxin injections?
☐ YES /☐ NO
If yes, how effective have they been?
☐ Excellent from beginning and still the same
☐ Excellent from beginning but lost some of the effect
☐ Moderate effect from the beginning
☐ Variable—no pattern

6. Some people with torticollis are able to reduce the severity of their torticollis by touching certain parts of their face or neck. This is called a "sensory trick." Have you ever been able to reduce the severity of your torticollis by touching certain parts of your face or neck?

☐ YES /☐ NO

If yes, then please proceed with question 7. If no, would you mind trying the following now?

With your hand (first right, then left hand), using either index or middle finger, please touch several points on your face and neck (first right side, then left side). Try a couple of points in each of the regions of the face, head, and neck (for reference, see question 9, below) on both right and left sides.

☐ Please check here if you do not feel like trying this now. You have completed this questionnaire. Thank you.

Did you notice that any of these actions brought some reduction or easing of torticollis symptoms, irrespective of the degree of improvement?

☐ YES / ☐ NO

If yes, please proceed to question 7. If no, thank you for your interest in this study.

7. When did you first notice your "sensory trick"?

☐ At the same time as the onset of my torticollis (within the same year)
☐ A few years later (please give approximate date, in years) _____
☐ Today

8. Is your sensory trick still effective in controlling your torticollis?

☐ YES / ☐ NO

If no, when did it stop being effective? (How many years ago?) _____

9. Touching of which part of the face or neck is/was effective?

(Please check all that apply, taking care about the side. If more than one part is effective, please put an asterisk (*) next to the one that brings the most relief.)

	Right	Middle	Left
Forehead	☐	☐	☐
Eye	☐		☐
Nose	☐	☐	☐
Cheek	☐		☐
Chin	☐	☐	☐
Earlobe	☐		☐
Top of the head	☐	☐	☐
Back of the head	☐	☐	☐
Front of the neck	☐	☐	☐
Back of the neck	☐	☐	☐
Shoulder	☐		☐
....	☐	☐	☐

(specify yourself)

10. What is your preferred hand for writing, holding spoon, cutting bread, waving good-bye?

☐ RIGHT ☐ LEFT ☐ DOESN'T MATTER

11. Does/did it matter which hand (left or right) you use/used to touch your face/neck?

☐ YES / ☐ NO

If yes, please go to question 13. If no, please continue.

12. Does/did it matter which part of the hand you use/used to touch your face/neck?

☐ YES / ☐ NO

13. Is/was the effect the same regardless of the hand/part of the hand used to touch the face/neck?

☐ YES / ☐ NO

14. Please specify the part(s) of the hand that are/were effective. If more than one part is effective, please put an asterisk (*) next to the one that is the most effective [please, take care about the side (left/right) also].

	Right	Left
Back of hand	☐	☐
Palm of hand	☐	☐
Thumb (1st finger)	☐	☐
Index finger (2nd)	☐	☐
Middle finger (3rd)	☐	☐
Fourth finger	☐	☐
Small finger (5th)	☐	☐

15. Which of these best describes the contact of your hand with your face/neck? (Please check the one that is appropriate.)
☐ light touch
☐ push
☐ pull

16. What is the exact timing of the relief of your torticollis when you use/were using your sensory trick? (Please check the one that is most appropriate.)
☐ Relief starts as soon as hand begins moving towards face
☐ Relief starts shortly before hand touches the face
☐ Relief starts as soon as hand touches face
☐ Relief starts shortly after hand touches faces

17. Does the effect last, or did it last, as long as you keep, or kept, the sensitive part of the face touched?
☐ YES / ☐ NO
If no, how long does/did the effect usually last? _____(approximate time)

18. Does/did touching the sensitive part of the face with some object (for example pen, cotton wool, or handkerchief) have/had a similar effect? (If you don't know, please try now, if possible.)
☐ YES / ☐ NO / ☐ Not possible to try now

19. Does someone else touching the sensitive part of your face/neck can produce a similar beneficial effect? (If you don't know, please try now, if possible.)
☐ YES / ☐ NO / ☐ Not possible to try now

20. Does/did merely thinking about (imagining that you are performing it in your mind's eye) the sensory trick brings/brought relief? (If you don't know, please try now.)
☐ YES / ☐ NO

21. How often is/was your sensory trick effective in reducing the severity of your torticollis?
(Check the one that applies.)
☐ Always (100% of time)
☐ Frequently (more than 75% of time)
☐ Unpredictably (about 50% of time)
☐ Occasionally (less than 50% of time)

☐ Rarely (less than 25% of time)

22. Is/was the effect of your sensory trick when present always the same or is/was it variable?
☐ Always the same   ☐ Variable

23. Botulinum toxin injections, if you are receiving them, might influence the effects of your sensory trick. (Please check the one statement that is most appropriate.)
☐ I am not receiving botulinum toxin (BT) injections.
☐ Since I started BT injections, I am not using my sensory trick anymore.
☐ BT injections are so effective that I hardly use my sensory trick anymore.
☐ I am still using my sensory trick and it is working as usual.
☐ I am still using my sensory trick but it is working less well than before.
☐ I am still using my sensory trick and it is now working better than before.
☐ I am still using my sensory trick but it is working much more unpredictably than before.

The next four questions are about the effectiveness of your sensory trick. This may vary with time and possibly with botulinum toxin treatment. Please answer them taking into account the period when the trick was most prominent and was expressed at its best.

24. What is your impression, to what extent does/did your sensory trick improve your torticollis in general? (Check the one that applies.)
☐ completely improves (100% better)
☐ greatly improves (about 75% better)
☐ moderately improves (about 50% better)
☐ mildly improves (less than 50% better)
☐ minimally improves (less than 25% better)

25. To what extent is/was your "sensory trick" helpful in correcting the position of your head, neck, and/or shoulder?
☐ Brings them back to the normal position completely.
☐ Reduces the abnormal position significantly (more than 75%), but not completely.

☐ Reduces the abnormal position to some extent (around 50%).

☐ Reduces the abnormal position to a small extent only.

☐ Does not have any impact on head, neck or shoulder position.

26. To what extent is/was your "sensory trick" helpful in restoring your neck and shoulder movements?

☐ Brings them back to the normal.

☐ Makes the movements significantly easier (more than 75%), but does not bring them back to normal completely.

☐ Makes the movements easier to some extent (around 50%).

☐ Eases the movements to a small extent only.

☐ Does not have any impact on neck or shoulder movements.

27. How much is your "sensory trick" helpful in relieving the feeling of tension, tenderness, and/or aching in your neck and/or shoulder?

☐ Abolishes it completely.

☐ Reduces them significantly (for about 75%).

☐ Reduces them to some extent (for about 50%).

☐ Reduces them a little (25% or less).

☐ Does nothing to them.

☐ Increases them.

You have now reached the end of our questionnaire. Thank you very much for your cooperation.

Dystonia 4: Advances in Neurology, Vol. 94. Edited
by Stanley Fahn, Mark Hallett, and Mahlon R.
DeLong. Lippincott Williams & Wilkins,
Philadelphia © 2004.

27

Executive Function in Dystonia

*Marjan Jahanshahi, †John Rowe, and ‡Rebecca Fuller

**Sobell Department of Movement Neuroscience and Movement Disorders, Institute of Neurology,
University College London, National Hospital for Neurology and Neurosurgery, Queen Square,
London, United Kingdom. †Department of Clinical Psychology, East London and The City Mental
Health Trust, Homerton Hospital, London, United Kingdom. ‡Maryland Psychiatric Research
Center, Outpatient Research Program, University of Maryland, Baltimore, Maryland*

According to the current pathophysiologic model of dystonia (1–4), the primary disorder is a result of overactivity in the direct pathway between the striatum, the internal section of the globus pallidus (GPi), thalamus, and cortex, which gives rise to excessively reduced inhibitory output from the GPi and disinhibition of thalamocortical activity, whereas symptoms such as bradykinesia in dystonia reflect overactivity in the indirect striatocortical pathway via the external section of the globus pallidus and the subthalamic nucleus. This model is supported by activation studies that have demonstrated frontostriatal dysfunction in patients with dystonia (5–7). For example, Ceballos-Baumann et al. (6) found that during freely selected joystick movements, dystonia patients showed greater activation than controls in the lateral premotor cortex (PMC), Brodmann area (BA) 8, anterior cingulate area 32, ipsilateral dorsolateral prefrontal cortex (DLPFC, BA 46), rostral supplementary motor area (SMA), and bilateral lentiform nuclei. In contrast, there was decreased activity relative to controls in the caudal SMA, bilateral sensorimotor cortex, posterior cingulate, and mesial parietal cortex.

The results of these imaging studies suggest that during movement or sensorimotor stimulation, the activation of prefrontal areas that are targets of striatal projections are significantly different in dystonia compared to normals. Some of these prefrontal areas such as the DLPFC are known to play a significant role in cognitive executive function and working memory. In humans, dysfunction of the DLPFC is associated with significant impairment on tests of executive function and working memory (8–10). Striatal dysfunction as in Parkinson's disease (10,11), Huntington's disease (12), or progressive supranuclear palsy and multiple system atrophy (13,14) also gives rise to similar deficits of executive function and working memory. The aim of this study was to investigate the functional significance of the prefrontal overactivation in dystonia by examining executive function and working memory in a sample of patients with primary dystonia.

METHOD

Design

A mixed between-groups and within-subjects design was used. Two groups of subjects, patients with primary dystonia and normal control subjects, completed a battery of tests of cognitive function.

Subjects

Ten patients (four male, six female) with a clinical diagnosis of primary dystonia according to the criteria of Marsden and Harrison (15) were tested. Their mean age was 47.3 years [standard deviation (SD) = 8.5]. Twelve age (mean 52.1, SD = 5.1 years) and gender (four male, eight female) matched healthy subjects with no history of neurologic, physical, or psychiatric illness or head injury were also tested. All but one patient and all control subjects were right handed. Three patients had generalized dystonia (arms, legs, trunk, and neck in all three, plus mouth and speech in two), seven had focal dystonia (five torticollis, two arm dystonia). The average age of onset was 33.7 years (SD = 13.5), and three patients had an age of onset before 20 (onset at ages 15, 18, and 19). The mean duration of illness was 13.6 years (SD = 7.7). None of the patients had Ashkenazi Jewish ancestry. One patient was on anticholinergic medication (4 mg Artane equivalent), while the remaining patients were on no medication and nine had received treatment with botulinum toxin injections. The severity of dystonia was rated by a neurologist using the Fahn and Marsden Scale for Primary Torsion Dystonia (16). On this scale, the patients had an average score of 14.8 (SD = 15.9) on the movement subscale and a mean score of 2.5 (SD = 3.0) on the disability subscale. Depression was assessed with the Beck Depression Inventory (BDI) (17). Informed consent was obtained from all patients.

Tests of Cognitive Function

Estimates of premorbid IQ were obtained using the National Adult Reading Test (18). A series of tests of executive function and working memory were administered, further details of which are provided in our previous publications (19,20). The tests included the following: (a) Word fluency (9): The first letter (F, A, S), category (animals), and alternating categories (boys names and fruits) versions of this test were completed, each for 60 seconds. (b) Wisconsin Card Sorting Test (21): This test assesses the subject's ability to develop, maintain, and shift mental set, as well as monitor one's responses and hold information "on line" in working memory. (c) Stroop Color Word Naming Test (22): This test assesses the subject's ability to maintain attention focused on one attribute of color words (ink) printed in color-incongruent ink and ignore/suppress the other (meaning of color words) while naming the color of the ink. (d) Missing Digit Test (23): This is a test of working memory. On each trial the subject was presented with a random sequence of nine of the numbers between 1 and 10 on the video display unit (VDU) at the rate of one digit every 2 seconds and had to identify the missing digit. (e) Self-ordered random number Sequences (23): On each trial, the subject is required to produce a random sequence of ten numbers using the numbers between 1 and 10, with the additional requirement of not missing any numbers or repeating any. Performance is paced with a visual pacing stimulus. (f) Random number generation (RNG) (24): Subjects were asked to say the numbers 1 to 9 in a random order for 100 trials and to synchronize the RNG with a pacing tone presented at the rate of once every 2 seconds. (g) Visual-visual conditional associative learning (25): The task requires the subject to learn and remember the arbitrary associations between six pairs of visual stimuli (abstract designs and colors) by trial and error. The arbitrary nature of the pairings reduces contextual discrimination. (h) Paced visual serial addition test (26): Subjects are presented with a series of 33 random single-digit numbers on the VDU and are to add the most recent number to the preceding one and provide the sum. Two versions of the task were used with digits presented on a VDU at the rate of one item every 2 or 4 seconds. (i) Dual-task performance (27): We used two motor tasks, tapping with the index finger and insertion of pegs into a pegboard. Each task was first performed alone with either the left or right hands, and then bimanually each time for 30 seconds. The tasks were then performed concurrently, each time for 30 seconds. Patients inserted pegs into the pegboard with the right hand and simultaneously tapped with the left hand and vice versa.

RESULTS

Given the number of between-group comparisons involved, an adjusted p value of .002 was used. There were no significant differences between the patient and control subjects in terms of age ($p > .05$) or National Adult Reading Test (NART) predicted estimates of premorbid IQ (patients: mean = 107.1, SD = 5.9; controls: mean = 112.7, SD = 7.9; $p > .05$). As expected, patients with dystonia had significantly higher self-reported depression scores (mean = 10.9, SD = 5.4) than the controls (mean = 6.4, SD = 5.1), but the difference was not significant ($p = .062$), and none of the subjects scored in the severe range (BDI score > 24) for depression.

Comparison of the mean scores on the various tests of executive function and working memory showed that on most measures the patients with dystonia had scores in the direction of lowered function compared to the controls (Table 27-1). However, very few significant group differences emerged. The group differences were significant for category ($p = .007$) word fluency, with the patients generating significantly fewer animals in 60 seconds than the normal controls. The patients and the controls did not differ significantly on the first letter ($p > .05$) or the alternating category ($p > .05$) versions of the word fluency task. The differences between the patients and the controls on all the other tests of cognitive executive function or working memory were not significant ($p > .05$).

The patients and the controls did not differ in terms of the unimanual or bimanual performance on the pegboard and tapping tasks ($p > .05$). For the bimanual peg insertion and tapping and the dual-task performance (concurrent tapping with one hand and peg insertion with the other) the scores are expressed as percentage change relative to unimanual performance of the pegboard or tapping tasks. The dystonia patients had a significantly greater drop in tapping with one hand ($p = .007$) when this was performed currently with peg insertion with the other hand. With the adjusted p value of .002, the patients and controls did not differ significantly on any of the measures.

DISCUSSION

The patients with dystonia and the controls were matched according to age, sex distribution, and estimates of premorbid verbal IQ. The patient group had higher self-reported depression than the control group, although the differences were not significant. This higher depression in the present sample of patients with primary dystonia is in agreement with the results of previous studies, which also found moderate-to-severe levels of self-reported depression in a proportion of these patients (28–31). The patients with primary dystonia did not differ from the normals on the majority of the tests of executive function and working memory used. The only significant differences between the two groups was that the patients had lower category fluency, and relative to single-task performance the patients showed a significantly greater drop in tapping with one hand when this was performed concurrently with peg insertion with the other hand. However, with a stringent significance level adjusting for the number of comparisons, even these differences were not significant.

Cognitive function in dystonia has been previously examined in three studies. The studies of Eldridge et al. (32) and Riklan et al. (33) were solely concerned with intellectual ability and are therefore not directly comparable with the present results, which focused on specific aspects of cognitive function, namely executive function and working memory. The aim of the

TABLE 27-1. *Means (and standard deviations) of scores on tests of cognitive function for dystonia patients and age-matched controls*

	Controls	Dystonia patients	
Word fluency			
First Letter (FAS)	44.7 (7.6)	37.7 (8.2)	
Category (animals)	21.6 (8.5)	13.2 (2.9)	*p = .007
Alternating categories	16.9 (2.2)	17.5 (3.4)	
Wisconsin card sort test			
Categories correctly sorted	5.3 (1.5)	5.0 (1.7)	
Nonperseverative errors	6.7 (6.4)	7.7 (6.4)	
Perseverative errors	2.0 (2.6)	3.2 (3.1)	
Percent perseverative errors	16.9 (18.0)	24.3 (14.8)	
Stroop color word naming test—time(s)			
Color naming–color words	38.9 (10.6)	33.9 (7.3)	
Color naming–rectangles	20.0 (4.6)	18.6 (5.1)	
Missing Digit (% correct)	60.8 (21.5)	53.7 (14.1)	
Self-ordered random number sequences			
Percent correct	35.4 (20.2)	38.1 (23.5)	
Missing items	14.9 (8.9)	14.0 (5.6)	
Repeated items	7.1 (4.7)	7.0 (5.9)	
Random number generation			
Count score 1	40.2 (26.6)	49.3 (24.5)	
Count score 2	45.3 (13.6)	52.2 (44.0)	
Median gap score	8.1 (0.43)	8.0 (0.62)	
Number of repetitions	2.5 (4.2)	0.6 (0.97)	
RNG index	0.34 (0.03)	0.37 (0.04)	
Visual-visual conditional associative learning			
Total number of trials	44.3 (17.0)	58.2 (22.8)	
Total number of errors	16.3 (9.5)	26.4 (16.7)	
Paced visual serial addition test—mean errors			
Fast rate	7.3 (5.9)	7.9 (7.3)	
Slow rate	2.9 (3.5)	2.2 (5.0)	
Tapping and pegboard			
Unimanual tapping	144.6 (30.4)	145.2 (20.8)	
Unimanual pegboard	14.8 (2.4)	14.2 (3.3)	
Bimanual tapping (% unimanual)	95.7 (10.5)	91.4 (6.9)	
Bimanual pegboard (% unimanual)	82.6 (6.7)	78.9 (9.6)	
Dual-task performance (percent of unimanual task performance)			
Pegboard concurrently with tapping	91.3 (12.9)	91.1 (10.5)	
Tapping concurrently with pegboard	87.2 (6.5)	73.9 (10.8)	*p = .007

*Significant differences.

study by Taylor et al. (34) was to examine the impact of high-dose anticholinergic medication used to treat the dystonic cramps on cognition. They pretested 55 patients on a baseline battery of neuropsychological tests and then pre-selected 20 patients "to insure absence of cognitive dysfunction," who then had more detailed neuropsychological assessment. Before starting medication, this preselected group of dystonia patients and the age- and IQ-matched controls did not differ on any of the tests of cognition used, which included tests of executive function. This is in agreement with the results of the present study.

Theoretical models (e.g., 35) consider the prefrontal cortex to act as the "supervisory attentional system," which would become engaged when strategic allocation of attention between two tasks is required as in dual-task performance. In the present study, concurrent performance of right-handed finger tapping with peg insertion with the other hand was associated with a significant drop in tapping for the patients with dystonia relative to the normals. Since the dystonia patients did not differ from the normals when the pegboard and finger tapping tasks were performed alone, this suggests a failure of the prefrontal cortex in its role as the supervisory attentional system overseeing the allocation of attention to the two tasks, maintaining better performance on the visually driven pegboard at the expense of finger tapping. An alternative explanation is also possible. Most patients with dystonia, particularly those with torticollis, have a *geste antagoniste* (GA) usually involving the use of the dominant hand to control the abnormal postures or muscle contractions associated with dystonia. The deterioration of tapping with one hand concurrently with peg insertion with the other hand may partly relate to the fact that under the dual-task condition, when the patients are using both hands, they cannot engage in their GA and may have to resort to controlling their dystonic postures/contractions through conscious effort, which would make further attentional demands and slow their performance relative to controls even though unimanual tapping or peg insertion was no different from controls. However, since change in bimanual tapping or bimanual peg insertion as a percentage of unimanual performance was not significantly different for the dystonia patients relative to the controls, the significant deterioration under dual-task conditions in dystonia cannot be simply due to the bimanual engagement and disruption of the GA, and the greater attentional demands of the dual-task condition must have also contributed to the poorer performance of the patients.

Dystonia is principally considered a motor disorder with little or no cognitive deficits. The present results confirm this clinical view and suggest that patients with dystonia do not show any significant deficits of executive function or working memory on neuropsychological assessment. This is in contrast to other movement disorders resulting from striatal dysfunction such as Huntington's disease, progressive supranuclear palsy, and Parkinson's disease, which are associated with frank dementia in all or a proportion of the sufferers and frontal-type deficits of executive function and working memory (10–14). These results suggest that in dystonia, the frontal dysfunction revealed in imaging studies, which takes

the form of "overactivation" of these areas relative to normals (6), is not associated with deficits in executive function, unlike the frontal "underactivation" observed in Parkinson's disease during performance of attention-demanding motor tasks (36), where concomitant deficits in executive function are also found on neuropsychological assessment (10,11).

Recently, surgical treatment of focal or generalized dystonia with pallidotomy or deep brain stimulation of the GPi or ventrolateral thalamic nucleus has been shown to be clinically effective (37–40). To date, the effects of such surgical procedures on cognition in dystonia patients has not been extensively reported. The present results have two implications for the assessment of cognitive function in patients with dystonia before and after surgery. First, given that cognitive function is largely intact in dystonia, preoperative screening of the patients does not need to be as extensive as that of patients with Parkinson's disease undergoing the same surgical procedures. However, since about a quarter to one third of patients with dystonia are moderately to severely depressed (28–31), depression and other disorders of mood should perhaps be a more primary focus of preoperative screening and more extensively investigated. Second, given the absence of any preoperative deficits in cognition prior to surgery in patients with dystonia, any alterations of cognition following surgery can be more directly related to the surgical intervention than in Parkinson's disease, where executive dysfunction is a feature of the disorder even preoperatively.

CONCLUSION

Dystonia is a movement disorder considered to result from basal ganglia dysfunction, and frontostriatal dysfunction has been found in patients with the disorder in imaging studies. Unlike other movement disorders, cognitive function in dystonia has been rarely studied. The aim of this study was to assess executive function and working memory in patients with dystonia. We assessed 10 patients with dystonia and 12 age- and IQ-matched normal controls on a battery of tests of executive function and working memory. The patients with dystonia did not significantly differ from the controls on any of the measures of executive function or working memory used other than category word fluency and the extent of decline in tapping with one hand under dual-task conditions when simultaneously inserting pegs with the other hand. These results suggest that unlike other movement disorders associated with frontostriatal dysfunction such as Parkinson's disease or Huntington's disease, dystonia is not associated with deficits on tests of executive function or working memory and can be considered to be primarily a motor disorder.

(*Note:* This chapter is an abbreviated version of a full article that will appear in Movement Disorders)

REFERENCES

1. De Long M. Primate models of movement disorders of basal ganglia origin. *Trends Neurosci* 1990;13:281–285.
2. Hallett M. Physiology of basal ganglia disorders: an overview. *J Can Sci Neurol* 1993;20:177–183.
3. Vitek JL, Chockkan V, Zhang JY, et al. Neuronal activity in the basal ganglia in patients with generalized dystonia and hemiballismus. *Ann-Neurol* 1999;46:22–35.
4. Vitek JL, Giroux M. Physiology of hypokinetic and hyperkinetic movement disorders: model for dyskinesia. *Ann Neurol* 2000;47(4 suppl 1):S131–140.
5. Tempel LW, Perlmutter JS. Abnormal cortical responses in patients with writer's cramp [published erratum appears in *Neurology* 1994;44(12):2411]. *Neurology* 1993; 43(11):2252–2257.
6. Ceballos-Baumann A, Passingham RE, Warner T, et al. Overactive prefrontal and underactive motor cortical areas in idiopathic dystonia. *Ann Neurol* 1995;37(3): 363–372.
7. Ibanez V, Sadato N, Karp B, et al. Deficient activation of the motor cortical network in patients with writer's cramp. *Neurology* 1999;53(1):96–105.
8. Milner B. Some effects of frontal lobectomy in man. In: Milner B, Warren JM, Akert K, eds. *The frontal granular cortex and behavior.* New York: McGraw-Hill, 1964:313–331.
9. Benton AL. Differential behavioral effects in frontal lobe disease. *Neuropsychologia* 1968;6:53–60.
10. Owen AM, Roberts AC, Hodges JR, et al. Contrasting mechanisms of impaired attentional set-shifting in patients with frontal lobe damage or Parkinson's disease. *Brain* 1993;116(pt 5):1159–1175.
11. Taylor AE, Saint-Cyr JA, Lang AE. Frontal lobe dysfunction in Parkinson's disease. *Brain* 1986;109: 845–883.
12. Lawrence AD, Weeks RA, Brooks DJ, et al. The relationship between striatal dopamine receptor binding and cognitive performance in Huntington's disease. *Brain* 1998;121(pt 7):1343–1355.
13. Pillon B, Dubois B, Ploska A, et al. Severity and specificity of cognitive impairment in Alzheimer's, Huntington's, and Parkinson's diseases and progressive supranuclear palsy. *Neurology* 1991;41(5):634–643.
14. Robbins TW, James M, Owen AM, et al. Cognitive deficits in progressive supranuclear palsy, Parkinson's disease, and multiple system atrophy in tests sensitive to frontal lobe dysfunction. *J Neurol Neurosurg Psychiatry* 1994;57(1):79–88.
15. Marsden CD, Harrison MJG. Idiopathic torsion dystonia (dystonia musculorum deformans): a review of forty-two patients. *Brain* 1974;97:793–810.
16. Burke RE, Fahn S, Marsden CD, et al. Validity and reliability of a rating scale for the primary torsion dystonias. *Neurology* 1985;35:73–77.
17. Beck AT, Ward C, Mendelson M, et al. An inventory for measuring depression. *Arch Gen Psychiatry* 1961;4: 561–567.
18. Nelson HC. *National Adult Reading Test (NART): test manual.* Windsor, UK: NFER-Nelson, 1982.
19. Jahanshahi M, Ardouin CM, Brown RG, et al. The impact of deep brain stimulation on executive function in Parkinson's disease. *Brain* 2000;123(pt 6):1142–1154.
20. Jahanshahi M, Rowe J, Saleem T, et al. Working memory and executive function in Parkinson's disease before and after unilateral pallidotomy. *J Cognitive Neurosci* 2002;14:298–310.
21. Nelson HE. A modified card sorting test sensitive to frontal lobe defects. *Cortex* 1976;12(4):313.
22. Stroop JR. Studies of interference in serial verbal reactions. *J Exp Psychol* 1935;18:643–662.
23. Petrides M, Alivisatos B, Meyer E, et al. Functional activation of the human frontal cortex during the performance of verbal working memory tasks. *Proc Natl Acad Sci USA* 1993;90(3):878–882.
24. Ginsburg N, Karpiuk P. Random generation: analysis of the responses. *Percept Motor Skills* 1994;79:1059–1067.
25. Petrides M. Deficits on conditional-associative learning tasks after frontal and temporal-lobe lesions in man. *Neuropsychologia* 1985;23:601–614.
26. Gronwall D, Wrightson P. Memory and information processing capacity after closed head injury. *J Neurol Neurosurg Psychiatry* 1981;44:889–895.
27. Brown RG, Jahanshahi M, Marsden CD. The execution of bimanual movements in patients with Parkinson's, Huntington's and cerebellar disease. *J Neurol Neurosurg Psychiatry* 1993;56(3):295–297.
28. Jahanshahi M, Marsden CD. Depression in torticollis: a controlled study. *Psychol Med* 1988;18(4):925–933.
29. Jahanshahi M, Marsden CD. Body concept, disability, and depression in patients with spasmodic torticollis. *Behav Neurol* 1990;3:117–131.
30. Jahanshahi M, Marsden CD. A longitudinal study of depression, disability and body concept in torticollis. *Behav Neurol* 1990;3:233–246.
31. Jahanshahi M. Psychosocial factors and depression in torticollis. *J Psychosom Res* 1991;35(4–5):493–507.
32. Eldridge R, Harlan A, Cooper IS, et al. Superior intelli-

gence in recessively inherited torsion dystonia. *Lancet* 1970;1(7637):65–67.

33. Riklan M, Cullinan T, Cooper IS. Psychological studies in dystonia musculorum deformans. *Adv Neurol* 1976;14:189–200.

34. Taylor AE, Lang AE, Saint CJ, et al. Cognitive processes in idiopathic dystonia treated with high-dose anticholinergic therapy: implications for treatment strategies. *Clin Neuropharmacol* 1991;14(1): 62–77.

35. Norman DA, Shallice T. Attention to action: willed and automatic control of behaviour. In: Davidson RJ, et al., eds. *Consciousness and self-regulation. Advance in research and theory.* New York: Plenum Press, 1986, pp. 1–18.

36. Jahanshahi M, Jenkins IH, Brown RG, et al. Self-initiated versus externally triggered movements. I. An in-vestigation using measurement of regional cerebral blood flow with PET and movement-related potentials in normal and Parkinson's disease subjects [see comments]. *Brain* 1995;118(pt 4):913–933.

37. Vitek JL, Zhang J, Evatt M, et al. GPi pallidotomy for dystonia: clinical outcome and neuronal activity. *Adv Neurol* 1998;78:211–219.

38. Kumar R, Dagher A, Hutchison W-D, et al. Globus pallidus deep brain stimulation for generalized dystonia: clinical and PET investigation. *Neurology* 1999;53(4): 871–874.

39. Vercueil L, Pollak P, Fraix V, et al. Deep brain stimulation in the treatment of severe dystonia. *J Neurol* 2001; 248(8):695–700.

40. Yoshor D, Hamilton W-J, Ondo W, et al. Comparison of thalamotomy and pallidotomy for the treatment of dystonia. *Neurosurgery* 2001;48(4):818–824.

Dystonia 4: Advances in Neurology, Vol. 94. Edited
by Stanley Fahn, Mark Hallett, and Mahlon R.
DeLong. Lippincott Williams & Wilkins,
Philadelphia © 2004.

28

Duration of Effectiveness of Botulinum Toxin Type B in the Treatment of Cervical Dystonia

Mark F. Lew

*Department of Neurology, Keck School of Medicine, University of Southern California,
Los Angeles, California*

Cervical dystonia is the most common form of focal dystonia, affecting 60,000 to 90,000 persons in the United States (1,2). It is an acquired neurologic syndrome of unknown etiology, and is characterized by involuntary contractions of the neck and shoulder muscles leading to sustained head deviation (3). Unlike other dystonias, cervical dystonia is often associated with significant musculoskeletal pain, and can interfere markedly with the ability to lead a normal life (4,5). Oral pharmacologic treatments, including anticholinergics, muscle relaxants, and anticonvulsant drugs, are generally inadequate. Surgical treatment is effective in some cases but does not routinely offer effective long-term improvement.

Botulinum toxin (BT) is currently the most effective treatment for the symptomatic relief of cervical dystonia (6). Studies with the type A toxin shows that it improves head position, pain, and disability in up to 90% of patients. Of the seven serotypes, types A, B, C, and F have been studied in the treatment of cervical dystonia; however, at the present time, only types A and B are available commercially. Botulinum toxin type B (BT-B) is an antigenically distinct serotype that inhibits the release of acetylcholine at the neuromuscular junction by a different mechanism than that of the BT-A. Antibodies to BT-A and BT-B do not cross-neutralize as documented with *in vivo* studies (7). The effectiveness of BT-B in re-

ducing pain and postural abnormalities in cervical dystonia has been substantiated by several controlled clinical trials, and extends to patients who are resistant to BT-A.

DURATION OF EFFECTIVENESS

The duration of effectiveness of a BT is a fundamental aspect of its use in therapy. BT is given by injection into the contracting muscles responsible for the symptoms of dystonia. The beneficial effects are transient, generally lasting 3 to 4 months and reversing over time, necessitating repeated injections to prevent recurrence of symptoms. On a molecular level, the cleavage of the soluble NSF (N-ethylmaleimide sensitive factor) attachment protein receptor (SNARE) complex by BT is irreversible; however, after a period of remodeling, the system recovers "normal" neuromuscular transmission (8). The precise neurobiology that underlies this recovery is still undetermined, but several factors have been identified, including initial changes in the sensitivity and ion distributions of the postsynaptic membrane, reactive collateral and noncollateral axonal sprouting, manufacture and transport of new intact vesicles, the reestablishment of transmission across the original synaptic cleft, and the regression of axonal sprouts.

The duration of efficacy of BT can depend on many factors. Other than the toxin itself, the duration of effectiveness may be related to the severity of the underlying disease, dose, or outcome measures used. With BT-A, clinical data and experience suggest that the effects of the toxin typically last 10 to 12 weeks in cervical dystonia (6,9). Therefore, it is generally recommended that the patient be reinjected no sooner than once every 3 months (10). Reinjection at this time-interval should maintain efficacy and, most importantly, minimize the risk for development of secondary resistance, which has been a growing concern. Using this approach, many patients treated with BT-A for up to 10 years have continued to respond to therapy.

In an early exploratory study, it was suggested that the duration of effect of BT-B was not as long-lasting as that of BT-A in a foot muscle (extensor digitorum brevis) model (11). This study suggested that BT-B may require shorter reinjection periods to maintain efficacy, which consequently would increase the risk for development of secondary resistance. However, this early study did not compare equivalent doses of the two toxins; that is, the peak effect was not equivalent, resulting in an invalid comparison. The following section evaluates the duration of effectiveness for BT-B by reviewing data from four clinical trials—two that were randomized, placebo-controlled trials (12,13), and two that were open-label (14,15).

STUDIES WITH BOTULINUM TOXIN TYPE B IN CERVICAL DYSTONIA

Data on the duration of effectiveness of BT-B were obtained from two placebo-controlled trials and compiled for two open-label trials in use for cervical dystonia. It should be noted that none of these trials was designed to primarily evaluate duration of efficacy. In the first placebo-controlled trial (12), patients who were responsive to BT-A treatment were randomly assigned to treatment with placebo, 5000 U or 10,000 U of BT-B. The second placebo-controlled study was similar in design but included only patients who were clinically resistant to BT-A [as confirmed by a unilateral frontalis injection of 15 U of BT-A with no weakness after 2 weeks (fluorescent treponemal antibody test [F-TAT])] (13). Patients were randomized to either placebo or 10,000 U of BT-B. All patients received only one dose of study medication and returned for evaluation at week 2, 4, 8, 12, and 16 (termination). To determine the duration of treatment effect, Kaplan-Meier survival analyses were conducted. The median time to return to the baseline total score of the Toronto Western Spasmodic Torticollis Rating Scale (TWSTRS) was estimated for each treatment group.

Compared with patients receiving placebo, patients treated with BT-B had a significantly longer duration of treatment effect. Based on Kaplan-Meier analyses for both studies, the median duration of BT-B treatment effect was 12 to 16 weeks. In the trial with BT-A responders, the estimated duration was 114 days with the 5000-U treatment group and 111 days with the 10,000-U treatment group. Comparatively, the estimated duration was 63 days with placebo ($p = .01$). In the trial with BT-A–resistant patients, the estimated duration of treatment effect was 112 days in the 10,000-U treatment group compared with 59 days in the placebo group ($p = .004$). In both studies combined, when assessed by the percentage of responders, at 12 and 16 weeks, the results showed that 30% and 14%, respectively, had a >20% decrease from baseline in TWSTRS total scores (Fig. 28-1).

In the first open-label study (14), 145 patients were enrolled sequentially and entered into three, forced dose-escalation, treatment phases with BT-B of 10,000, 12,500, and 15,000 U. For each treatment phase, patients were injected with study drug on day 1, and then returned at weeks 2 and 4, and every 4 weeks thereafter until the investigator judged that the patient had returned to baseline cervical dystonia status. Once a patient returned to baseline status, dose-escalation occurred irrespective of the response to treatment, provided significant adverse events did not prevent continuation in the study. The last visit for each previous treatment phase was the day 1 visit for the subsequent treatment phase. The TW-

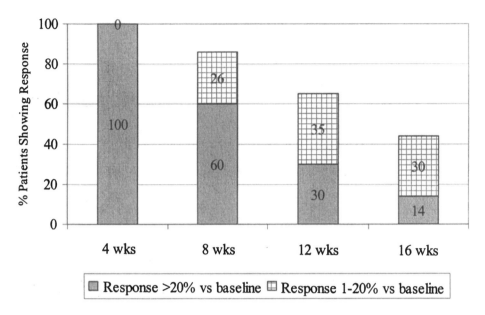

FIG. 28-1. Placebo-controlled studies: duration of effect by percentage of responders [based on change in the Toronto Western Spasmodic Torticollis Rating Scale (TWSTRS) total scores versus baseline].

STRS total score was the primary measure of treatment effect in this open-label study.

The majority of patients (>70%) in each dosing phase returned to baseline cervical dystonia status between 12 and 16 weeks (Fig. 28-2). The size of the mean TWSTRS-total improvement at 2 and 4 weeks after treatment was similar for the three treatment phases and was not related to escalating doses. However, there was evidence that the higher doses of BT-B may maintain effect longer than the lower dose. In responsive patients, the duration of effect was variable, ranging from 12 weeks to as long as 48 weeks in one patient. Overall, the effect of treatment for most patients was 12 to 16 weeks.

The second open-label study was a multicenter, outpatient, open-label extension study for those patients who had participated in earlier phase 2 and phase 3 studies with BT-B (15). The study also included a limited number of patients who were toxin-naive, postsurgical, or who had received phenol injections, and patients who failed the frontalis injection (i.e., had weakness with injection of BT-A) in the second placebo-controlled study (13). In

this study, 393 of the 427 patients enrolled had prior exposure to BT-B. For the first dosing session (session 1), all patients received up to 10,000 U of BT-B. Patients then returned to the clinic 4 weeks after their initial injection for a follow-up visit. Subsequently, patients were to be evaluated and reinjected after they had returned to baseline session 1 status or experienced bothersome return of symptoms and after at least 12 weeks had passed since their treatment session.

Several factors make it difficult to interpret the duration of efficacy within this study. First, it should be noted that enrollment in the study was staggered over a period of almost 4 years; therefore, some patients may have received more sessions of BT-B than other patients, depending on when they were enrolled in the study. (Note: The study was closed after BT-B was approved by the U.S. Food and Drug Administration for the treatment of cervical dystonia in December 2000.) In addition, some patients received an injection every 12 weeks regardless of whether they had returned to the session 1 baseline status.

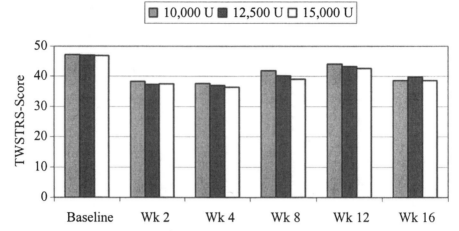

FIG. 28-2. Open-label study 1: TWSTRS (Toronto Western Spasmodic Torticollis Rating Scale) total scores by dose and visits through week 16.

Results show that repeated dosing with BT-B was effective, as measured by a decrease in TWSTRS scores following each treatment session (Fig. 28-3). There was also a decrease in baseline TWSTRS total scores at each session compared with session 1 baseline. This correlates with the fact that most patients were reinjected before returning to session 1 baseline. These findings also reflect an overall long-term duration of effect, as seen by the persistent reduction in baseline at the reinjection visit. This finding is consistent with a maintenance effect and continued benefit.

DISCUSSION

BT-B (Myobloc) is an antigenically distinct serotype available as a ready-to-use injectable solution, and is available in three dosing volumes: 2500, 5000, and 10,000 U. Clinical trials

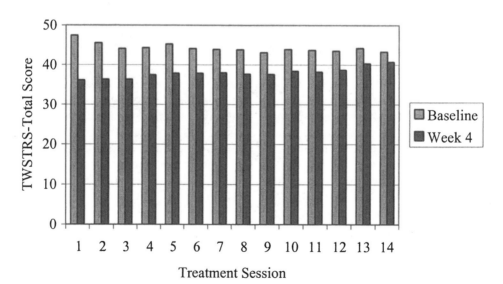

FIG. 28-3. Open-label study 2: mean TWSTRS (Toronto Western Spasmodic Torticollis Rating Scale) scores at baseline and week 4 of each treatment session. (Based on change in TWSTRS total scores versus baseline.)

have demonstrated its efficacy and safety in the treatment of cervical dystonia. This analysis of the duration of effect shows that BT-B produces a long-lasting benefit of 12 to 16 weeks, which is comparable to that of BT-A. In addition, it is worth mentioning a recent study, using surface electromyographic (EMG) recording in a nonhuman primate model, that evaluated the duration of paralysis in the trapezius muscle of the cynomolgus monkey, directly comparing BT-B and BT-A (16). By using doses of the toxins adjusted to produce equivalent initial effects (i.e., 70% denervation), the study found that the duration of effect is related to the dose and initial level of induced paralysis: the greater the initial paralysis, the longer the duration of denervation. There was no difference in the duration of effect produced by BT-B or BT-A toxins when dosed for equivalent denervation.

Clearly, a long duration of effectiveness is important in terms of BT therapy because it impacts patient satisfaction and cost of therapy, it determines the frequency of injections, and it may have an impact on immunogenicity. Based on data from two large placebo-controlled studies and two open-label studies, the duration of effectiveness of BT-B is between 12 and 16 weeks. Additional data will emerge from ongoing, multicenter, long-term cervical dystonia trials that will provide more information on the incidence of resistance and efficacy of BTs.

REFERENCES

1. Fahn S. The varied clinical expressions of dystonia. *Neurol Clin* 1984;2:541–554.
2. Nutt JG, Muenter MD, Aronson A, et al. Epidemiology of focal and generalized dystonia in Rochester, Minnesota. *Mov Disord* 1988;3:188–194.
3. Chan J, Brin MF, Fahn S. Idiopathic cervical dystonia: clinical characteristics. *Mov Disord* 1991;6:119–126.
4. Jankovic J, Leder S, Warner D, et al. Cervical dystonia: clinical findings and associated movement disorders. *Neurology* 1991;41:1088–1091.
5. Muller J, Kemmler G, Wissel J, et al. The impact of blepharospasm and cervical dystonia on health-related quality of life and depression. *J Neurol* 2002;249:842–846.
6. Dauer WT, Burke RE, Greene P, et al. Current concepts on the clinical features, aetiology and management of idiopathic cervical dystonia. *Brain* 1998;121:547–560.
7. Callaway JE, Arezzo JC, Grethlein AJ. Botulinum toxin type B: an overview of its biochemistry and preclinical pharmacology. *Semin Cut Med Surg* 2001;20:127–136.
8. Ahnert-Hilger G, Bigalke H. Molecular aspects of tetanus and botulinum neurotoxin poisoning. *Prog Neurobiol* 1995;46:83–96.
9. Odergren T, Hjaltason H, Kaakkola S, et al. A double blind, randomised, parallel group study to investigate the dose equivalence of Dysport and Botox in the treatment of cervical dystonia. *J Neurol Neurosurg Psychiatry* 1998;64:6–12.
10. Greene P, Fahn S, Diamond B. Development of resistance to botulinum toxin type A patients with torticollis. *Mov Disord* 1994;9:213–217.
11. Sloop RR, Cole BA, Escutin RO. Human response to botulinum toxin injection: type B compared with type A. *Neurology* 1997;49:189–194.
12. Brashear A, Lew MF, Dykstra DD, et al. Safety and efficacy of NeuroBloc (botulinum toxin type B) in type A-responsive cervical dystonia. *Neurology* 1999;53:1439–1446.
13. Brin MF, Lew MF, Adler CH, et al. Safety and efficacy of NeuroBloc (botulinum toxin type B) in type A-resistant cervical dystonia. *Neurology* 1999;53:1431–1438.
14. Cullis PA. Safety and efficacy of botulinum toxin type B: an open-label, dose-escalation study. *J Neurol Sci* 2001;187(suppl 1):1258(abst).
15. Data on file (Myobloc Study 351), Elan Pharmaceuticals, San Diego, California.
16. Arezzo JC, Litwak MS, Meyer KE, et al. The duration of paralysis in the trapezius muscle induced by botulinum toxins in the cynomolgus monkey. Abstract presented at the *Movement Disorder Society's 7th International Congress of Parkinson's Disease and Movement Disorders*, Miami, November 11–14, 2002.

Dystonia 4: Advances in Neurology, Vol. 94. Edited by Stanley Fahn, Mark Hallett, and Mahlon R. DeLong. Lippincott Williams & Wilkins, Philadelphia © 2004.

29

Is Phenotypic Variation of Hereditary Progressive Dystonia with Marked Diurnal Fluctuation/Dopa-Responsive Dystonia (HPD/DRD) Caused by the Difference of the Locus of Mutation on the GTP Cyclohydrolase 1 (GCH-1) Gene?

*Masaya Segawa, *Yoshiko Nomura, *Shoko Yukishita, †Nobuyoshi Nishiyama, and ‡Masayuki Yokochi

Segawa Neurological Clinic for Children, Tokyo, Japan. †Graduate School of Pharmaceutical Sciences, The University of Tokyo, Tokyo, Japan. ‡Department of Neurology, Tokyo Metropolitan Ebara Hospital, Tokyo, Japan

Hereditary progressive dystonia (HPD) with marked diurnal fluctuation or autosomal-dominant guanosine triphosphate (GTP) cyclohydrolase I (AD-GCH-I) deficiency is a dopa-responsive dystonia (DRD) caused by mutation of the gene of *GCH-I* located on 14q22.1 to q22.2. Clinically, HPD is characterized by a generalized postural dystonia with diurnal fluctuation, which has onset in childhood and shows an age-related course (1). Although HPD has been shown to have intra- and inter-familial variation, mainly depending on the ages at onset (2), after the discovery of the causative gene (3) a broad phenotypic variation was shown (4,5). On the other hand, the more than 80 loci of the mutation detected in this disease differ among families except for a few exceptions, and the ratio of mutant messenger RNA (mRNA) to wild mRNA of the *GCH-I* gene was shown to differ depending on the loci (6,7). This chapter evaluates phenotypes of 32 gene-proven patients and assesses the cause of the variation.

PATIENTS AND METHODS

Thirty-two patients from 16 families were studied. The ages of the patients at the time of study ranged from 18 to 82 years, and they were followed for 1 to 32 years. All patients and 20 parents provided informed consent to have gene analyses performed. We assessed the incidence and the pattern of familial occurrence, gender difference, ages at onset, and clinical phenotypes, and correlated these factors with the locus of mutation. Familial occurrence was assessed in three generations, including the parents' and grandparents' generation of the proband.

RESULTS

The locus of mutation of these families is shown in Table 29-1. All families had a different mutation, except for two unrelated families with mutation in intron 3. There were one nonsense, six missense mutations, and nine early truncations. Of the latter,

TABLE 29-1. *Mutation of guanosine triphosphate (GTP) cyclohydrolase I in patients with hereditary progressive dystonia (HPD) dopa-responsive dystonia (DRD)*

Domain of mutation	Family	Mutation	No. of patients
Exon 1	Sa	3 ins GG	2
	Ya	Leu 79 Pro	1
	Ka	Arg 88 Trp	2
	Is	Met 102 Arg	1
	Ik	200 ins 4 bp	2
	Oh	276 del C	2
Exon 2	Su	Asp 134 Val	3
	Mo	Cys 141 Arg	5
Intron 3	Ta	+1 G > A	4
	Sk	+1 G > A	1
	Ku	del +1– +4	2
Exon 4	It	511 del 13 bp	1
	Sh	Gln 180 stop	1
Exon 5	Na	Gly 201 Glu	2
	Yg	547 ins G	2
Exon 6	Nk	Met 230 Ile	1

three with mutations in intron 3 had skipping of exon 3.

The 32 patients showed marked female predominance: 27 females and 5 males (Table 29-2). This predominance was observed in each domain. Analysis of 20 parents revealed seven maternal and 12 paternal transmissions and one de novo case. Four of seven mothers and 10 of 12 fathers were asymptomatic carriers (Table 29-2).

As shown in Table 29-3, in five of the 16 families there were no other affected members in any of the three generations. Of these five families, two (including one de novo case) had a mutation in exon 1, two had a mutation in exon 4, and one had a mutation in exon 6. Of 11 families with affected individu-

als, six had affected members in the same generation including five with sibling occurrences, and eight had affected members in different generations including four parent–child occurrences. Three of these families also had sibling occurrence in one of the generations, one each in exon 1, intron 3, and exon 5.

The ages at onset were in childhood, ranging from 1 year 4 months to 13 years, except for one male with onset at 58 years, and most (30/32) were under 10 years (Fig. 29-1). Although they were not examined personally, there was one individual with ages at onset in the 20s and two with ages at onset in the 40s. These late-onset patients in the upper generation were observed in families with mutation in exon 2 (Mo) and intron 3 (Su, Ku), whereas

TABLE 29-2. *Profiles of patients (1): gender and transmission*

Locus of mutation	No. of families	No. of patients	Gender		Transmission		
			Female	Male	Mother	Father	Unknown
Exon 1	6	10	8	2	1(1)	1(0)	8(1)
Exon 2	2	8	7	1	2(1)	5(1)	1
Intron 3	3	7	6	1	2(0)	4(1)	1
Exon 4	2	2	2	0	1(0)	1(0)	0
Exon 5	2	4	3	1	1(1)	1(0)	2
Exon 6	1	1	1	0	0	0	1
Total	16	32	27	5	7(3*)	12(2*)	13(1**)

*Symptomatic individuals.
**De novo case.

TABLE 29-3. *Profiles of patients (2): familial occurrence*

Locus of mutation	No. of families	Familial occurrence		Same generation (sibling)	Different generation (parent–child)
		(−)	(+)		
Exon 1	6	2*	4	3(3)	2**(1)
Exon 2	2	0	2	1(0)	2(1)
Intron 3	3	0	3	2(1)	2**(1)
Exon 4	2	2	0	0(0)	0(0)
Exon 5	2	0	2	1(1)	2**(1)
Exon 6	1	1	0	0(0)	0(0)
Total	16	5	11	6(5)	8(4)

*One with de novo mutation.
**One had sibling occurrence in one generation.

patients with mutations in other domains had onset at under 10 years of age without any relation to the generation (Fig. 29-1). In families with mutation in exon 1 (Sa, Ka) and exon 2 (Su, Mo), the ages at onset tended to be earlier in the younger generation; however, in two families, one with mutation in exon 2 (Mo) and two in exon 5 (Na, Yg) the ages at onset were later in the younger generation.

Table 29-4 shows the initial symptoms and symptoms commonly observed. In most patients (29/32) the initial symptom was dystonia of one leg with gait disturbance. Two patients, a female with mutation in intron 3 (Ta) and a male with mutation in exon 5 (Na), started with dystonia at 8 years of age on the right and left upper extremity, respectively. The female also had action tremor and diffi-

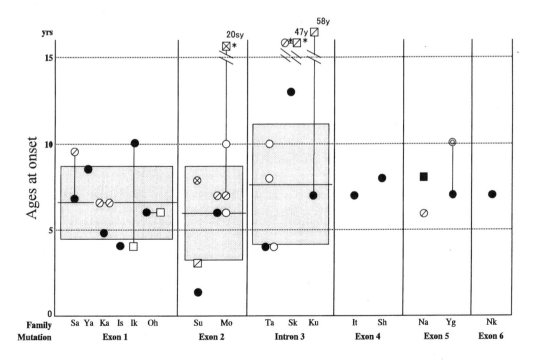

FIG. 29-1.

TABLE 29-4. *Clinical symptoms (1)*

| Locus of mutation | No. of patients | Initial symptom | | | Postural dystonia with LE predominance | Diurnal fluctuation | Postural tremor | Asymmetry | Low body length |
| | | Dystonia | | Tremor | | | | | |
		LE	UE						
Exon 1	10	10	0	0	10	10	5 (>10 yrs)	10	10
Exon 2	8	8	0	0	8	8	4 (>14 yrs)	8	7
Intron 3	7	5	1*	2*	6	6	2 (11, 58 yrs)	7	5
Exon 4	2	2	0	0	2	2	2 (9 yrs)	2	2
Exon 5	4	3	1	0	4	4	3 (>11 yrs)	4	3
Exon 6	1	1	0	0	1	1	1 (10 yrs)	1	1
Total	32	29	2	2	31	31	18 (ages at onset)	32	28

LE, lower extremity; UE, upper extremity.
*One started with dystonia and action tremor of a hand.

culty in getting dressed and undressed. The patient with onset at 58 years of age started with postural tremor of one hand.

The main symptoms were postural dystonia with lower extremity predominance in all except the one with onset at age 58. Diurnal fluctuation of symptoms was also observed in all patients except the adult-onset patient. Postural tremor was observed in 17 patients. The tremor appeared in one hand after 9 years of age, and in most in the second decade. In four L-dopa naive adult female patients with clinical histories of more than 30 years, the tremor was observed in all extremities including trunk muscles. No patient who started L-dopa before 9 years showed tremor. It was a predominant symptom of the adult-onset patient. Asymmetry of symptoms was observed in all patients. Shortness of body length including stagnation of growth was observed in all patients except four who had onset at around 10 years or later in adulthood.

As for less frequent symptoms, we observed action dystonia in four patients, oculogyric crisis in two, dystonic spasm in five, and torticollis in four (Table 29-5). However, one of two patients (exon 1) with oculogyric crisis, and two of five patients (exon 1 and 2) with dystonic spasm showed these symptoms after L-dopa. Except for patients with mutation in exon 1, oculogyric crisis and torticollis were observed in patients with action dystonia. No patients showed focal dystonia. In addition to these patients, one with de novo mutation in exon 1 showed myoclonic movement of one lower extremity and one each with mutation in exon 1 and exon 4 showed movement-induced aggravation of dystonia. One patient with mutation in exon 1 (Ya) had a depressive state and one in intron 3 (Ta) had migraine.

All patients responded to L-dopa markedly, the effects of which were sustained without any unfavorable side effects. However, patients with action dystonia with mutation in intron 3

TABLE 29-5. *Clinical symptoms (2)*

Locus of mutation	No. of patients	Action dystonia	Oculogyric crisis	Dystonic spasm	Torticollis
Exon 1	10	0	(1)	3(1)	1
Exon 2	8	1	0	(1)	1*
Intron 3	7	2	1*	0	1*
Exon 4	2	0	0	0	0
Exon 5	4	0	0	1	0
Exon 6	1	1	0	0	1*
Total	32	4	2(1)	5(2)	4

(): developed after L-dopa.
*Patient with action dystonia.

and exon 6 showed aggravation of action retrocollis and oculogyric crisis with initial doses of L-dopa, and one patient of family Oh with mutation in exon 1 demonstrated severe L-dopa–induced dyskinesia that necessitated stereotactic thalamotomy for treatment.

DISCUSSION

HPD/DRD or AD-GCH-I deficiency was first discovered by one of us (M.S.) (8), and, after accumulation of patients, its clinical characteristics were defined as follows: autosomal-dominant inheritance, onset in childhood (1–9 years), with gait disturbance due to dystonic posture of one leg, postural dystonia with lower limb predominance, postural tremor of hand, exaggeration of deep tendon reflexes with ankle clonus but without Babinski sign, asymmetry of symptoms, diurnal fluctuation, female predominance, and stagnation of body length (9,10). These symptoms are shown in Table 29-4. Symptoms shown in Table 29-5 are those that we excluded from the classic HPD/DRD (9,10).

We also postulated the age dependency of these symptoms, that is, postural tremor develops later, after 10 years, and the diurnal fluctuation is reduced with the passage of years. Additionally, there is a subsidence of progression of dystonia, while postural tremor expands to all extremities and trunk muscles by the fourth decade (9,10). The stagnation of body length is observed in childhood with development of dystonia. This is improved by L-dopa administrated before puberty and is not observed in patients with age at onset after the second decade.

Nomura and Segawa (2) evaluated their 22 patients and 43 reported patients with HPD, and confirmed the age-related variations of symptoms. Furthermore, they reported three adult-onset patients who started with hand tremor, whereas tremor did not develop if L-dopa was started in childhood (2). A patient with onset in his 20s (Mo) started with postural tremor and dystonia, but the dystonia was mild and showed no apparent progression. Two patients with onset in their 40s (Su)

started with postural tremor, which progressed with the course of the illness similarly to the postural tremor observed in the patient with onset at 58 years.

Patients with action dystonia and oculogyric crisis were considered to differ from patients with classic HPD because of differences in pathophysiology evaluated by clinical and neurophysiologic studies in two patients (11). However, we detected mutation of the *GCH-I* gene in these patients, one in intron 3 and the other in exon 6 (12). With reference to early-onset autosomal-dominant torsion dystonia [dystonia type 1 (DYT-1)], which has action and postural dystonia depending on the family, and focal dystonia in parents of the probands with action dystonia (13), we postulate that mutation of *GCH-I* could cause action as well as postural dystonia by the involvement of different neuronal pathways (12). Because torticollis as well as oculogyric crisis was observed in patients with action dystonia, these symptoms and focal dystonia might be caused by the pathophysiologic mechanisms involving action dystonia, which differ from those for postural dystonia (12).

Depressive state and migraine are symptoms caused by hypofunction of the serotonin [5-hydroxytryptamine (5-HT)] neurons, which could occur in AD-GCH-I deficiency with partial deficiency of tetrahydrobiopterin (BH4). Involvement of the 5-HT neurons was suggested from the necessity of using BH4 in addition to L-Dopa for complete recovery (14). Hypotonia and delay in walking and in language observed in patients with compound heterozygosity (5) are considered as symptoms caused by early 5-HT hypofunction.

L-dopa–induced dyskinesia observed in a female of family Oh had already been published by one of the authors (M.Y.) (15). It developed with a high dose of plain L-dopa of more than 60 mg/kg/day (the maximum optimal dose for HPD is 20 mg/kg/day). The histochemistry revealed a decrease of tyrosine hydroxylase and dopamine only in the striatum (15); however, her neuropathology showed gliosis and Lewy body–like structure in the substantia nigra (15,16).

Thus, for phenotypical variation in HPD/DRD or AD-GCH-I deficiency, at least three factors are considered to be involved: age (current age of the patient and age at onset), the difference in pathophysiology or in the involved neuronal circuit in the basal ganglia, and the presence or absence of hypofunction of the 5-HT neurons. The age factor might depend on the structural and functional maturation of the nigrostriatal dopamine neurons and the neuronal pathways related to the striatum (17,18). However, for the second and third factors, particularly for the second, the loci of the mutation might be involved.

In addition to these variations observed in our patients, there are other phenotypical variations reviewed by Bandmann et al. (4) and Müller et al, (19). Recently another phenotype with myoclonus was reported (20). The exact mechanism for AD-GCH-I mutation remains unclarified (19). It is necessary to clarify how the early BH4 hypofunction causes dysfunction of a certain neuron or neurons producing specific phenotypes, and why there is female predominance and age dependence of symptoms, and to demonstrate the roles of the loci of mutation. Evaluation of changes of the structure of the mutated GCH-I protein (21) should be assessed in addition to identification of the mutation itself.

ACKNOWLEDGMENTS

This study was partly supported by the Ministry of Health and Welfare of Japan. We extend sincere thanks to Dr. Hiroshi Ichinose for his advice and to Miho Tamaki, Junko Abe, and Makiko Ishikawa for preparation of this manuscript.

REFERENCES

1. Segawa M, Hosaka A, Miyagawa F, et al. Hereditary progressive dystonia with marked diurnal fluctuation. In: Eldridge R., Fahn S, eds. *Advances in Neurology,* vol 14. New York: Raven Press, 1976:215–233.
2. Nomura Y, Segawa M. Intrafamilial and interfamilial variations of symptoms of Japanese hereditary progressive dystonia with marked diurnal fluctuation. In: Segawa M, ed. *Hereditary progressive dystonia with marked diurnal fluctuation.* New York: Parthenon, 1993:73–96.
3. Ichinose H, Ohye T, Takahashi E, et al. Hereditary progressive dystonia with marked diurnal fluctuation caused by mutations in the GTP cyclohydrolase I gene. *Nat Genet* 1994;8:236–242.
4. Bandmann O, Valente EM, Holmans P, et al. Dopa-responsive dystonia. A clinical and molecular genetic study. *Ann Neurol* 1998;44:649.
5. Furukawa Y, Kish SJ, Bebin EM, et al. Dystonia with motor delay in compound heterozygotes for GTP-cyclohydrolase I gene mutations. *Ann Neurol* 1998;44:10–16.
6. Hirano M, Yanagihara T, Ueno S. Dominant negative effect of GTP cyclohydrolase I mutations in Dopa-responsive hereditary progressive dystonia. *Ann Neurol* 1998;44:365–371.
7. Hirano M, Ueno S. Mutant GTP cyclohydrolase I in autosomal dominant dystonia and recessive hyperphenylalaninemia. *Neurology* 1999;52:182–184.
8. Segawa M, Ohmi K, Itoh S, et al. Childhood basal ganglia disease with remarkable response to l-dopa. Hereditary basal ganglia disease with marked diurnal fluctuation [in Japanese]. *Shinryo* 1971;24:667–672.
9. Segawa M. Hereditary progressive dystonia with marked diurnal fluctuation (HPD) (in Japanese). *Adv Neurol Sci* 1981;25:73–81.
10. Segawa M, Nomura Y, Kase M. Diurnally fluctuating hereditary progressive dystonia. In: Vinken PJ, Bruyn GW, eds. *Handbook of clinical neurology. Extrapyramidal disorders,* vol 5(49). Amsterdam: Elsevier, 1986:529–539.
11. Segawa M, Nomura Y, Tanaka S, et al. Hereditary progressive dystonia with marked diurnal fluctuation. Consideration on its pathophysiology based on the characteristics of clinical and polysomnographical findings. In: Fahn S, Marsden CD, Calne DB, eds. *Advances in neurology,* vol 50. New York: Raven Press, 1988:367–376.
12. Segawa M, Hoshino K, Hachimori K, et al. A single gene for dystonia involves both or either of the two striatal pathways. In: Nicholson, Faull, eds. *The basal ganglia VII.* New York: Kluwer Academic/Plenum Press, 2002:155–163.
13. Nomura Y, Ikeuchi T, Tsuji S, et al. Two phenotypes and anticipation observed in Japanese cases with early onset torsion dystonia (DYT1)—pathophysiological consideration. *Brain Dev* 2000;22(suppl 1):92–101.
14. Ishida A, Takada G, Kobayashi Y, et al. Involvement of serotonergic neurons in hereditary progressive dystonia: clinical effects of tetrahydrobiopterin and 5-hydroxytryptophan [in Japanese]. *No To Hattatsu* 1988;20:195–199.
15. Yokochi M, Narabayashi H, Izuka R, et al. Juvenile parkinsonism—some clinical, pharmacological and neuropathological aspects. In: Hassler RG, Christ JF, eds. *Advances in neurology,* vol 40. New York: Raven Press, 1984:407–413.
16. Gibb WR, Narabayashi H, Yokochi M, et al. New pathologic observations in juvenile onset parkinsonism with dystonia. *Neurology* 1991;41:820–822.
17. Segawa M. Development of the nigrostriatal dopamine neuron and the pathways in the basal ganglia. *Brain Dev* 2000;22(suppl 1):1–4.
18. Segawa M. Hereditary progressive dystonia with

marked diurnal fluctuation. *Brain Dev* 2000;22(suppl 1):65–80.

19. Müller U, Steinberger D, Topka H. Mutation of GCH1 in Dopa-responsive dystonia. *J Neural Transm* 2002;109:321–328.

20. Leuzzi V, Antonozzi I. Autosomal dominant GTP-CH deficiency presenting as a dopa-responsive myoclonus-dystonia syndrome. *Neurology* 2002;59:1241–1243.

21. Maita N, Okada K, Hatakeyama K, et al. Crystal structure of the stimulatory complex of GTP cyclohydrolase I and its feedback regulatory protein GFRP. *Proc Natl Acad Sci USA* 2002;99(3):1212–1217.

Dystonia 4: Advances in Neurology, Vol. 94. Edited by Stanley Fahn, Mark Hallett, and Mahlon R. DeLong. Lippincott Williams & Wilkins, Philadelphia © 2004.

30

Focal Task-Specific Dystonia in Musicians

Steven J. Frucht

Department of Neurology, Columbia University, New York, New York

HISTORICAL PERSPECTIVE

By definition, focal task-specific dystonia (FTSD) affects one part of the body and occurs only during performance of a specific activity. Many different forms of FTSD have been described, and the disorder has attracted the interest of important neurologists of the nineteenth and twentieth centuries. Even subtle symptoms of musicians' dystonia are sufficient to derail a professional career, and unlike other forms of FTSD, the disorder is both visible and audible. For musicians, performance is integrally tied to the psyche, and the diagnosis of FTSD is a watershed event in a musician's life.

Although Sir Charles Bell was the first to report a patient with FTSD in 1830, Gowers' (1) 1888 account of writer's cramp remains unsurpassed. His insights on the clinical phenomenology, natural history, and treatment of FTSD apply not only to writer's cramp but to musicians' dystonia as well:

The affection [writer's cramp] is very much more common in males...doubtless because comparatively few women are engaged in occupations that involve a large amount of writing....It is a disease of the active period of adult life, very rarely commencing under twenty or after fifty....The affection sometimes follows local disease or injury....In many recorded instances some painful affection of a finger has preceded the onset....The occurrence of the disease is influenced less by the amount than by the manner of writing....It is the mode in which the pen is moved that chiefly determines the occurrence of the disease....The smaller the muscles employed, the greater must be the relative degree of contraction to produce a given movement of the pen, the greater is the amount of fatigue produced, and the more readily does cramp occur....The best and freest method is to write from the upper arm and shoulder, with no fixation of the arm....Writer's cramp is practically unknown among...shorthand writers. The speed required and the style needed for forming shorthand characters compels a very free style of writing, generally from the shoulder...and the result is that they have an almost complete immunity from the disease.

The commencement [of symptoms] is almost always gradual....After writing for some time the patient finds something unusual about his writing....In very rare instances the affection comes on in an acute manner....The spasm is almost always tonic in character...often accompanied by some tremor....The spasm may be limited to the act of writing, and other actions, even such as involve delicate muscular coordination, may be performed without the slightest difficulty. It is not uncommon, for instance, for the patient to be able to shave himself or to play the piano with perfect facility.

The symptoms continue and usually increase as long as the patient perseveres in the attempt to write....The sufferer who finds himself unable to write with one hand often learns to write with the other. After he has acquired the needful facility, and has written with the left hand for a long time, similar symptoms may develop in this hand, and they then usually progress more quickly than in the arm first affected....The tendency, often seen, for the other hand to be affected, affords additional evidence that the disease is essentially central....A patient, when he tried to write with his left hand, found his right fingers performing slow movements of flexion and extension.

The disease, when well developed, is one in which the prognosis is always uncertain, and often unfavorable....For the affection itself, treatment, to be effective, should be early. The commencing symptoms often pass away with a brief rest; a month's abstinence from writing at the onset will do more than a year's rest if the disease has continued for six months.

Among other occupations which have been known to lead to the development of cramp and have given names to special varieties, are those of...pianoforte players, violin players, seamstresses, telegraphists, smiths, harpists, artificial flower makers, turners, watchmakers, knitters, engravers, masons, compositors, enamellers, cigarette makers, shoemakers, milkers, money counters and zither players.

Although Gowers mentions FTSD affecting musicians, Poore (2) published the first large series of musicians with professional disability in 1887. His report describes 21 professional pianists with impaired performance, but careful review reveals that virtually none of these cases would meet the criteria for FTSD. Most had very prominent pain, likely from overuse or frank entrapment neuropathy. Poore recognized this fact:

You will have noticed that, although the act of piano-playing was most seriously affected, there was usually some general disability of the limb as well, which accompanied the "professional" trouble in almost every case. You are aware that, with regard to "writers' cramp," it is often asserted that, with the exception of the act of writing, there is nothing wrong. Although I cannot quite endorse the statement with regard to "writers' cramp," still I must admit that these cases of pianists' trouble offer a contrast to "writer's cramp" in the large amount of disability which generally existed for acts other than piano-playing.

Poore elegantly summarized the importance of professional impairment to the performing musician:

When I use the word "minor," please remember that they are minor only to our eye, and in a pathological sense; they are often of maximum importance to the sufferer, who possibly sees his livelihood in jeopardy, because his hand has forgotten its cunning.

Until the later part of the twentieth century, musicians' dystonia was generally regarded as a curiosity. The American pianist Gary Graffman's public announcement in 1981 that he was afflicted with FTSD in his right hand (3) sparked a surge of interest in performing arts medicine. Over the next decade Drs. Brandfonbrener, Lederman, Hochberg, and Charness reported large series of musicians with FTSD (4–7), and in the last 5 years neurophysiology and functional imaging approaches have been applied to patients with musicians' dystonia.

This chapter reviews the clinical problem of FTSD in musicians, addressing six questions:

1. What is the prevalence of FTSD in musicians?
2. Who is at risk for developing FTSD?
3. What triggers the onset of symptoms of FTSD in musicians?
4. Is musical performance a risk factor for development of dystonia?
5. Why does FTSD affect the hand?
6. How should musicians with FTSD be managed?

QUESTION 1: WHAT IS THE PREVALENCE OF FOCAL TASK-SPECIFIC DYSTONIA IN MUSICIANS?

Of the five studies published on the epidemiology of writer's cramp (8–11), prevalence rates vary from 7 per million for Northern England to 69 per million for the United States. The largest study conducted by the European Collaborative Group revealed a prevalence of 14 per million (12). Although there are no comparable data for musicians, the prevalence of musicians' dystonia can be estimated from clinical series of performing arts medicine centers in the United States. Performing artists are usually loath to seek medical attention, preferring to battle out their difficulties in the practice room. Once they do seek attention, appropriate diagnosis may be delayed due to failure of the clinician to recognize the disorder. Even so, in these clinical series the percentage of patients with FTSD ranged from 5% to 14% (4–6). Assuming that

10% of patients evaluated at performing arts clinics are affected with FTSD, and assuming also that 2% of professional musicians might seek medical evaluation during this period, the prevalence among professional musicians might be as high as 0.2%. Altenmuller (personal communication) estimated the prevalence of FTSD among musicians to be as high as 0.5% of 10,000 performing German musicians, based on his personal series of 179 musicians diagnosed with FTSD.

QUESTION 2: WHO IS AT RISK FOR DEVELOPING FOCAL TASK-SPECIFIC DYSTONIA?

FTSD has been reported in players of virtually every instrument, including strings (violin, viola, cello), keyboard (piano, accordion, organ, harpsichord), plectrum instruments (guitar, banjo, lute, mandolin), woodwinds (flute, clarinet, saxophone, oboe, bassoon), and brass (trumpet, French horn, trombone, tuba). Men outnumber women in most clinical series. Symptoms of musicians' dystonia usually begin in the fourth decade, similar to Gowers' description of writer's cramp. Musicians usually begin their formal training between the ages of 4 and 10, and most elements of their technique are fully formed by age 20. Thus, FTSD rarely occurs during the period when fine motor skills are acquired but rather during the period of peak professional output. Most musicians with FTSD do not have a family history of dystonia, and the *DYT1* gene mutation has not been found in several small series of musicians with FTSD (13). Both amateur and professional musicians are at risk for FTSD.

QUESTION 3: WHAT TRIGGERS THE ONSET OF SYMPTOMS OF FOCAL TASK-SPECIFIC DYSTONIA IN MUSICIANS?

Several case series have commented on the association of injury or overuse with the onset of dystonic symptoms. Patients often date the onset of dystonia to an increase in practice time, change in technique, or an attempt to tackle a challenging repertoire. However, many patients with FTSD cannot recall exactly when their symptoms began, similar to Gowers' description of patients with writer's cramp. Musicians tend to relate the onset of their symptoms to a particular event, in the hope that identifying a trigger may help treat their symptoms.

Although rare, peripheral trauma may trigger FTSD. Charness et al. (7) reported a series of patients whose dystonic flexion of the fourth and fifth fingers was associated with an ipsilateral ulnar neuropathy. The presence of ulnar neuropathy strongly predicted the pattern of dystonic movements, and in some patients symptoms of FTSD improved when the ulnar neuropathy was surgically corrected (7). Two other musicians have been reported with FTSD following peripheral trauma (14), suggesting that peripheral injury can trigger a central movement disorder.

QUESTION 4: IS MUSICAL PERFORMANCE A RISK FACTOR FOR THE DEVELOPMENT OF DYSTONIA?

Nonhuman primate studies by Byl et al. (15) and others have suggested that focal dystonia results when a limb is subjected to repetitive, attended, fine movements. If true, one might expect that among musicians, the hand that performs the more complex task would be more likely to develop FTSD. Although there are no prospective studies to answer this question, pooling of available case series of musicians with FTSD (4–7) confirms this impression. Among 129 musicians reported in the literature with FTSD in which information was available about their instrument and hand involvement, the right hand was affected in 64%. Among keyboard players, 75% involved the right hand ($n = 61$), and plectrum instruments had a similar predisposition for the right hand (79%, $n = 19$). In most keyboard pieces, the demands placed on the right hand far exceed those placed on the left, and similarly the complexity of plucking six strings outweighs the demands placed on a guitarist's left hand.

Among string players (violin, viola, and cello) the situation is reversed, with 71% of reported patients (n = 24) affected on the left. Compared to the demands placed on the bow arm, the fingers of the left hand perform a far more complex task in negotiating fingering and shifting of positions. If this hypothesis is correct, one might also expect that woodwind players should not show a hand preference for FTSD, as both right and left hands perform tasks of equal difficulty in depressing the keys. Although the numbers are small, published examples of flutists and clarinetists with FTSD (n = 25) support this hypothesis, with 44% involving the left hand and 54% the right.

If the nature and complexity of the motor task is related to the development of FTSD, one might also expect that the pattern of dystonic hand movements should reflect these demands, i.e., that certain patterns of hand movements would be associated with certain instruments. Several dystonic hand patterns have been described, including flexion of the fourth and fifth fingers in pianists (4,7), flexion of the third finger in guitarists, and extension of the third finger in clarinetists (4). However, many different patterns of dystonia have been reported among performers of the same instrument, and the same stereotyped pattern of dystonic movements may be seen in a wide range of different instruments. One possible explanation is that while the demands of the instrument may influence the pattern of dystonia, the complexity and large number of degrees of freedom inherent in hand and finger movements make this association a loose one.

QUESTION 5: WHY DOES FOCAL TASK-SPECIFIC DYSTONIA AFFECT THE HAND?

This question might seem absurd—after all, musicians use their hands to play their instruments. However, Lederman (5) and Brandfon-brener (6) first reported several woodwind and brass instrumentalists with dystonia of the lips and face. In a recent paper, my colleagues and I reviewed the natural history of embouchure dystonia in 26 professional brass and woodwind performers (16). This series has been expanded to include 57 patients, the largest series of such patients reported.

The embouchure refers to the pattern of muscles of the lower face, tongue, and jaw used to control the force and direction of airflow into the mouthpiece of a woodwind or brass instrument. Just as string and keyboard instrumentalists spend their adult lives learning to control rapid fine hand movements, brass and woodwind players devote similar attention to developing exquisite control of the embouchure. Patients with embouchure dystonia were strikingly similar to musicians with FTSD of the hand. Symptoms began in the fourth decade, an average of 25 years after inception of musical study. Only one patient had a first-degree relative with dystonia, and only two had experienced an oral trauma immediately prior to the onset of dystonic symptoms. Five of 57 patients also developed a coincident writer's cramp, suggesting a possible genetic predisposition to the development of FTSD.

Symptoms of dystonia began in one register (74%) and with one technique (56%), and remained register-specific (65%) and technique-specific (38%) at the time of evaluation. Only 12% of patients had experienced prior difficulties with their embouchure, and pain was distinctly uncommon (18%). Unlike dystonia of the hand, each patient could be categorized into one of four groups by the phenomenology of their movements: embouchure tremor (a fine, fast tremor of the lips), lip-pulling (lateral or upward movement of one or both lips), lip-lock (involuntary clamping together of the lips), and jaw movement (lateral movement or jaw clenching). Patients who played high-register brass instruments (trumpet and French horn) were much more likely to develop embouchure tremor or lip-pulling, while all patients affected with lip-lock dystonia played low-register brass instruments, trombone or tuba. Eight of 11 patients with jaw dystonia were woodwind players, and five patients with jaw involvement during playing experienced spread of dystonia to other oral activities, such as speaking or eating.

QUESTION 6: HOW SHOULD MUSICIANS WITH FOCAL TASK-SPECIFIC DYSTONIA BE MANAGED?

Historical therapies for FTSD included treatment with cod-liver oil, strychnine, arsenic, atropine, morphine, belladonna extract, cocaine, electricity, tenotomy, and even putting an affected hand into the belly of a slaughtered animal, which were of questionable benefit (and sanitary concern!). Modern approaches to treatment include injections of botulinum toxin (17,18), instrument modification and retraining, and rehabilitation approaches aimed at modifying the cortical representation of the affected limb, including limb immobilization (see Chapter 33) (19,20). Botulinum toxin offers a safe and effective technique for inhibiting excessive spasms, but often at the cost of excessive weakness. It also does not improve the subjective feeling of incoordination or lack of control of fine hand movements that may be very frustrating for the patient. Preliminary results from rehabilitation techniques are promising but require larger trials to confirm their initial success.

Perhaps the most important point in caring for musicians with FTSD is to understand their expectations and needs. Unlike other patients with dystonia, therapy of FTSD is of little use to a performing artist unless it produces virtually 100% recovery. For many musicians, being able to play their instrument is intimately tied to their sense of self-worth, and the diagnosis of FTSD carries profound psychological and financial implications. To address the needs of musicians with FTSD, Glen Estrin and I founded a program, Musicians with Dystonia, in January 2000 as part of the Dystonia Medical Research Foundation. The organization was formed with three major goals: to offer practical support to musicians afflicted with dystonia, to raise awareness of dystonia in the musical community and in the community at large, and to facilitate research collaborations into the cause and treatment of focal dystonia in musicians. Interested patients and researchers may contact the foundation at the website: *www.dystonia-foundation.org*, or by e-mail, *musicians@dystonia-foundation.org*.

REFERENCES

1. Gowers WR. *A manual of diseases of the nervous system.* Philadelphia: P. Blakiston, 1888.
2. Poore GV. Clinical lecture on certain conditions of the hand and arm which interfere with the performance of professional acts, especially piano-playing. *Br Med J* 1887;1:441–447.
3. Graffman G. Doctor, can you lend an ear? *Med Probl Perform Art* 1986;1:3–6.
4. Newmark J, Hochberg FH. Isolated painless manual incoordination in 57 musicians. *J Neurol Neurosurg Psychiatry* 1987;50:291–295.
5. Lederman RJ. Focal dystonia in instrumentalists: clinical features. *Med Probl Perform Art* 1991;6:132–136.
6. Brandfonbrener AG. Musicians with focal dystonia: a report of 58 cases seen during a ten-year period at a performing arts medicine clinic. *Med Probl Perform Art* 1995;10:121–127.
7. Charness ME, Ross MH, Shefner JM. Ulnar neuropathy and dystonic flexion of the fourth and fifth digits: clinical correlation in musicians. *Muscle Nerve* 1996;19:431–437.
8. Nutt JG, Muenter MD, Aronson A, et al. Epidemiology of focal and generalized dystonia in Rochester, Minnesota. *Mov Disord* 1988;3:188–194.
9. Sempere AP, Duarte J, Coria F, et al. Prevalence of idiopathic focal dystonia in the province of Segovia, Spain. *J Neurol* 1994;241:S124.
10. Nakashima K, Kusumi M, Inoue Y, et al. Prevalence of focal dystonias in the western area of Trottori prefecture in Japan. *Mov Disord* 1995;10:440–443.
11. Duffey POF, Butler AG, Hawthorne MR, et al. The epidemiology of the primary dystonias in the North of England. In: Fahn S, Marsden CD, DeLong M, eds. *Advances in neurology, dystonia 3.* Philadelphia: Lippincott-Raven, 1998:121–125.
12. Warner TT. A prevalence study of primary dystonia in eight European countries. *J Neurol* 2000;247:787–792.
13. Friedman JR, Klein C, Leung J, et al. The GAG deletion of the *DYT1* gene is infrequent in musicians with focal dystonia. *Neurology* 2000;55:1417–1418.
14. Frucht S, Fahn S, Ford B. Focal task-specific dystonia induced by peripheral trauma. *Mov Disord* 2000;15:348–350.

15. Byl NN, Merzenich MM, Cheung S, et al. A primate model for studying focal dystonia and repetitive strain injury: effects on the primary somatosensory cortex. *Phys Ther* 1997;77:269–284.
16. Frucht SJ, Fahn S, Greene PE, et al. The natural history of embouchure dystonia. *Mov Disord* 2001;16: 899–906.
17. Cole RA, Cohen LG, Hallett M. Treatment of musician's cramp with botulinum toxin. *Med Probl Perform Art* 1991;6:137–143.
18. Ross MH, Charness ME, Sudarsky L, et al. Treatment of occupational cramp with botulinum toxin: diffusion of toxin to adjacent noninjected muscles. *Muscle Nerve* 1997;20:593–598.
19. Candia V, Elbert T, Altenmuller E, et al. Constraint-induced movement therapy for focal hand dystonia in musicians. *Lancet* 1999;353:42.
20. Priori A, Pesenti A, Cappellari A, et al. Limb immobilization for the treatment of focal occupational dystonia. *Neurology* 2001;57:405–409.

Dystonia 4: Advances in Neurology, Vol. 94. Edited by Stanley Fahn, Mark Hallett, and Mahlon R. DeLong. Lippincott Williams & Wilkins, Philadelphia © 2004.

31

Brain Mapping in Musicians with Focal Task-Specific Dystonia

*Michael E. Charness and †Gottfried Schlaug

*Department of Neurology, Harvard Medical School; Department of Neurology, Brigham and Women's Hospital; and Neurology Service, Veterans Affairs Boston Healthcare System, Boston, Massachusetts. †Department of Neurology, Harvard Medical School; and Beth Israel Deaconess Medical Center, Boston, Massachusetts

FOCAL TASK-SPECIFIC DYSTONIA IN MUSICIANS: A DISORDER OF SKILL

Focal task-specific dystonia (FTSD) in musicians is a disorder of skill. Though sometimes unable to play music at the most elementary level, musicians with FTSD may function normally in all other respects. Once considered a psychogenic disorder, FTSD is associated with a variety of physiologic abnormalities, even when subjects do not perform any movements. Physiologic studies of patients with FTSD provide evidence for reorganization of sensorimotor cortex, decreased cortical inhibition, reduced suppression of competing movements, altered planning of movement, and impaired integration of sensory and motor processes (1–8).

FTSD arises primarily in those musicians with high levels of skill and develops rarely during the acquisition of the skill (9). Therefore, FTSD may emerge through an alteration of the plastic neural processes that accompany the rehearsal of highly skilled movements. Because FTSD occurs in a minority of musicians, it is clear that experience-related neural plasticity is not a sufficient condition for the emergence of this disorder. This chapter examines brain mapping studies in musicians with FTSD and in patients with writer's cramp, a related FTSD;

explores the experience-dependent neural plasticity that accompanies the acquisition and maintenance of motor skill in normal musicians; and speculates on additional genetic and environmental factors that might trigger the onset of FTSD.

PHYSIOLOGICAL ALTERATIONS IN MUSICIANS WITH FOCAL TASK-SPECIFIC DYSTONIA

Patients with FTSD show abnormalities in sensory processing and sensorimotor integration. For example, sensory input to the resting limb of patients with FTSD can provoke dystonic limb contraction (10–12). Vibration-induced muscle contraction in patients with FTSD can be diminished by small doses of locally injected lidocaine that reduce muscle spindle afferent activity without causing paralysis (11). Vibration of the affected or the unaffected hand produced significantly less activation of the contralateral sensorimotor cortex and supplementary motor area (SMA) in the FTSD patients than in normal controls (13,14). Yoneda et al. (15) found that perception of the tonic vibration reflex was reduced at multiple levels of the nervous system in patients with FTSD. These studies provide evidence for widespread abnormalities in the processing of muscle spindle afferents in FTSD.

INCREASED CORTICAL EXCITATION AND DECREASED CORTICAL INHIBITION

One apparent locus for the loss of reciprocal inhibition is the motor cortex. Siebner et al. (16) used repetitive transcranial magnetic stimulation (rTMS) to study the excitability of motor cortex in patients with FTSD and in controls. They found that rTMS caused a significant increase in motor unit potentials in dystonic patients, but a significant decrease in those of controls. They concluded that corticomotor excitation is significantly greater in patients with FTSD than in controls. Using TMS, Ikoma et al. (17) also found evidence of increased cortical excitability in patients with FTSD. Increased cortical excitability may result from reduced intracortical inhibition, as suggested by physiologic studies using a paired pulse TMS paradigm (18). Subthreshold, low-frequency rTMS diminished the excitability of motor cortex in patients with writer's cramp and produced a concomitant, transient improvement in writing (19). Evidence from magnetic resonance spectroscopy suggests that decreased cortical inhibition in FTSD may be the result of decreased levels of cortical γ-aminobutyric acid (GABA) (20). The observation of increased cortical excitability in patients with FTSD is interesting in light of similar findings in some studies of nondystonic subjects after the learning of new motor skills (see below).

Patients with FTSD show alterations in the organization of the motor cortex as well as its excitability. Using TMS, Byrnes et al. (21) mapped the corticomotor projections to the abductor pollicis brevis (APB) and first dorsal interosseus (FDI) in patients with writer's cramp and in normal controls. Patients with writer's cramp showed displacement of the maps for the APB and FDI, which normalized transiently following treatment with botulinum toxin. Abnormal maps were sometimes evident in clinically unaffected muscles, consistent with a generalized abnormality of motor control in patients with FTSD. The magnitude of displacement of the corticomotor maps was a function of the duration and severity of the FTSD. The plasticity of cortical maps following botulinum toxin injection suggests that the abnormal cortical maps arise from altered sensory feedback from dystonic muscles.

There is also evidence that FTSD is associated with abnormalities in the planning of movement. Deuschl et al. (22) studied movement-related cortical potentials in a self-paced finger abduction task. The amplitude of the early portion of the negative slope peak, the Bereitschaftspotential, was reduced in patients with simple or dystonic writer's cramp. Because this activity precedes electromyographic activity, the authors concluded that patients with FTSD have a deficiency in motor cortex activation just prior to movement.

ABNORMALITIES IN SENSORY MAPS

Frank distortions in the cortical representations of the digits have also been identified by brain imaging in patients with FTSD. Elbert et al. (23), using magnetic source imaging [magnetoencephalography (MEG)], found that the distance between the cortical sensory representation of digit pairs was smaller in musicians with FTSD than in nondystonic musicians or in normal controls. Interestingly, four of seven dystonic musicians also showed fusion of the cortical digital representation contralateral to the nondystonic hand, consistent with the presence of a generalized disorder of sensory organization. Bara-Jiminez et al. (24), mapping with somatosensory evoked responses, observed fusion of the cortical representation of the digits in primary somatosensory cortex (S1) as well as inversion of the position of the thumb and little finger in patients with FTSD (including one musician) compared to the typical sensory homunculus of healthy controls. Meunier et al. (25) found more prominent fusion of the cortical representation of the digits contralateral to the normal hand than contralateral to the dystonic hand. They speculated that physiologic adaptations to the FTSD helped normalize somatosensory maps contralateral to the FTSD. These data are consistent with observations in monkeys that alterations of sensory input can lead to a reorganization of the sensory cortex (26,27). Indeed, patients with FTSD showed a defect in the discrimination of temporally and spatially related sensory input to the hand (4,5).

Functional magnetic resonance imaging (fMRI) has been employed to study patterns of brain activation in musicians with FTSD. Pujol et al. (28) employed a specially constructed guitar that could be played in the MRI scanner. Playing the guitar in normal subjects activated the somatosensory cortex contralaterally and the premotor area (PMA), SMA, and posterior parietal lobe bilaterally. In contrast, dystonia-inducing guitar playing resulted in a greatly reduced activation of the PMA and a significantly increased activation of the primary sensorimotor cortex. Charness and Schlaug (29) compared brain activation during paced tapping of the little finger among concert pianists, pianists with FTSD, and nonmusicians. Although the tapping task was performed similarly among the three groups, the concert pianists showed increased activation of the dorsolateral precentral gyrus and a tendency for reduced activation of SMA and parietal regions compared with the nonmusicians. Pianists with FTSD showed a pattern of activation that was more similar to that of the nonmusicians than to that of the concert pianists. These findings imply that concert pianists can control finger movements by activating neural networks that are smaller than those activated in nonmusicians. In contrast, the loss of skill in pianists with FTSD was associated with a regression toward the activation pattern of the less skilled nonmusicians.

EXPERIENCE-RELATED NEUROPLASTICITY AND MOTOR LEARNING

If FTSD is a disorder of skill, then experience-related neuroplasticity may be a neces-

sary, but not sufficient, condition for the development of FTSD. Motor learning in humans is associated with short-term and long-term neural plasticity, each component mediated by different neural networks (30–32). Initial learning of a motor task engages the sensorimotor cortex and the prefrontal cortex. Within hours, strengthening and stabilization of the motor program is associated with a shift in regional brain activation to the PMA, cerebellum, and posterior parietal cortex. Using TMS, Pascual-Leone et al. (33) showed that corticomotor output is potentiated during the learning of a five-finger scale. Functional MRI also demonstrates increased movement-induced activation of the motor cortex after motor training (34). Cortical plasticity may be extremely rapid; reversible changes in the motor representation of thumb movements can be demonstrated by TMS after 15 to 30 minutes of training, and in a few cases in as little as 5 to 10 minutes (35). This rapid and reversible plasticity may reflect a reduction in GABA-mediated cortical inhibition (36), and precedes the more permanent changes in cortical representation that characterize motor learning (31,32,34).

FUNCTIONAL AND STRUCTURAL REORGANIZATION OF THE BRAIN IN MUSICIANS

If motor training alters brain circuitry, then movement of the fingers should activate the brain differently in instrumental musicians than in nonmusicians. Jancke et al. (37) observed a decrease in the activation of presupplementary motor area, cingulate motor area (CMA), and primary motor cortex (M1) during a tapping task in two pianists compared with a larger group of controls. Using a different task and larger experimental groups, Krings et al. (38) found a significantly smaller number of activated voxels for the primary sensorimotor cortex (SM1), SMA, and PMA in pianists compared to nonmusicians. Hund-Georgiadis and von Cramon (39) observed changes in the activation patterns between pianists and nonmusicians during the 35-minute course of learning a complex finger tapping task. At the beginning of the learning period, pianists showed reduced activation of secondary motor areas, whereas at the end, they showed increased activation of contralateral M1. Taken together, these fMRI studies suggest that the advanced training of pianists allows them to control complex finger movements through increased activation of M1 but reduced activation of secondary motor areas, compared with nonmusicians.

The manual skills of musicians are dependent on the integration of somatosensory and motor information. Musical training might therefore lead to changes in sensorimotor organization. Elbert et al. (40) used MEG to study the organization of the somatosensory cortex in string players. The dipole localization for the somatosensory representation of the second and fifth digits after applying a vibratory stimulus was significantly further apart in string players than in controls, but there were no significant group differences for the right digits. The magnitude of these changes was inversely correlated with the age at which musical lessons began. The playing of a bowed string instrument places asymmetric demands on the digits of the left and right hands. These data indicate that unique patterns of hand and finger activity in musicians shape the functional organization of the nervous system, particularly when musical training begins early.

Brain development is influenced by neuronal activity; hence, it is possible that musical training alters brain morphology as well as brain function. Studies in musicians suggest that early musical training influences the volume of selective brain regions. Schlaug et al. (41) showed that the anterior half of the corpus callosum was significantly larger in musicians with early training than in musicians with late training or in nonmusicians. Enlargement of other portions of the corpus callosum has also been reported in musicians compared with controls (42). The absolute and percentage volume of the cerebellum in male musicians was 5% larger than that of male nonmusicians, and there was a significant correlation between practice intensity and cerebellar volume (43). Amunts et al. (44) measured the intrasulcal length of the posterior precentral gyrus (ILPG) as a gross anatomic marker of primary motor cortex size in musicians and in nonmusicians. The ILPG was larger in a dorsal subregion of the motor cortex of both hemispheres in musicians compared to nonmusicians. This study also found a correlation between the enlarged ILPG and early commencement of musical training. In addition, the ILPG was less asymmetrical in musicians than in nonmusicians, which was due to an enlargement of the ILPG of the nondominant hand in keyboard players.

Overall, these data indicate that early musical training alters both the functional organization and the structure of the brain. In considering the contribution of motor learning to the development of FTSD, one important point is that the acquisition and maintenance of motor skill is associated with a reduction in cortical inhibition and an increase in cortical excitability. These changes are associated with an expansion of the representational area of fingers as well as movements, physiologic changes also observed in FTSD. This experience-related neural plasticity may predispose to FTSD, although additional factors must also be involved, because most musicians are unaffected.

FUNCTIONAL REORGANIZATION OF THE BRAIN AFTER INJURY AND OVERUSE

The search for factors that trigger FTSD in musicians should include an examination of the events that are associated with its onset. Although the onset of FTSD is insidious and uneventful in some musicians, others develop FTSD in the setting of nerve entrapment, soft tissue injury, overuse, learning of a second musical instrument, stress, or alterations in musical technique (9). To the extent that some of these conditions induce cortical plasticity, they might also contribute to the onset of FTSD. For example, some musicians develop FTSD for their primary instrument while learning to play a second instrument (9). For these patients, FTSD may be triggered when learning the second instrument lowers cortical inhibition below a critical threshold that is approached after learning to play the primary instrument. Musicians must also alter long-standing motor patterns to play while recovering from a soft tissue injury, to avoid pain, or to compensate for weakness. Like learning to play a second instrument, learning these alterations in technique might impose a sufficient reduction in cortical inhibition to trigger FTSD.

Nerve, tendon, and other soft tissue injuries occur commonly after prolonged playing in instrumental musicians (45–47). These injuries can also lead to reorganization of the sensorimotor cortex. Section of the median nerve in adult monkeys causes an expansion of the somatosensory cortical representation of the radial and ulnar cutaneous territory into the territory of the previous median representation (48). Injury to the facial nerve, a purely motor nerve, results in enlargement of the cortical representation of the hand into regions that normally subserve movement of the face (49). Therefore, it is possible that common nerve entrapments in musicians, such as carpal tunnel syndrome or cubital tunnel syndrome, induce plastic changes that predispose to FTSD.

Many musicians with dystonic flexion of the little and ring fingers have an ipsilateral ulnar neuropathy, and in some the severity of the dystonia and the ulnar neuropathy fluctuate in parallel (9). Interestingly, patients with ulnar neuropathy and no FTSD show the same pattern of co-contraction in agonist and antagonist muscles as patients with FTSD (50,51). Although patients with isolated ulnar neuropathy have reduced reciprocal inhibition of the H reflex and decreased spinal inhibition, they do not exhibit the increased cortical excitation observed in patients with FTSD (51). What triggers the transition from ulnar neuropathy to FTSD is unknown. Conceivably, constitutively low levels of cortical inhibition predispose some musicians to develop FTSD after the onset of ulnar neuropathy. Ulnar nerve injury might selectively increase the cortical representation of the median superficial flexors, predisposing to flexion dystonia of the little and ring fingers.

Repetitive movements of the hands, even in the absence of nerve or tendon injury, can lead to cortical reorganization. Byl and colleagues (26) trained New World owl monkeys to perform a repetitive grasping task. With time, there was a decline in the accuracy of the performance of the task, and dystonic-appearing grasping movements appeared. Cortical mapping with penetrating electrodes revealed reorganization of the somatosensory cortex, with enlargement and overlap of receptive fields. This model might be relevant to some musicians who develop FTSD in the setting of overuse, such as a large increase in the number of their customary repetitive movements.

Learning an advanced motor skill is common to all musicians, and upper extremity injuries occur at some time during the careers of most musicians (52); hence, additional factors must account for the development of FTSD in a minority. Genetic factors may play a role, because FTSD occurs with increased frequency among first-degree relatives of patients with Oppenheim's dystonia *(DYT1)*, and in one series, 25% of patients with focal dystonia had relatives with dystonia (53). One reported family with mutations in the *DYT1* gene comprised multiple members with writer's cramp, including one with guitarist's cramp (54). A study of 18 consecutive musicians with FTSD did not reveal any with mutations in the *DYT1* gene, although one small family was encountered that included two sibling musicians with FTSD (55). Thus, while mutation of the *DYT1* gene is not a common cause of FTSD in musicians, other genetic abnormalities might still play a role.

The nature of what might be inherited in FTSD is unknown. It is noteworthy that many patients with unilateral FTSD have bilateral abnormalities on physiologic or brain mapping studies (18,21,23,25,56–58). It remains unclear whether these abnormalities precede and predispose to the development of FTSD or reflect the physiologic events that follow the onset of FTSD. The emergence of FTSD may require "multiple hits." For example, FTSD might occur in a musician with ulnar neuropathy and genetically determined low levels of cortical GABA, but not in a musician with ulnar neuropathy and normal levels of GABA. FTSD is more prevalent in males than in females (9,59), consistent with the possibility that male or female hormones modulate the expression of FTSD.

Although mutations in the *DYT1* gene are rare in FTSD, Oppenheim's dystonia is an instructive model of a genetic disorder in which clinical expression appears to require multiple hits. Oppenheim's dystonia is an autosomal-dominant disorder, yet clinical penetrance is only 30% to 40% (60–62). Positron emission tomographic (PET) studies comparing patients with Oppenheim's dystonia to normal subjects reveal different patterns of brain activation during dystonic movement and at rest (63). Manifesting *DYT1* carriers exhibit increased metabolic activity in the cerebellum, thalamus, and midbrain during dystonic movement, but not during sleep, when involuntary movements cease. In contrast, both manifesting and nonmanifesting *DYT1* carriers show increased activity in the lenticular nuclei, cerebellum, and SMA while at rest compared with normal controls (63). These findings suggest that mutations in the *DYT1* gene are commonly associated with abnormalities in regional brain metabolism, but additional genetic or environmental factors are required for clinical expression of the disorder. As is true for FTSD, the triggering events in Oppenheim's dystonia are unknown.

It is conceivable that FTSD is a genetic disorder with extremely low penetrance. If so, brain mapping may help identify an inherited physiologic predisposition to develop FTSD. Mapping during dystonic movements will reveal patterns of brain activation in neural circuits that mediate the execution of dystonic movements. In contrast, imaging during nondystonic movements, sensory mapping, or mapping of the rest condition will reveal more about the physiologic substrate that engenders dystonia. If one or more susceptibility genes predispose to the development of FTSD, one might find nonaffected family members who manifest the same patterns of brain activation in the rest condition as patients with FTSD. In this way, brain mapping may help identify nonmanifesting carriers of a gene abnormality that could then be identified through linkage analysis.

ACKNOWLEDGMENTS

This work is supported in part by the Medical Research Service, Department of Veterans Affairs, and the Milton Foundation.

REFERENCES

1. Panizza ME, Hallett M, Nilsson J. Reciprocal inhibition in patients with hand cramps. *Neurology* 1989;39(1):85–89.
2. Panizza M, Lelli S, Nilsson J, et al. H-reflex recovery curve and reciprocal inhibition of H-reflex in different kinds of dystonia. *Neurology* 1990;40(5):824–828.
3. Hallett M. Is dystonia a sensory disorder? [editorial]. *Ann Neurol* 1995;38(2):139–140.
4. Bara-Jimenez W, Shelton P, Sanger TD, et al. Sensory discrimination capabilities in patients with focal hand dystonia. *Ann Neurol* 2000;47(3):377–380.
5. Bara-Jimenez W, Shelton, Hallett M. Spatial discrimination is abnormal in focal hand dystonia. *Neurology* 2000;55(12):1869–1873.
6. Mink JW. The basal ganglia: focused selection and inhibition of competing motor programs. *Prog Neurobiol* 1996;50(4):381–425.
7. Sommer M, Ruge D, Tergau F, et al. Intracortical excitability in the hand motor representation in hand dystonia and blepharospasm. *Mov Disord* 2002;17(5):1017–1025.
8. Sanger TD, Pascual-Leone A, Tarsy D, et al. Nonlinear sensory cortex response to simultaneous tactile stimuli in writer's cramp. *Mov Disord* 2002;17(1):105–111.
9. Charness ME, Ross MH, Shefner JM. Ulnar neuropathy and dystonic flexion of the fourth and fifth digits: clinical correlation in musicians. *Muscle Nerve* 1996;19(4):431–437.
10. Kaji R, Kohara N, Katayama M, et al. Muscle afferent block by intramuscular injection of lidocaine for the treatment of writer's cramp. *Muscle Nerve* 1995;18(2):234–235.
11. Kaji R, Rothwell JC, Katayama M, et al. Tonic vibration reflex and muscle afferent block in writer's cramp. *Ann Neurol* 1995;38(2):155–162.
12. Kaji R, Shibasaki H, Kimura J. Writer's cramp: a disorder of motor subroutine? [editorial; comment]. *Ann Neurol* 1995;38(6):837–838.
13. Tempel LW, Perlmutter JS. Abnormal vibration-induced cerebral blood flow responses in idiopathic dystonia. *Brain* 1990;113(Pt 3):691–707.

14. Tempel LW, Perlmutter JS. Abnormal cortical responses in patients with writer's cramp [published erratum appears in *Neurology* 1994;44(12):2411]. *Neurology* 1993; 43(11):2252–2257.

15. Yoneda Y, Rome S, Sagar HJ, et al. Abnormal perception of the tonic vibration reflex in idiopathic focal dystonia. *Eur J Neurol* 2000;7(5):529–533.

16. Siebner HR, Auer C, Conrad B. Abnormal increase in the corticomotor output to the affected hand during repetitive transcranial magnetic stimulation of the primary motor cortex in patients with writer's cramp. *Neurosci Lett* 1999;262(2):133–136.

17. Ikoma K, Samii A, Mercuri B, et al. Abnormal cortical motor excitability in dystonia. *Neurology* 1996;46(5): 1371–1376.

18. Ridding MC, Sheean G, Rothwell JC, et al. Changes in the balance between motor cortical excitation and inhibition in focal, task specific dystonia. *J Neurol Neurosurg Psychiatry* 1995;59(5):493–498.

19. Siebner HR, Tormos JM, Ceballos-Baumann AO, et al. Low-frequency repetitive transcranial magnetic stimulation of the motor cortex in writer's cramp. *Neurology* 1999;52(3):529–537.

20. Levy LM, Hallett M. Impaired brain GABA in focal dystonia. *Ann Neurol* 2002;51:93–101.

21. Byrnes ML, Thickbroom GW, Wilson SA, et al. The corticomotor representation of upper limb muscles in writer's cramp and changes following botulinum toxin injection. *Brain* 1998;121(pt 5):977–988.

22. Deuschl G, Toro C, Matsumoto J, et al. Movement-related cortical potentials in writers cramp. *Ann Neurol* 1995;38(6):862–868.

23. Elbert T, Candia V, Altenmuller E, et al. Alteration of digital representations in somatosensory cortex in focal hand dystonia. *Neuroreport* 1998;9(16):3571–3575.

24. Bara-Jimenez W, Catalan MJ, Hallett M, et al. Abnormal somatosensory homunculus in dystonia of the hand. *Ann Neurol* 1998;44(5):828–831.

25. Meunier S, Garnero L, Ducorps A, et al. Human brain mapping in dystonia reveals both endophenotypic traits and adaptive reorganization. *Ann Neurol* 2001;50(4): 521–527.

26. Byl NN, Merzenich MM, Jenkins WM. A primate genesis model of focal dystonia and repetitive strain injury: I. Learning-induced dedifferentiation of the representation of the hand in the primary somatosensory cortex in adult monkeys. *Neurology* 1996;47(2):508–520.

27. Topp KS, Byl NN. Movement dysfunction following repetitive hand opening and closing: anatomical analysis in owl monkeys. *Mov Disord* 1999;14(2):295–306.

28. Pujol J, Roset-Llobet J, Rosines-Cubells D, et al. Brain cortical activation during guitar-induced hand dystonia studied by functional MRI. *Neuroimage* 2000;12(3): 257–267.

29. Charness ME, Schlaug G. Cortical activation during finger movements in concert pianists, dystonic pianists, and non-musicians. *Neurology* 2000;54(suppl 3):A221.

30. Pascual-Leone A, Grafman J, Hallett M. Modulation of cortical motor output maps during development of implicit and explicit knowledge [see comments]. *Science* 1994;263(5151):1287–1289.

31. Shadmehr R, Holcomb HH. Neural correlates of motor memory consolidation. *Science* 1997;277(5327): 821–825.

32. Karni A, Meyer G, Rey-Hipolito C, et al. The acquisition of skilled motor performance: fast and slow experience-driven changes in primary motor cortex. *Proc Natl Acad Sci USA* 1998;95(3):861–868.

33. Pascual-Leone A, Nguyet D, Cohen LG, et al. Modulation of muscle responses evoked by transcranial magnetic stimulation during the acquisition of new fine motor skills. *J Neurophysiol* 1995;74(3):1037–1045.

34. Karni A, Meyer G, Jezzard P, et al. Functional MRI evidence for adult motor cortex plasticity during motor skill learning. *Nature* 1995;377(6545):155–158.

35. Classen J, Liepert J, Wise SP, et al. Rapid plasticity of human cortical movement representation induced by practice. *J Neurophysiol* 1998;79(2):1117–1123.

36. Levy LM, Ziemann U, Chen R, et al. Rapid modulation of GABA in sensorimotor cortex induced by acute deafferentation. *Ann Neurol* 2002;52:755–761.

37. Jancke L, Shah NJ, Peters M. Cortical activations in primary and secondary motor areas for complex bimanual movements in professional pianists. *Brain Res Cogn Brain Res* 2000;10(1–2):177–183.

38. Krings T, Topper R, Foltys H, et al. Cortical activation patterns during complex motor tasks in piano players and control subjects. A functional magnetic resonance imaging study. *Neurosci Lett* 2000;278(3):189–193.

39. Hund-Georgiadis M, von Cramon DY. Motor-learning-related changes in piano players and non-musicians revealed by functional magnetic-resonance signals. *Exp Brain Res* 1999;125(4):417–425.

40. Elbert T, Pantev C, Wienbruch C, et al. Increased cortical representation of the fingers of the left hand in string players. *Science* 1995;270(5234):305–307.

41. Schlaug G, Jancke L, Huang Y, et al. Increased corpus callosum size in musicians. *Neuropsychologia* 1995;33 (8):1047–1055.

42. Ozturk AH, Tascioglu B, Aktekin M, et al. Morphometric comparison of the human corpus callosum in professional musicians and non-musicians by using in vivo magnetic resonance imaging. *J Neuroradiol* 2002;29(1):29–34.

43. Schlaug G. The brain of musicians: a model for functional and structural adaptation. *Ann NY Acad Sci* 2001;930:281–299.

44. Amunts K, Schlaug G, Jancke L, et al. Motor cortex and hand motor skills: structural compliance in the human brain. *Human Brain Mapp* 1997;5:206–215.

45. Lederman RJ, Calabrese LH. Overuse syndromes in instrumentalists. *Med Probl Perform Art* 1986;1:7–11.

46. Lederman RJ. Nerve entrapment syndromes in instrumental musicians. *Med Probl Perform Art* 1986;1:45–48.

47. Charness ME. Unique upper extremity disorders of musicians. In: Millender LH, Louis DS, Simmons BP, eds. *Occupational disorders of the upper extremity.* New York: Churchill Livingstone, 1992:227–252.

48. Merzenich MM, Kaas JH, Wall JT, et al. Progression of change following median nerve section in the cortical representation of the hand in areas 3b and 1 in adult owl and squirrel monkeys. *Neuroscience* 1983;10:639–665.

49. Rijntjes M, Tegenthoff M, Liepert J, et al. Cortical reorganization in patients with facial palsy. *Ann Neurol* 1997;41(5):621–630.

50. Ross MH, Charness ME, Lee D, et al. Does ulnar neuropathy predispose to focal dystonia? *Muscle Nerve* 1995;18(6):606–611.

51. Girlanda P, Quartarone A, Battaglia F, et al. Changes in spinal cord excitability in patients affected by ulnar neuropathy. *Neurology* 2000;55(7):975–978.

52. Fishbein M, Middlestadt SE, Ottati V, et al. Medical problems among ICSOM musicians: overview of a national survey. *Med Probl Perform Art* 1988;3:1–8.

53. Waddy HM, Fletcher NA, Harding AE, et al. A genetic study of idiopathic focal dystonias. *Ann Neurol* 1991; 29(3):320–324.

54. Gasser T, Windgassen K, Bereznai B, et al. Phenotypic expression of the DYT1 mutation: a family with writer's cramp of juvenile onset [see comments]. *Ann Neurol* 1998;44(1):126–128.

55. Friedman JR, Klein C, Leung J, et al. The GAG deletion of the DYT1 gene is infrequent in musicians with focal dystonia. *Neurology* 2000;55(9):1417–1418.

56. Tempel LW, Perlmutter JS. Abnormal cortical responses in patients with writers cramp. *Neurology* 1993;43(11): 2252–2257.

57. Chen RS, Tsai CH, Lu CS. Reciprocal inhibition in writer's cramp. *Mov Disord* 1995;10(5):556–561.

58. Grunewald RA, Yoneda Y, Shipman JM, et al. Idiopathic focal dystonia: a disorder of muscle spindle afferent processing? *Brain* 1997;120(pt 12):2179–2185.

59. Lederman RJ. AAEM minimonograph #43: neuromuscular problems in the performing arts. *Muscle Nerve* 1994;17(6):569–577.

60. Bressman SB, de Leon D, Brin MF, et al. Idiopathic dystonia among Ashkenazi Jews: evidence for autosomal dominant inheritance. *Ann Neurol* 1989;26(5): 612–620.

61. Pauls DL, Korczyn AD. Complex segregation analysis of dystonia pedigrees suggests autosomal dominant inheritance. *Neurology* 1990;40(7):1107–1110.

62. Opal P, Tintner R, Jankovic J, et al. Intrafamilial phenotypic variability of the DYT1 dystonia: from asymptomatic TOR1A gene carrier status to dystonic storm. *Mov Disord* 2002;17(2):339–345.

63. Eidelberg D, Moeller JR, Antonini A, et al. Functional brain networks in DYT1 dystonia. *Ann Neurol* 1998;44 (3):303–312.

Dystonia 4: Advances in Neurology, Vol. 94. Edited by Stanley Fahn, Mark Hallett, and Mahlon R. DeLong. Lippincott Williams & Wilkins, Philadelphia © 2004.

32

Three-Dimensional Movement Analysis as a Promising Tool for Treatment Evaluation of Musicians' Dystonia

Hans-Christian Jabusch and Eckart Altenmüller

Institute of Music Physiology and Musicians' Medicine, University of Music and Drama, Hanover, Germany

Focal dystonia in musicians, also referred to as musicians' cramp, is a task-specific movement disorder that presents itself as a loss of voluntary motor control in extensively trained movements (1,2). Involuntary flexion or extension of individual fingers fundamentally impairs technical skills on the instrument, and affected musicians may suffer dramatic impact on their musical careers (1,2).

In the past, the extent of focal dystonia in affected musicians has mainly been estimated by means of visual inspection (3) and rating procedures (4–6) employing rating scales such as the Arm Dystonia Disability Scale (7), which includes the following subscale for musicians: 0 for normal, 1 for mild difficulty in playing, 2 for moderate difficulty in playing, and 3 for marked difficulty in playing. Alternatively, the Tubiana and Chamagne Scale (8) was applied, which more specifically focuses on motor skills in a musical context. However, especially within the range between "normal" and "moderate difficulty in playing," none of the available scales provided fine resolution. A quantification tool for objective measurement of the extent of musicians' cramps having a high precision and being independent of rating methods has not been available. Follow-up examinations

after treatment of musicians' dystonia were mainly accomplished by subjective comparison of videographic documents (5,6). Moreover, reliable evaluation of different therapies for musicians' cramp was not possible. Since focal dystonia in musicians is task-specific (1,2), any quantification approach has to be performed while the patient is playing the instrument. Tests away from the instrument might not provide the desired information.

Therefore, a computer-based three-dimensional movement analysis system has been utilized to objectively measure the extent of focal hand dystonia while musicians are playing their instruments. The principle of the measurement is based on the phenomenology of dystonic movements. In musicians with from focal hand dystonia, involuntary flexion or extension of individual fingers can be observed (9,10). Adjacent fingers tend to compensate for the dysfunction of the dystonic finger by performing exaggerated movements in the opposite (antidystonic) direction (11). By means of three-dimensional movement analysis, path acceleration of dystonic fingers and of adjacent fingers has been measured in antagonistic movements while musicians were carrying out standardized movements on their instruments. This chapter discusses the results of the three-dimensional movement analysis of fingers in a flutist with focal dystonia compared to those of six healthy flutists. Finger movements were recorded during execution of simple five-tone exercises. Finally, results of a follow-up examination in the dystonic flutist are presented, which were yielded after treatment with botulinum toxin A.

PARTICIPANTS AND METHODS

Patient and Controls

A 34-year-old female flutist with focal hand dystonia was recruited from the outpatient clinic of the Institute of Music Physiology and Musicians' Medicine of the Hanover University of Music and Drama. She underwent complete neurologic examination and was diagnosed by one of the authors (E.A.). She was suffering from focal dystonia in her right hand that presented itself as involuntary flexion of the ring finger in the metacarpophalangeal joint while she was playing the flute. A pattern of compensatory movements occurred in the middle finger that showed exaggerated extension. The onset of the movement disorder had been 3 years before the time of the study and had forced her to interrupt her career as an orchestral musician. She did not display dystonic movement patterns in any other activity. There was no evidence for any other neurologic disorder or a secondary dystonia. The group of healthy controls consisted of four female and two male professional flutists aged 29 ± 9.0 years either graduated or in advanced stages of training.

Methods

Prior to the test, colored markers were attached to the regions of interest, i.e., fingertips of the middle finger (third finger, D3) and ring finger (fourth finger, D4) of the right hand. For the test, a series of ten sequences of a five-tone exercise (c–d–e–f–g and back) was played on the flute. The sequences were played in 16th notes, and the tempo was standardized at 120 beats per minute for a quarter note and paced by a metronome. The movements of the affected hand were captured by three digital video cameras, which were connected to a computer and recorded 50 images per second. Movement analysis was carried out using commercially available software (SIMI Motion 3D, SIMI Reality Motion Systems GmbH, Unterschleissheim, Germany). Movements of the third and fourth finger were tracked, and path velocity and path acceleration of the fingertips were analyzed. Maximum path acceleration of all flexion and extension movements was derived. Average maximum path acceleration of flexion (a_f) and extension (a_e) was calculated; a_f was divided by a_e, indicating the balance between flexion and extension movements for each finger. The asymmetry index (I_A) was defined as $(a_f/a_e)_{D4}/(a_f/a_e)_{D3}$, reflecting the asymmetry of acceleration behavior between both adjacent fingers. An asymmetry index of $I_A = 1$ would reflect the same acceleration behavior in both fingers. Alterations in acceleration behavior according to the above-mentioned dystonic and compensatory movement patterns were expected to result in an increased asymmetry index ($I_A > 1$).

The same procedure of three-dimensional movement analysis was performed with the reference hands of the healthy flutists.

Follow-Up After Therapy

The flutist with flexion dystonia in the fourth finger of the right hand underwent injection therapy with botulinum toxin A after taking part in the study. Because the dystonic movement of the fourth finger presented itself as flexion in the metacarpophalangeal joint with additional extension in the proximal and distal interphalangeal joints, a total dose of 5 units of Dysport (Ipsen Ltd., Berkshire, United Kingdom) was injected into the interosseus and lumbrical muscles of the fourth finger under electromyographic guidance. The same muscles were reinjected three times after periods of 49, 48, and 49 days, respectively, using the same total dose of Dysport each time. A follow-up examination was carried out using movement analysis on day 162 after the first injection.

RESULTS

Path velocity and path acceleration of an individual finger in a healthy flutist are displayed in Fig. 32-1. In this example, graphs are shown for the fourth finger of the right hand during execution of one sequence of the five-tone exercise. Within this sequence, the fourth finger performed one extension movement and one flexion movement. In the photographs 1 to 4, the motion sequence is split into four sections: 1, finger resting on the key; 2, finger during extension movement; 3, finger resting in the extended position; and 4,

finger during flexion movement. In the graphs for path velocity and path acceleration, vertical lines indicate the sections 1 to 4. Path acceleration for the third and fourth fingers of a healthy flutist playing several sequences of the five-tone exercise is given in Fig. 32-2. The parts of the graph highlighted by the frames reflect the movements during one sequence as shown in Fig. 32-1. Upward arrows indicate extension movements, and downward arrows indicate flexion movements. In both fingers, maximum path acceleration of the flexion movement was slightly higher compared to the extension movement. This was observed in all sequences. The ratio between average maximum path acceleration of flexion and extension movements (a_f/a_e)

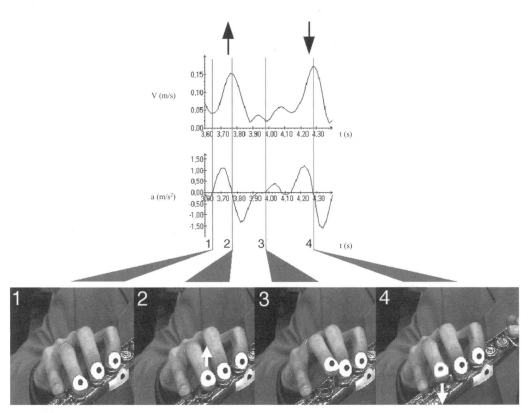

FIG. 32-1. Path velocity (V) and path acceleration (a) for the fourth finger of the right hand in a healthy flutist playing one sequence of the five-tone exercise (c–d–e–f–g and back). *Vertical lines* in the diagram indicate the different sections: *1,* finger resting on the key; *2,* finger during extension movement; *3,* finger resting in the extended position; *4,* finger during flexion movement.

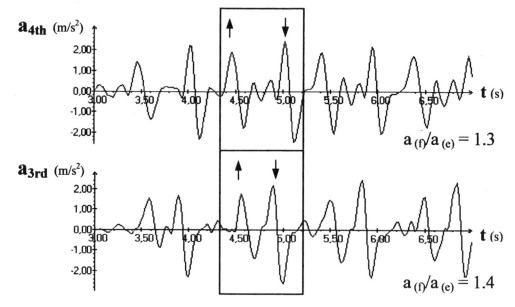

FIG. 32-2. Path acceleration for the third (a_{3rd}) and fourth (a_{4th}) fingers of the right hand in a healthy flutist playing several sequences of the five-tone exercise. Frames highlight one sequence. *Arrows* indicate movement direction. *Upward arrow:* extension. *Downward arrow:* flexion. $a_{(e)}$: average maximum path acceleration in all extension movements; $a_{(f)}$: average maximum path acceleration in all flexion movements.

was 1.4 for the third finger and 1.3 for the fourth finger, demonstrating a similar acceleration behavior in both adjacent fingers. This finding was consistent for all healthy participants. Figure 32-3 displays the situation for the flutist suffering from focal dystonia. Before treatment, maximum path acceleration of the fourth (dystonic) finger was much higher during the flexion (dystonic) movement than during extension. Compensation of the third finger was reflected by more accelerated extension movements as opposed to flexion. After treatment with botulinum toxin, the follow-up examination carried out 162 days later revealed a markedly higher acceleration of the extension movement in the dystonic fourth finger than before treatment. Compensatory extension of the third finger was slightly less accelerated. The ratio between average maximum path acceleration of flexion and extension movements (a_f/a_e) was 0.6 for the third finger and 2.2 for the fourth finger before treatment, indicating oppositional accelera-

tion behavior of both adjacent fingers. After treatment, this ratio was 0.5 for the third finger and 1.3 for the fourth finger. The asymmetry index (I_A) reflected the asymmetry of acceleration behavior between the third and fourth fingers. In the group of healthy flutists, this asymmetry index was $I_A = 1.1 \pm 0.5$, indicating similar acceleration behavior in both adjacent fingers (Fig. 32-4). In the patient with dystonia, an elevated asymmetry index of $I_A = 3.7$ reflected oppositional acceleration behavior of the dystonic and the compensating fingers. After treatment, I_A was clearly reduced ($I_A = 2.6$).

DISCUSSION

Three-dimensional movement analysis has been used for examination of a flutist with focal hand dystonia, with the aim of precise quantification of the disorder and objective identification of subtle differences in the symptomatology such as in follow-up exami-

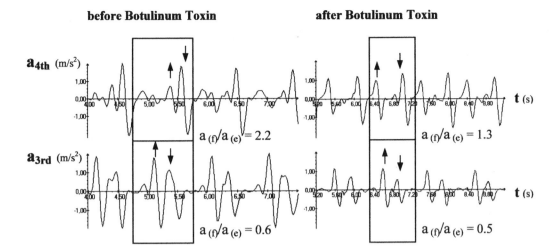

FIG. 32-3. Flutist with dystonic flexion of the fourth finger and compensatory extension of the third finger of the right hand. Path acceleration for the third (a_{3rd}) and fourth (a_{4th}) fingers during execution of several sequences of the five-tone exercise before and after therapy. Frames highlight one sequence. *Arrows* indicate movement direction. ↑: extension. ↓: flexion. $a_{(e)}$: average maximum path acceleration in all extension movements; $a_{(f)}$: average maximum path acceleration in all flexion movements.

nations during treatment. Taking place at the instrument, this method takes into consideration the crucial fact that focal dystonia is task-specific and occurs while the patient is playing the instrument. In dystonic hands, a mechanism of compensatory movements has been described; involuntary flexion of dystonic fingers is accompanied by compensatory extension of adjacent fingers (11). In the flutist examined in the present study, involuntary flexion of the fourth finger of the right hand was accompanied by compen-

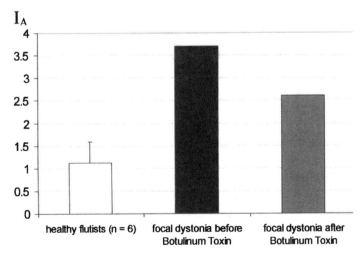

FIG. 32-4. Asymmetry index (I_A) indicating asymmetry of acceleration behavior of the third and fourth fingers in healthy flutists and in a flutist with focal dystonia before and after treatment with botulinum toxin.

satory extension of the third finger. As an indirect measure of the extent of the disorder, the asymmetry index $I_A = (a_f/a_e)D_4/(a_f/a_e)D_3$, has been introduced, indicating the asymmetry of acceleration behavior of the third and fourth fingers. An asymmetry index of $I_A = 1$ would reflect the same acceleration behavior in both adjacent fingers. In the group of healthy flutists, the asymmetry index was $I_A = 1.1 \pm 0.5$, indicating similar acceleration behavior in both fingers. However, in the dystonic flutist, three-dimensional movement analysis revealed oppositional acceleration behavior of the dystonic and the compensating fingers, resulting in an elevated asymmetry index of $I_A = 3.7$. After four injections of botulinum toxin A within a period of approximately half a year, the condition improved markedly. Although symptoms were still present to a certain extent, the patient was able to play technically demanding music, which had not been possible before treatment, and she returned to playing in an orchestra. At the follow-up examination, relief of symptoms could be objectified; three-dimensional movement analysis yielded an asymmetry index of $I_A = 2.6$.

To quantify flexion dystonia of the fourth finger with compensatory extension of the third finger, the asymmetry index was defined as $I_A = (a_f/a_e)D_4/(a_f/a_e)D_3$. Correspondingly, in focal hand dystonia affecting other fingers, the following calculation of the asymmetry index is suggested:

$$I_A = \frac{\left(\dfrac{a_{dystonic\ movement}}{a_{antidystonic\ movement}}\right)_{dystonic\ finger}}{\left(\dfrac{a_{movement\ in\ dystonic\ direction}}{a_{movement\ in\ antidystonic\ direction}}\right)_{compensating\ finger}}$$

In the case of flexion dystonia, "dystonic movement" refers to flexion and "antidystonic movement" to extension. For the compensating finger, "movement in dystonic direction" means flexion and "movement in antidystonic direction" means extension. As discussed for the special situation with the fourth dystonic finger and the third compensating finger, the general formula would also

result in an elevated asymmetry index ($I_A > 1$) in the case of alterations in the acceleration behavior of other dystonic and compensating fingers according to the patterns discussed.

Concerning therapy with botulinum toxin, injections into the intrinsic hand muscles hold several advantages over injections into the long flexor and extensor muscles of the forearm. There is a lower risk of impairing movement in adjacent fingers due to either diffusion of the botulinum toxin solution or the intermingling of muscular fascicles of different fingers. The required dosage is small, which lowers the risk of antibody development. In the case of overdosage, serious paresis impairing the function of dystonic fingers is less frequent and is more easily compensated for by the functionally intact long flexors and extensors. However, injections should be performed only into those intrinsics, which are not required to perform rapid lateral movements of the fingers on the instrument. In woodwinds, most of the instruments equipped with the Boehm system (e.g., flute, saxophone, clarinet) almost exclusively demand such lateral movements in the right and left little fingers. According to our experience, injections into the involved interosseus and lumbrical muscles, therefore, should be administered in all cases of flexion or extension dystonia in the index, middle, or ring finger of woodwind instrumentalists. It is a safe and effective treatment as demonstrated by the described three-dimensional movement analysis.

CONCLUSION

The results of the present study suggest that the asymmetry index based on three-dimensional movement analysis is a useful parameter for objective quantification of focal dystonia in flutists and for monitoring the development of the disorder in follow-up examinations during and after treatment. Additional investigations are required to evaluate the method in a larger number of healthy and dystonic flutists as well as in musicians playing other instruments. In further studies, objective quantification using three-dimensional movement analysis may be helpful for evaluation of different treatment approaches to optimize therapeutic possibilities for focal dystonia in musicians.

REFERENCES

1. Altenmüller E. Causes et traitements de la dystonie de fonction chez les musiciens. *Med Arts* 2001;36:19–27.
2. Jankovic J, Shale H. Dystonia in musicians. *Semin Neurol* 1989;9(2):131–135.
3. Frucht SJ, Fahn S, Greene PE. The natural history of embouchure dystonia. *Mov Disord* 2001;16(5):899–906.
4. Cole RA, Cohen LG, Hallett M. Treatment of musician's cramp with botulinum toxin. *Med Probl Perform Art* 1991;6:137–143.
5. Byl NN, McKenzie A. Treatment effectiveness for patients with a history of repetitive hand use and focal dystonia: a planned prospective follow-up study. *J Hand Ther* 2000;13:289–301.
6. Priori A, Pesenti A, Cappellari A, et al. Limb immobilization for the treatment of focal occupational dystonia. *Neurology* 2001;57:405–409.
7. Fahn S. Assessment of primary dystonias. In: Munsat TL, ed. *Quantification of neurologic deficit.* Boston: Butterworths, 1989:241–270.
8. Tubiana R, Chamagne P. Les affections professionnelles du membre supérieur chez les musiciens. *Bull Acad Natl Med* 1993;177:203–216.
9. Charness ME, Ross MH, Shefner JM. Ulnar neuropathy and dystonic flexion of the fourth and fifth digits: clinical correlation in musicians. *Muscle Nerve* 1996;19(4):431–437.
10. Lederman RJ. Focal dystonia in instrumentalists: clinical features. *Med Probl Perform Art* 1991;6:132–136.
11. Candia V, Schaefer T, Taub E, et al. Sensory motor retuning: a behavioral treatment for focal hand dystonia of pianists and guitarists. *Arch Phys Med Rehabil* 2002;83:1342–1348.

Dystonia 4: Advances in Neurology, Vol. 94. Edited
by Stanley Fahn, Mark Hallett, and Mahlon R.
DeLong. Lippincott Williams & Wilkins,
Philadelphia © 2004.

33

Limb Immobilization for Occupational Dystonia: A Possible Alternative Treatment for Selected Patients

Alessandra Pesenti, Sergio Barbieri, and Alberto Priori

*Department of Neurological Sciences, IRCCS Ospedale Maggiore di Milano, University of Milan,
Milan, Italy*

Because current treatments including botulinum toxin or drugs often yield disappointing results, focal occupational dystonia is a challenging issue in neurologic practice, especially in certain professional categories such as musicians. Although not a life-threatening disorder, it can severely impair a patient's social life and destroy a professional career.

Although the various forms of focal occupational upper-limb dystonia are customarily termed cramps (for example, writer's cramp, musician's cramp), this usage is confusing. The term *cramp* indicates a brisk, involuntary, painful muscle contraction relieved by muscle stretch, and most frequently arising from excessive activity of motor axons or spinal motoneurons (1). True muscle cramps arise from metabolic or neuromuscular disorders. Focal occupational dystonia of the upper limb is not related to true muscle cramps (2); however, for historical reasons some forms of occupational upper-limb dystonia related to specific occupations are still referred to as cramp. Since the earliest reports, occupational dystonia has been causally related to motor activities involving repetitive hand or finger movements and overuse (3,4).

The general principle of rest as a treatment for human disease was first introduced by Hippocrates. During the past two centuries several neurologists have observed that rest or immobilization can be helpful in treating focal occupational dystonia (Table 33-1) [see references in Lanska (5)]. For this purpose, various therapeutic devices have been proposed (5,6).

Although morphologic neuroimaging studies rarely disclose anatomic or structural abnormalities of the brain in patients with focal occupational dystonia, neurophysiology suggests brain dysfunction. In an experimental model of dystonia in nonhuman primates and in patients, several reports describe a disorganization of the somatosensory map in the cerebral cortex (3) and motor cortical hyperexcitability (7,8). The cortical representations of the dystonic fingers and hands lose their spatial segregation. In addition, in dystonic patients the somatosensory input is temporally and spatially disinhibited (9,10).

PHYSIOLOGIC EFFECTS OF IMMOBILIZATION

In healthy subjects, motor inactivity of a limb dramatically influences several physiologic and anatomic factors. When a limb is immobilized, the nails stop growing (11).

TABLE 33-1. *Historical background*

Reference	Author	Description
1865: Lectures on Scrivener's palsy: lecture III. *Lancet* 1865;1:113–115.	Solly S	2 months of "entire rest from the occupation that has produced the disease"
1885: The neural disorders of writers and artisans. In: Pepper W, Starr L, eds. *A system of practical medicine,* vol. 5. Philadelphia: Lea & Prothers, 1885–1886: 504–543.	Lewis MJ	"Forced rest by fastening the hand upon a splint"
1885: "Writers' cramp" and its treatment, with the notes of several cases. *Am J Med Sci* 1885;89:452–462.	Robins RP	"Your patient must have absolute rest, not necessarily of the whole body, but absolutely and entirely of the affected muscles, as far as those particular movements of coordination are concerned, whose abuse has brought on the attack.... In some cases I have been accustomed to order the arm to be carried in a sling for a week or so, to remind the patient that all writing is to be shunned."
1888: *A manual of diseases of the nervous system,* vol II. London: J&A Churchill, 1888:657–674.	Gowers WR	Rest is beneficial, especially if begun early: "The commencing symptoms often pass away with a brief rest; a month's abstinence from writing at the onset will do more than a year's rest if the disease has continued for six months."
1892: *The principles and practice of medicine, designed for the use of practitioners and students of medicine.* New York: D. Appleton, 1892:963–965.	Osler W	"Rest is essential. No measures are of value without this." (7)

From reference 5, Lanska.

Effects on Skeletal Muscle Properties

Although empirical observations show that the long-term immobilization of a limb leads to muscle atrophy, strength reduction, and functionality loss, only limited systematic information is available on the effects of immobilization in healthy subjects. Studies conducted on the immobilization of the lower limb in healthy volunteers (12,13) demonstrated changes in skeletal muscle properties. Immobilization alters the proportion of fast and slow muscle fibers. Hortobagyi and colleagues (13) reported a significant reduction of type I and II muscle fibers, but a statistically significant increase in type IIx fibers (type IIa fibers were not affected), after 3 weeks of immobilization of the knee joint in healthy subjects. These data correlate with a dysregulation in myosin heavy chain gene expression in the atrophic muscles; immobilization downregulates the expression of the myosin heavy chain in type I fiber messenger RNA (mRNA), and, conversely, upregulates type IIx fiber mRNA expression. Seki at al. (14) demonstrated alterations of the muscle contractility properties in human immobilized upper limbs. The decrease in maximal tetanic force occurs as a consequence of muscular atrophy, whereas the twitch force is enhanced significantly, maybe as a consequence of an alteration in the excitation–contraction coupling mechanism: reuptake of Ca^{2+} by sarcoplasmic reticulum occurs more slowly during immobilization; a slower Ca^{2+} release would induce a slower dissociation of calcium from the myofibrillar protein, which, in turn, enhances cross-bridge formation. In the lower limb, after immobilization, a significant reduction of eccentric, concentric, and isometric force is observed with loss of strength (on average 50%); an almost complete recovery with a spontaneous muscle activity restoration is observed 2 weeks after cast removal (12,13). When the cast is removed, the knee extension and flexion torque is decreased significantly (12) and the mean endurance time is increased (15). Joint immobilization also influences surface electromyographic (EMG) activity; the amount of EMG activity, as well as the pattern of EMG bursts (a transient decrease in the number of turns and in mean amplitude of the EMG of the disused muscle), is modified after immobilization in association with changes in the contractile properties of skeletal muscle (15,16). Less information is available on the effects of immobilization in animals. An impairment of muscular sarcolemmal excitability in immobilized rat skeletal muscles is indicated by a reduction in resting membrane potential, a decline in frequency of miniature end-plate potentials, and a decrease of [^{3}H]ouabain binding (17).

The immobilization-related changes affecting nails, joints, bones, and skeletal muscles probably also arise from disuse and metabolic dysfunction secondary to reduced blood circulation.

Effects on Spinal Motoneurons

Because motoneuronal activity is responsible for EMG activity, immobilization should in theory also affect motoneuronal properties during voluntary contractions. Yet, little evidence indicates a relationship between immobilization-induced changes in motoneuronal activity and changes in the contractile properties of the muscle. In a study investigating the alterations in contractile properties of human skeletal muscle induced by joint immobilization, Seki et al. (18) suggested that the motor system might adapt to limb immobilization in two ways: by restricting motoneuron firing to the lower rates and by enhancing the force exerted at low firing rates. The frequency restriction after immobilization could arise from a reduced afferent input to motoneurons during immobilization.

Effects on Motor Cortex

In nondystonic subjects, prolonged limb immobilization causes the motor cortical representation of the immobilized limb to shrink, as demonstrated by Liepert et al. (19,20) using cortical focal transcranial magnetic stimulation (TMS) in patients undergoing constraint-induced movement therapy of the healthy upper limb after stroke. In a recently published study, Facchini and colleagues (21) showed that the sensorimotor restriction of two fingers with short-term immobilization in healthy subjects induces an early decrease of cortical excitability, possibly at the cortical level, which involves not only the immobilized muscle but also muscles with overlapping neural representations.

Several experimental studies on adult monkeys have shown that when input from peripheral somatosensory receptors is reduced by cutting a peripheral nerve or amputating a digit, maps of the body surface in the somatosensory cortex reorganize. The cortical reorganization, probably owing to the altered sensory experiences, could be explained by various mechanisms, including divergence of preexisting connections, expression of latent synapses, and sprouting of new (22).

EFFECTS OF IMMOBILIZATION IN DYSTONIA

Patients often report that sustained or prolonged motor activity worsens their dystonia and that dystonia becomes progressively more severe after several minutes of exercise. This observation suggests that rather than being a fixed unchangeable condition, focal occupational dystonia can be altered, albeit transiently, by the motor activity itself. Thus focal occupational dystonia could be envisaged not simply as a fixed, hardwired dysfunction of the motor system, but as a condition potentially affected by environmental factors, including motor activity itself. Muscle fatigue is the decrease in muscle force output induced by prolonged and sustained muscle contraction. The decrease originates at several motor system levels, from muscle tissue to the brain (23). Interestingly, after a prolonged maximum fatiguing voluntary contraction, musicians with dystonia often report a mild but consistent improvement lasting a couple of minutes or so (24). After this short respite, dystonia again affects their voluntary movements.

If muscle fatigue during a sustained muscle contraction (i.e., overactivity) affects dystonia, then so could the lack of activity after limb immobilization (i.e., hypoactivity). Interestingly, whereas in patients with focal dystonia the motor area of the cerebral cortex is enlarged and hyperexcitable, in subjects undergoing prolonged limb immobilization the cortical representation of the immobilized muscles shrinks and is hypoexcitable. In a preliminary open study in eight patients, Priori et al. (25) found that after 4 to 5 weeks of upper limb immobilization, the benefit of therapy on dystonia varied: four patients obtained a good improvement, three a mild improvement, and one patient no improvement at all. After limb immobilization the patients complained of minor and short-lasting side-effects: clumsiness, inability to control the hand (all the patients, for about a week), weakness of the immobilized arm (all the patients, immediately after the splint was removed, and lasting for 7 to 10 days), minor local subcutaneous edema, and pain (complete resolution within 3 to 6 days); in about 50% of the patients nail growth stopped during splinting. All the patients had some degree of muscle atrophy that disappeared within 2 to 3 weeks. Interestingly, two patients were professional musicians who had stopped their activity because of dystonia, but who resumed playing after limb immobilization. Hence, we proposed immobilization as a possible alternative therapeutic approach to focal dystonia in selected patients. Despite these encouraging results, our patients' responses varied widely. Unfortunately, the small sample size prevented us from identifying the clinical profile of the best candidate for immobilization therapy.

We now report the effects of immobilization in a larger group of patients with focal occupational dystonia of the upper limb. Most of the patients were musicians. We also reviewed our data to identify clinical features that would distinguish patients likely to respond best to immobilization therapy for focal occupational upper-limb dystonia.

PATIENTS AND METHODS

Nineteen patients [17 men and two women; age 34.5 ± 2.6 years (mean $\pm$ standard error of the mean, SEM)], four affected by writer's cramps and 15 by musician's cramp, were immobilized (Table 33–2). After immobilization, patients were instructed to progressively resume their normal professional motor activity in 3 months, as reported elsewhere (25). As previously described (25), all patients underwent at least six visits (before they had the arm splinted, on the day of splint removal, and 1, 4, 12, and 24 weeks later). Clinical changes were quantified by the self-rating score (SRS) (25). This score gives results similar to those from objective evaluations [Arm Dystonia Disability Scale (ADDS) and Tubiana and Chamagne Scale (TCS)], or even slightly underestimates the clinical effect of immobilization. For the analysis, the study group was arbitrarily subdivided into responders (improvement $\geq 35\%$) and nonresponders (improvement $<35\%$). The two subgroups were

TABLE 33-2. *Patients' features*

Splinting age (mean $\pm$ SE)	34.5 ± 2.6 years (range 21–61)
Dystonia duration (mean $\pm$ SE)	4.1 ± 0.6 years (range 1–10)
Age of onset (mean $\pm$ SE)	30.5 ± 2.4 years (range 18–51)
Overuse syndrome	65%
Residual function (see text)	$16.0 \pm 3.9\%$ (range 0–50)
Pure focal hand dystonia	76.5%
Number of joints involved (mean $\pm$ SE)	2.6 ± 0.3 (range 1–6)
Hand-grip test (Pesenti et al., 2001)	$21.5 \pm 5.5\%$ (range 0–85)
Splinting duration (mean $\pm$ SE)	4.4 ± 0.1 weeks (range 4–6)
Previous botulinum toxin treatment	12%
Flexion/extension dystonia	50%

SE, standard error.

then compared for the following clinical variables: age at treatment, duration of illness, duration of treatment (from 4 to 6 weeks), previous treatment with botulinum toxin, the severity of dystonia (residual function percent), the onset of dystonia (sudden or slowly progressive) and its association with an "overuse syndrome," the number of joints involved and the presence of a posture mainly in flexion or extension, and the response to the hand-grip test (24).

Differences in the clinical variables were tested by the Student's t-test and checked by the Mann-Whitney nonparametric test in the two subgroups. Unless otherwise specified, all values are expressed as mean ± SEM; p <.05 was considered to indicate statistical significance.

RESULTS

Limb immobilization had a highly variable outcome, ranging from marked improvement to no improvement at all (Fig. 33–1). On average, improvement appeared from the 12-week visit after the splint was removed and reached maximum at the 24-week visit. The mean follow-up in the 19 patients is now 23.0 ± 2.0 months (range 6–33 months), and the patients who showed a motor improvement at the 24-week visit have remained stable or have obtained a further slight improvement. None worsened or had severe or persistent side effects. Transient side effects were weakness, clumsiness, inability to control the hand, local subcutaneous edema, pain, and a reduction of nail growing during splinting.

Several of the clinical variables assessed at baseline (before treatment) differed between responders and nonresponders. The most important differences were that the responder group had more severe dystonia at the onset and a larger number of joints involved; a shorter disease duration (<5 year from the onset of the first symptom); a transient improvement after a fatiguing contraction (hand-grip test >20%); but also a younger age (<35–37 years), an onset related to overuse, and possibly no previous treatment with botulinum toxin (Fig. 33–2). Patients who had a good response generally fulfilled all these criteria; conversely, those who had no response fulfilled only some or none.

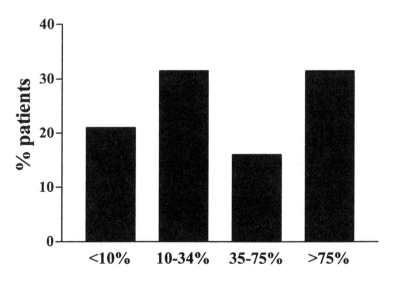

FIG. 33-1. The distribution of the patients (percentage of the total group) in four subgroups according to the degree (percentage) of improvement after limb immobilization.

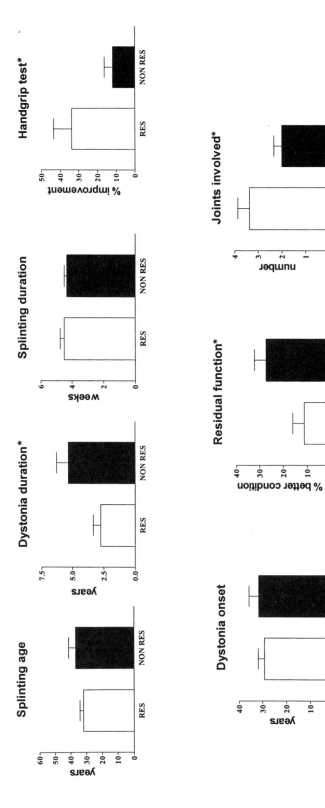

FIG. 33-2. Clinical variables in responder and nonresponder patients. *Open bars*, responders (improvement ≥35% according to the subjective rating scale (SRS, see text); *solid bars*, nonresponders (improvement <35%, according to the SRS; error bars are 1 standard error of the mean (SEM). Note that the duration of dystonia, the severity of illness (residual function), the number of joints involved, and the effect of the fatiguing task (handgrip test) differ significantly in responders and nonresponders (*p <.05, Mann-Whitney test). The age at onset of dystonia and the age at treatment differed in the two groups, although not significantly.

DISCUSSION

Despite the wide variability in our patients' responses, in most of our patients (79%) immobilization of the affected arm led to some improvements in focal occupational dystonia, and in some patients (31.5%) improvement was marked. None of our patients worsened or had serious or persistent side effects. Immobilization therapy could have several advantages over botulinum toxin injections and other pharmacologic approaches, at least in some patients. First, it induces few, and only minor, adverse reactions. Second, whereas botulinum toxin injections need to be repeated regularly, splinting apparently maintains its therapeutic benefits over time. Third, unlike other treatments, immobilization leads at least in some cases to restoring the patient's motor performance to a professional level. The botulinum toxin injection (one of the current treatments for hand dystonia) has also been used with some success in musicians' cramp, but the management of the treatment in these patients is difficult because the "therapeutic window" is very narrow. In fact, there is a fine line between administering not enough Botox and too much of it, which may weaken the muscles and impair their control (26). Finally, botulinum toxin treatment, although a relief from excessive muscle contraction, cannot correct the loss of coordination associated with dystonia, and dystonic musicians often consider the therapeutic effect of botulinum toxin inadequate for professional performances (27).

Although we hypothesize that immobilization improves dystonia by reshaping the abnormal motor map (25), other mechanisms acting at various levels of the motor system may be important, notably changes at the muscular or spinal level. Assuming cortical reshaping as a possible mechanism of immobilization, this treatment could be associated with specific rehabilitative programs for focal occupational dystonias (28), boosting their effects. Ideally, whereas immobilization might "erase" cortical dysplasticity responsible for focal occupational dystonia, specific rehabilitation protocols could help to properly rewire cortical connection, thereby allowing correct

movement. Hence, a preliminary immobilization treatment could be useful in patients undergoing specific rehabilitative treatments.

The variability in our patients' clinical responses to limb immobilization is intriguing. Does it imply that various subtypes of focal dystonia exist? Why do responses differ? Both questions await more data for definitive answers. One explanation is that although the clinical manifestations of focal occupational dystonia remain stable over time, the pathophysiologic substrate changes. Whereas at its onset the disorder is still reversible, in the later stages it progresses until stable irreversible hardwired motor system dysfunction ultimately sets in. If so, then at-risk categories such as musicians should be educated in advance about the risk of occupational dystonia so that they can recognize the condition in its early stages. Thus to achieve the best response, those selected for treatment should be immobilized before the disease advances.

In this study, we identified several clinical features that seem likely to predict a good response to immobilization therapy for focal upper-limb dystonia. Further studies are needed to identify other, still unrecognized, variables that may also be important for patient selection.

CONCLUSION

Our experience to date suggests that limb immobilization, though not a first-choice treatment for all patients, can be an appropriate alternative, safe, initial treatment in selected patients in the early stages of focal occupational dystonia. The new data from this study in a larger sample of patients suggest that the therapy probably works best in young patients with a recent onset of a severe illness related to an overuse syndrome and involving at least three joints, whose dystonic symptoms improve transiently by more than 20% in the hand-grip test.

REFERENCES

1. Kimura J. *Electrodiagnosis in diseases of nerve and muscle: principles and practice.* Philadelphia: FA Davis, 1989.
2. Marsden CD, Harrison MJ, Bundey S. The natural his-

tory of idiopathic torsion dystonia. In: Eldridge R, Fahn S, eds. *Dystonia. Advances in neurology,* vol 14. New York: Raven Press, 1976:177–187.

3. Byl NN, Merzenich MM, Jenkins WM. A primate genesis model of focal dystonia and repetitive strain injury: I. Learning-induced dedifferentiation of representation of the hand in the primary somatosensory cortex in adult monkeys. *Neurology* 1996;47:508–520.

4. Topp KS, Byl NN. Movement dysfunction following repetitive hand opening and closing: anatomical analysis in owl monkeys. *Mov Disord* 1999;2:225–306.

5. Lanska DJ. Limb immobilization for the treatment of focal occupational dystonia [letter]. *Neurology* 2002;58 (2):991.

6. Candia V, Elbert T, Altenmuller E, et al. Constraint-induced movement therapy for focal hand dystonia in musicians [letter]. *Lancet* 1999;353:42.

7. Berardelli A, Rothwell JC, Hallett M, et al. Pathophysiology of dystonia. *Brain* 1998;121:195–212.

8. Nordstrom MA, Butler SL. Reduced intracortical inhibition and facilitation of corticospinal neurons in musicians. *Exp Brain Res* 2002;144:336–342.

9. Frasson E, Priori A, Bertolasi L, et al. Somatosensory disinhibition in dystonia. *Mov Disord* 2001;16(4): 674–682.

10. Tinazzi M, Priori A, Bertolasi L, et al. Abnormal central integration of a dual somatosensory input in dystonia. Evidence for sensory overflow. *Brain* 2000;123:42–50.

11. Dawber R. The effect of immobilization on fingernail growth. *Clin Exp Dermatol* 1981;6(5):533–535.

12. Veldhuizen JM, Verstappen FTJ, Vroemen JPAM, et al. Functional and morphological adaptation following four weeks of knee immobilization. *Int J Sports Med* 1993;14:283–287.

13. Hortobagyi T, Demsey L, Fraser D, et al. Changes in muscle strength, muscle fiber size and myofibrillar gene expression after immobilization and retraining in humans. *J Physiol* 2000;524.1:293–304.

14. Seki K, Taniguchi Y, Narusawa M. Effects of joint immobilization on firing rate modulation of human motor units. *J Physiol* 2001;530.3:507–519.

15. Semmler JC, Kutzscher DV, Enoka RM. Limb immobilization alters muscle activation patterns during a fatiguing isometric contraction. *Muscle Nerve* 2000;23: 1381–1392.

16. Fuglsang-Frederiksen A, Scheel U. Transient decrease in number of motor units after immobilisation in man. *J Neurol Neurosurg Psychiatry* 1978;41(10):924–929.

17. Zemkova H, Teisinger J, Almon RR, et al. Immobilization atrophy and membrane properties in rat skeletal muscle. *Pflugers Arch* 1990;416:126–129.

18. Seki K, Taniguchi Y, Narusawa M. Alterations in contractile properties of human skeletal muscle induced by joint immobilization. *J Physiol* 2001;530.3:521–532.

19. Liepert J, Tegenthoff M, Malin JP. Changes of cortical motor area size during immobilization. *Electroenceph Clin Neurophys* 1995;97:382–386.

20. Liepert J, Miltner WHR, Bauder H, et al. Motor cortex plasticity during constraint-induced movement therapy in stroke patients. *Neurosci Lett* 1998;250:5–8.

21. Facchini S, Romani M, Tinazzi M, et al. Time-related changes of excitability of the human motor system contingent upon immobilization of the ring and little finger. *Clin Neurophysiol* 2002;113:367–375.

22. Jones EG. Cortical and subcortical contributions to activity-dependent plasticity in primate somatosensory cortex. *Annu Rev Neurosci* 2000;23:1–37.

23. Gandevia SC. Neural control in human muscle fatigue: changes in muscle afferents, motoneurons and motor cortical drive. *Acta Physiol Scand* 1998;162:275–283.

24. Pesenti A, Priori A, Scarlato G, et al. Transient improvement induced by motor fatigue in focal occupational dystonia: the hand-grip test. *Mov Disord* 2001; 16:1143–1147.

25. Priori A, Pesenti A, Cappellari A, et al. Limb immobilization for the treatment of focal occupational dystonia. *Neurology* 2001;57:405–409.

26. Lim VK, Altenmuller E, Bradshaw JL. Focal dystonia: current theories. *Hum Mov Sci* 2001;20:875–914.

27. Karp BI, Cole RA, Cohen LG, et al. Long-term botulinum toxin treatment of focal hand dystonia. *Neurology* 1994;44:70–76.

28. Tubiana R, Chamagne P. Prolonged rehabilitation treatment of musician's focal dystonia. In: Tubiana R, Amadio PC, eds. *Medical problems of the instrumentalist musician.* London: Martin Dunitz, 2000;19:369–378.

Dystonia 4: Advances in Neurology, Vol. 94. Edited by Stanley Fahn, Mark Hallett, and Mahlon R. DeLong. Lippincott Williams & Wilkins, Philadelphia © 2004.

34

Review of 113 Musicians with Focal Dystonia Seen Between 1985 and 2002 at a Clinic for Performing Artists

*Alice G. Brandfonbrener and †Chester Robson

*Medical Program for Performing Artists, Rehabilitation Institute of Chicago, Chicago, Illinois.
†Department of Family Medicine, La Grange Memorial Hospital, La Grange, Illinois

This chapter discusses the demographics, manifestations, treatments, and effect on playing and on the careers of 113 musicians diagnosed with focal dystonias and followed for 1 to 12 years.

The diagnosis of focal dystonia in musicians carries the most serious implications for their careers of any occupationally induced medical problems they may face. Although among musicians as a whole this diagnosis is relatively uncommon, physicians who specialize in the field recognize that it is far from rare.

The Medical Program for Performing Artists of the Rehabilitation Institute of Chicago was founded at Northwestern University in 1985 to provide multidisciplinary evaluation and treatment of performers in general, but with particular emphasis on instrumentalists. Between 1985 and March 2002, approximately 2,400 instrumental musicians have been seen for a wide variety of medical problems that in one way or another affect their ability to play. This chapter concerns 113 of these musician patients, or approximately 5%, who had findings typical of focal dystonias, the majority of these being focal hand dystonias. Also included are 16 brass and woodwind players whose dystonia affected the facial and other muscles comprising their embouchures. An additional 19 patients seen during this period had probable dys-

tonias but are excluded from this report because of something atypical in their presentation.

The demographics of these 113 patients are similar to those reported in other series. Seventy-four percent are men, and 77% are professional musicians. The age at initial presentation peaked in the fourth decade (45%), and the remainder are reasonably distributed in a bell-shaped curve. Forty-four percent of these patients were seen initially during the first year they became aware of their symptoms, or, perhaps more accurately, after they acknowledged the problematic nature of these symptoms. Another 20% were seen 5 years or longer after the onset of symptoms, and although most had previously consulted one or more physicians, a significant number did not have a prior accurate diagnosis. In fact, several had undergone to surgical procedures, most commonly carpal tunnel release in the absence of typical clinical presentations or documentation of the diagnosis through electrodiagnostic testing, and without postoperative relief of symptoms. The single most troubling surgery performed was an extensor tendon transplantation for an alleged ruptured tendon without clinical evidence supporting such a diagnosis and again without symptomatic relief following the surgical procedure.

The instrumental distribution among those with hand dystonias was 34 keyboard players, 35 strings, of which 15 were bowed and 20 were plucked, 26 woodwinds, and five percussionists. All 13 brass players included had embouchure dystonias, as did three flute players.

Among the keyboard players 74% had right-hand symptoms, but two whose initial symptoms were in the right-hand fingers later also developed dystonias in their left hands, approximately 2 and 6 years, respectively, after the first symptoms in the right hand.

Among the bowed strings 60% had left-hand dystonias, while 19 of 20 of the plucked strings had right-hand dystonias. While their number is too small to be of great significance, nine of the ten flute players had left-hand dystonias, while five of eight clarinetists had right-hand problems. There were only five percussionists seen whose affected hands divided 3:2 right vs. left. The hands affected by dystonias in each type of instrumentalist correlate with the hands affected by other medical problems of lesser severity seen in musicians playing these instruments.

Patients are routinely queried regarding possible risks or precipitants to the development of the dystonia, including trauma, family history of movement disorders, recent changes in instrumental technique, a new or altered instrument, and increased level of stress. In 67%, no clear-cut risk or immediate precipitant could be identified, and in very few was there a history of significant past trauma or pain, related or unrelated to music making, involving the affected extremity. History of movement or other neurologic disorders in close relatives was likewise negative, except for one patient whose father had torticollis and another whose father had Parkinson's. Most remarkable in terms of family history are two sets of identical twins who played the same instrument, had studied with the same music teachers, and were highly successful professional musicians. One pair played piano, the other pair viola, and in each case only one twin has focal dystonia. In the case of the pianist twins, the senior author has

been in a position to follow both the affected and unaffected twin for many years, both prior to and following the onset of the dystonia.

Telephone contact was attempted with all patients who had not been seen for more than 1 year previous to this report. Contact was made with 54 patients in all, of whom 14 were patients whose initial visit had been 12 or more years previously. Thirty-six of the 54 are professional musicians of whom 19 are still playing, albeit mostly with significant changes to their technique and/or repertoire. Seventeen professionals no longer play, ten found new careers, and two chose early retirement. Two patients are deceased (one of whom had developed Alzheimer's disease), but both had been forced to discontinue playing years prior to their deaths due to the dystonia.

Several who had been primarily performers as well as those who were already teachers are currently teaching. In no patient have the symptoms resolved or significantly improved; typically the symptoms have stabilized and in a minority have progressed, including the two pianists who have developed bilateral dystonias. A variety of treatments were used, none of which were felt to be of significant help. Only two of these patients had had Botox treatment, and neither was satisfied with the results. Most of these patients at some point delved into a variety of alternative therapies, again with results they found disappointing.

No one who knows or has cared for musicians affected with focal dystonias can fail to feel not only empathy but also great frustration with being so ineffective in providing significant help, and even less effective at providing a permanent solution. Granted, however, that progress has and is being made to an extent that only a few years ago seemed unimaginable. With the growing sophistication of brain science and the fact that there are now so many investigators dedicated to finding fundamental answers to the etiology as well as to the treatment of this difficult and fascinating problem, there are grounds for cautious optimism.

Dystonia 4: Advances in Neurology, Vol. 94. Edited by Stanley Fahn, Mark Hallett, and Mahlon R. DeLong. Lippincott Williams & Wilkins, Philadelphia © 2004.

35

The Impact of Focal Dystonia on the Working Life of Musicians in the United Kingdom

*Anthony G. Butler, †Philip O. F. Duffey, ‡Maurice R. Hawthorne, and §Michael P. Barnes

*Dystonia Epidemiologist, Durham, United Kingdom. †York District Hospital, York, United Kingdom. ‡The North Riding Infirmary, Middlesbrough, United Kingdom. §Department of Neurological Rehabilitation, University of Newcastle, Hunters Moor Rehabilitation Centre, Newcastle-upon-Tyne, United Kingdom

Although something is known about the prevalence of dystonia around the world (1–4), there was originally little reliable evidence about the incidence of individual types of dystonia in musicians. However, during the Epidemiological Survey of Dystonia (ESD) carried out in northeast England over the past 9½ years, since May 1993 (see Chapter 13), a small number of musicians were identified with different forms of focal dystonia.

The principal author, an ex-professional musician himself from 1965 until 1980, addressed a conference organized by the British Association of Performing Arts Medicine in York, England, in March 1997 (5). By the time of this conference, the author recognized the sense of isolation felt by most people with dystonia, which had never been previously measured, and as the disorder is predominantly visual in presentation, a number of sufferers felt severe social and psychological pressure to remain hidden from public view (6). Social isolation in patients breeds a lack of diagnostic skill in general practitioners (family physicians), which in turn leads to nondiagnosis or misdiagnosis, thus increasing the isolation felt by most people with dystonia (7). Therefore, the onset of dystonia for a musician can have a particularly debilitating effect, especially if the musician develops a task-specific focal dystonia affecting the hands or the neck.

This chapter describes the classification of the five male musicians currently involved in the ESD study. Although the ESD has shown that dystonia is twice as prevalent in females as in males, we have yet to find a female musician with dystonia. The five case histories involve a professional rock guitarist, a semiprofessional club guitarist and singer, an amateur classical pianist, a world-renowned accordionist, and an ex–lead singer with a well-known vocal quartet. The case histories of these individuals show how the onset of dystonia has affected the working (playing) life of each musician, together with the results and the effectiveness of botulinum toxin therapy in the treatment of primary focal dystonia of the hands or neck in musicians.

The impact of focal dystonia makes no distinction between primary and secondary dystonia because an abnormal posture or involuntary muscle spasm presents in exactly the same way in both cases. If the subjects become unemployed due to their dystonia, it does not matter if it was induced, genetically inherited, or idiopathic—they are still economically vulnerable.

CASE HISTORIES

The first case involves a professional guitarist in a rock band. He is currently 38 years of age; his dystonia onset was in 1991 but was not diagnosed until two years later. It started with the fifth finger of his left (keyboard) hand, thus forcing him to re-finger chords. Eventually the fourth finger began to flex and the third finger developed such pressure that it would break open the skin under the nail. By 1994 his other hand developed a dystonic tremor, but his left hand is the one that causes him the most problems. After several years of "musical hell" (his own words) he was referred in 1993 for botulinum toxin therapy. He has been receiving this treatment ever since, initially every 3 months, but recently the techniques of his injections have improved, so he now goes every 6 months or so. In his opinion, he is now back to about 90% of where he was playing-wise before the onset of dystonia. He states, "I have met a number of other dystonia patients at the injection clinic and, in my opinion, I have a less obvious disability than any of them; nevertheless dystonia has created a severe handicap and had an extremely debilitating effect on my life as a musician."

The second case involves a semiprofessional singer/guitarist, age 58 years, who began playing in the 1960s. He developed spasmodic torticollis in 1985, which might be secondary to his alcohol abuse. He is a confirmed alcoholic, but has not had a drink for many years. He was diagnosed with dystonia in 1991, and has been receiving botulinum toxin therapy ever since, which still works well for him. His neck turns to the right, making it very difficult for him to sing or play with a normal posture. He also found it difficult to stand for long periods on stage. He, therefore, had given up playing by the time that I met him in 1993. However, to quote from a recent message from him:

> Three months before Millennium night, we were requested by a good friend to get the five original members of the band to re-form to play a Millennium gig [one night stand], which we did. We went down so well, we have decided to carry on. Originally in the 1960s, I was one of the front men who used to do a lot of jokes and patter [talking]. I now find this embarrassing and stand on the right of the stage looking out to the audience as my head turns to the right. I find it extremely difficult on the vocal side, as I have to have the microphone tilted to one side to suit my neck position. However, I must say this time around how much I am enjoying playing music again, but I must limit myself to one or, at the most, two nights per week. When walking onto a dark stage, I have to be very, very careful of cables, etc. as my balance is also badly affected by my dystonic posture. Although I still love playing music, I find it very difficult indeed—but I am prepared to pay the price for the love of playing music.

The third case is a person who has taken a long time to come to terms with his dystonia. He is currently 58 years old and has also had one of the hardest musical times because, although an amateur, he used to play some of the most difficult classical pieces composed for the piano.

He developed action-induced dystonia in the third, fourth, and fifth fingers of his right hand. The first indications occurred in 1981, but were not diagnosed until 1995, i.e., 14 years later. At first, he developed exercises to counter this trait, which initially worked at the expense of his speed of movement. He received botulinum toxin therapy in 1995 to help him, but it became ineffective in 1998. He has now developed his clarinet playing as a way of countering his dystonic fingers, which are still problematic, but less so than while playing the piano. In his own words:

> This coordination problem has meant that I have lost the facility to play comfortably the music that gave me the deepest satisfaction— any Mozart or Haydn piano sonata, Scarlatti, Bach's *Goldberg Variations*—linear music. I still have not accepted in every way that this happened to me and I often sit down to play feeling that I might play naturally this time.

The fourth case was referred to us by the largest botulinum toxin clinic in the United Kingdom, Hunters Moor Regional Rehabilitation Centre in Newcastle. The patient is currently 73 years old and he has been a professional accordion player, gaining a silver medal in a competition in 1957 in Moscow.

His initial onset of symptoms was in 1999, but he was not diagnosed until 2 years later, in 2001. He has action-induced dystonia of the fourth and fifth fingers of his right hand. He had his first set of botulinum toxin injections in April 2002 and has already started playing again after a layoff of several months. In his own words:

> During the past four years I noticed a decline in my right hand ability, which I just put down to my advancing years. Towards the end of 1999, my fourth and fifth fingers started to curl in, but only when I was playing. The condition deteriorated until my fingernails were leaving a mark on my palm. My doctor had no idea what was causing this problem, as my fingers were fine until I played the accordion.

The fifth case is a 49-year-old man who has had much difficulty, having been the lead singer with an internationally renowned vocal quartet. He developed spasmodic dysphonia (laryngeal dystonia) in 1991, while working in different venues all over the world. He feels as if he "went through hell," not just because his dystonia interfered with his singing fine harmonies, but also because of a particularly unsympathetic fellow band member. He eventually had to give up a brilliant career in 1999, although he was not formally diagnosed until 2000. He is currently obtaining botulinum toxin therapy from an ear, nose, and throat consultant in Middlesbrough, and this is working well for him, but not well enough for him to resume his singing career.

DISCUSSION

These five case histories show that there can be music after dystonia, but it depends on the age of onset and how soon after the onset effective treatment is obtained.

Musicians make up less than 0.4% of the 1,337 dystonia patients currently registered in the ESD. Therefore, if they are not specifi-

cally sought by investigators, they may not present themselves in a general survey, such as the ESD.

In Germany, Eckart Altenmueller (see Chapter 32) has been treating a large number of musicians for several years. The United States has also progressed in its treatment of musicians, with the establishment of the Musicians with Dystonia program of the Dystonia Medical Research Foundation. There seems, however, to be a lack of research involving musicians with dystonia in the United Kingdom. Therefore, I propose extending the ESD in an attempt to find out how many musicians are affected in the United Kingdom. This will be accomplished using two separate organizations. As a member of the British Musician's Union since 1964, I propose to inform union members of dystonia and its treatments, and thus establish a dystonia bank of musicians. I will also use the British Association of Performing Arts Medicine as another vehicle to try to establish the number of musicians in the UK who have any form of dystonia. I shall report these findings to the next international symposium.

REFERENCES

1. Defazio G, Livrea P. Epidemiology of primary blepharospasm. *Mov Disord* 2002;17:7–12.
2. Nakashima K, Kusumi M, Inoue Y, et al. Prevalence of focal dystonias in the western area of Tottori Prefecture in Japan. *Mov Disord* 1995;10;440–443.
3. Nutt JG, Muenter MD, Aronson A, et al. Epidemiology of focal and generalized dystonia in Rochester, Minnesota. *Mov Disord* 1983;3:188–194.
4. The Epidemiological Study of Dystonia in Europe Collaborative Group. A prevalence study of primary dystonia in eight European countries. *J Neurol* 2000;247:787–792.
5. Butler AG, Duffey POF. The impact of focal dystonia on the working life of musicians. *Perform Arts Med News BAPAM* 1997;G1.16–G1.24
6. Butler AG. The social and economic implications of dystonia. *Eur Neurol* 1996;3:79.
7. Butler AG, Duffey POF. The epidemiological survey of dystonia in the North East of England. *Eur Neurol* 1996;3:28.

Dystonia 4: Advances in Neurology, Vol. 94. Edited by Stanley Fahn, Mark Hallett, and Mahlon R. DeLong. Lippincott Williams & Wilkins, Philadelphia © 2004.

36

Long-Term Outcome of Focal Dystonia in Instrumental Musicians

Stephan U. Schuele and Richard J. Lederman

Department of Neurology and Medical Center for Performing Artists, The Cleveland Clinic Foundation, Cleveland, Ohio

Dystonia is defined as a syndrome of sustained muscle contractions, frequently causing twisting and repetitive movements or abnormal posture (1). In musicians, dystonia is usually confined to the hand or arm or to the muscles of embouchure, often experienced only with certain activities (focal task-specific dystonia, FTSD) (2). FTSD affects between 5% and 14% of instrumental musicians who seek medical attention for playing-related problems in performing art medical centers (3–7). Involvement is mostly instrument specific, affecting the limb in string, percussion, and piano players, and primarily the embouchure in brass instrumentalists. It can, however, affect the limb or the embouchure in woodwind instrumentalists.

In several larger series describing the clinical characteristics of various forms of focal dystonia in instrumentalists, symptoms often persisted over many years and only limited benefit was seen with treatment (7–9). Compared to other medical problems afflicting instrumental musicians, including musculoskeletal and nerve compression syndromes, the prognosis in focal dystonia appears unfavorable (10). Cross-sectional data on 179 musicians with FTSD demonstrated long-term improvement with botulinum toxin injections, anticholinergic drugs, and ergonomic changes in 34 patients, but also no benefit from any therapy in 42 patients, and 26 patients had

abandoned their careers as performing artists at initial presentation (11). A recent review of 111 musicians with FTSD included follow-up data in 51 patients of at least 1 year's duration; of 33 professional performers, 17 had stopped playing (12).

Systematic studies regarding long-term outcome of FTSD in musicians are limited. We are presenting the results of a survey on treatment and long-term outcome in 45 instrumental musicians—21 violin and viola players and 24 woodwind players. Because FTSD can affect the fingering hand or the bowing arm in string players and the limb or the embouchure in woodwind players (13,14), we will compare treatment options and long-term outcome in these subgroups separately.

PATIENTS AND METHODS

Forty-five bowed string and woodwind instrumentalists with a diagnosis of focal dystonia were seen between 1985 and 2001 at our Medical Center for Performing Artists. All patients underwent a thorough history and physical examination on initial visit, including observation while playing their instruments. Many patients underwent ancillary studies, including blood analysis, x-ray, and electrodiagnostic testing. A small number of patients had computed tomographic or magnetic resonance imaging scans of the head performed.

The violin and viola instrumentalists were contacted by phone and the woodwind players were contacted by mail. Both groups were asked to answer a standardized questionnaire. The questions included a self-rating of the current level of performance compared with the time before onset of symptoms, the current and previous status as musicians, interim physician visits, additional diagnostic tests performed, suggested alternative diagnoses, and treatment attempts including the benefit from each individual treatment. The study was approved by The Cleveland Clinic Institutional Review Board (IRB 5638).

RESULTS

Demographics

The group of violin and viola instrumentalists included 18 men and three women. Mean age at onset of symptoms was 34 years (range 22–68, median 31 years). Fifteen musicians played the violin, and six played the viola. Seventeen were professional instrumentalists actively performing, two were mainly teachers, and two were music students. Mean duration of symptoms at presentation was 4.7 years (range 0.6–21, median 3 years). Eighteen musicians responded to the questionnaire (86%). The questionnaire was administered on average 10.4 years (range 0.6–21, median 11.5 years) after the initial evaluation at our center, and information on long-term outcome was available on average 15.3 years after the onset of symptoms (range 1–36, median 15 years). The results are summarized in Table 36-1.

The group of woodwind instrumentalists included 15 men and nine women. Mean age of onset was 34 years (range of 18–56, median 32.5 years). Ten musicians played the clarinet, five played the flute, four played bagpipes, three played the oboe, and two played the bassoon. At the time of evaluation, 20 were professional musicians actively performing, two were in graduate studies, one was a college student, and one was an amateur. Mean duration of symptoms at presentation was 3.6 years (range 1–22, median 2 years). Fifteen (63%) musicians responded to the written questionnaire. The questionnaire was administered on average 7.7 years (range 1–13, median 7 years) after the initial evaluation, and information on long-term outcome was available on average 12.1 years after the onset of symptoms (range 1–33, median 9 years).

Clinical Presentation

The main complaints in both instrument groups were loss of control and involuntary movements. All patients were questioned during the first visit for risk factors that might have predisposed them to develop dystonia. No patient was exposed to neuroleptics or had

TABLE 36-1. *Demographics, clinical characteristics, and long-term outcome*

	String instrumentalists: violin (15), viola (6)		Woodwind instrumentalists: clarinet (10), bagpipes (4), bassoon (2), flute (5), oboe (3)	
Dystonic muscles	Fingering hand (16)	Bow arm (5)	Limb (18)	Embouchure (6)
Mean age at onset (range)	32 years (22–45)	39 years (25–68)	32 years (22–49)	42 years (36–56)
Initial status	14 professionals	3 professionals	14 professionals	6 professionals
Trigger	8	4	8	4
Other activities	4 (25%)	1 (20%)	4 (22%)	2 (33%)
Abnormal posture	13 (81%)	5 (100%)	14 (78%)	5 (83%)
Response	13 (81%)	5 (100%)	10 (56%)	6 (83%)
Follow-up symptom onset	15.6 years	14.6 years	13.4 years	9.4 years
Remaining performing artists (of those responding)	5/11 (45%)	0/3 (0%)	5/9 (55%)	3/6 (50%)

a family history of dystonia or, specifically, involuntary movements or abnormal posture; 50% in the woodwind group and 57% in the string players recalled some event preceding the onset of symptoms, most often a change in technique, instrument, or teacher, an increase in practice time, or a minor trauma. Between 20% and 33% of musicians noted difficulties with other activities. Eleven patients complained about mild initial pain or discomfort. No sensory deficits were reported. In most cases the dystonic symptoms had an insidious onset and gradual progression over a period of less than 1 year. Symptoms tended to plateau afterward without major fluctuations. Some musicians felt that they had slow and mild spontaneous improvement over the following 5 to 10 years.

Among the bowed string instrumentalists, 16 (76%) had symptoms affecting their fingering hand and five (24%) had problems with the bowing arm. The musicians with bowing arm symptoms were on average 7 years older at onset of symptoms than the group with fingering hand problems. In all but three patients, abnormal posture could be noted while playing their instrument (86%). One right-handed violinist initially presented with symptoms in the left fingering hand and learned to play the violin using the left hand to bow. He developed similar symptoms in his right fingering hand with a delay of 11 years. Eleven patients showed involuntary flexion mostly of their fourth or fifth digit; only one patient demonstrated extension of the interphalangeal joint associated with flexion of the wrist. The movements of the bowing arm were less predictable, ranging from forced pressure on the fingerboard to involuntary wrist flexion, forearm pronation, and tremor.

In the group of woodwind instrumentalists, 18 (75%) had symptoms affecting the upper limb and six (25%) had problems with the embouchure. The musicians with embouchure dystonia were on average 10 years older than the group with limb dystonia. Fourteen musicians with limb dystonia (78%) showed abnormal posturing while playing, in nine associated with flexion of the interphalangeal joints

and in five with involuntary extension. In four patients, loss of motor control could be appreciated without definite abnormal posture allowing only a presumptive diagnosis of focal dystonia. Certain patterns of involvement were seen in the musicians with limb dystonia: in seven of eight clarinetists, and in all three oboe players the right hand was affected. Three of five flutists had left hand involvement. Three bagpipers had symptoms only on the left hand and one had bilateral symptoms, although there was a 14-year delay from onset in the right hand until the left hand symptoms emerged. Five patients (83%) with embouchure dystonia showed clinical signs, including tremulous movements of the jaw, lateral pulling of the chin, and involuntary jaw closure and tongue protrusion. Embouchure dystonia was seen in the two bassoon players as well as in two clarinetists and two flutists. Detailed clinical characteristics of these patients are published elsewhere (13).

Treatment and Long-Term Outcome

Our patients employed a wide range of treatments, including most of the options previously outlined (Table 36-2). Among the 21 string players, 11 underwent nerve conduction studies and electromyography, in seven with normal results. Four patients showed findings suggestive of entrapment neuropathy, including the median nerve at the wrist, the median nerve at the proximal forearm, the ulnar nerve

TABLE 36-2. *Treatment of focal dystonia in instrumentalists*

Abstinence from playing
Physical exercise
Biofeedback
Psychotherapy
Body awareness technique
Alteration in playing technique
Change of instrument
New teacher
Slow practice/relearning
Medication (anticholinergic, dopaminergic, other)
Surgery (nerve entrapment)
Botulinum toxin
Splinting/immobilization
Sensory motor retuning/constraint-induced therapy

at the elbow, and the posterior interosseus branch of the radial nerve at the forearm. The musician with median neuropathy at the wrist underwent surgical release without benefit. Other treatment attempts included physical therapy, retraining, and medication (in most cases, trihexyphenidyl). In selected patients with hand but also with bow arm dystonia we offered botulinum toxin injections or splint devices. For all these options the response varied from none to mild or moderate improvement, mostly insufficient to maintain their high level as professional performers. Five of 11 patients with hand dystonia were able to continue their performing career, three by altering their technique and refingering certain passages. One musician changed from first desk to a section position and stabilized with a combination of medication, botulinum injections, tapping, and refingering exercises. The fifth musician who had dystonic movements limited to one distal interphalangeal joint had an excellent recovery after surgical immobilization of his distal finger. Overall, five of 14 professional performers (36%) responding to our questionnaire, among them none with bowing arm dystonia, were able to stay in their professional careers. The majority either became instrument teachers or entirely changed their professional field.

Among the woodwind instrumentalists with limb dystonia, 14 underwent nerve conduction studies and electromyography, in ten with normal results. Four patients showed results consistent with mild median neuropathy at or distal to the wrist. Three patients had nerve decompressive surgery—carpal tunnel release in one, ulnar nerve decompression at the elbow in another, and decompression of both nerves of one limb in the third. No patient experienced significant improvement. One musician had good results with anticholinergic treatment (trihexyphenidyl) and two (including one amateur) responded to a combination of trihexyphenidyl and botulinum toxin injections. Three indicated benefit from immobilizing their fingers with a splint device while playing. Two of the three were only mildly affected at baseline, and the third had persistent moderate-to-marked im-

pairment, but was able to continue playing with his self-designed splints. Another musician with only mild impairment had a temporary immobilization of his affected limb after a fracture and noticed improvement in his playing afterward. Of the six musicians with embouchure dystonia, the two patients with lateral pulling of their chin and jaw experienced very good results with rebuilding the embouchure, one with additional acupuncture treatment. The rebuilding of the embouchure included changes in size, configuration, and placement of the mouthpiece, but also correction and retraining of the embouchure with "buzzing" exercises. The two patients with complex tongue protrusions and jaw closing also affecting other oral activities stopped playing their instrument. The flutist with lip and cheek tremors declined treatment and concentrated on teaching. One musician who was only mildly affected at baseline, was stabilized with retraining and using a different flute. Overall, eight (53%) of the 15 woodwind instrumentalists responding to our survey were able to remain professional performers, among them five of nine musicians with limb dystonia and three of six musicians with embouchure dystonia.

DISCUSSION

We report the treatment attempts and long-term outcome of 45 instrumental musicians with FTSD. In our series, 33 (73%) of the musicians were male and 12 (27%) female. The increased risk of male musicians to develop focal dystonia is evident, especially considering that among all woodwind players seen at our center, females outnumber males by 2:1 (a total of 179 musicians, of whom 119 are female and 60 male). In a recent report on 111 musicians with focal dystonia, Brandfonbrener and Robson. (12) also described a significant male predominance (75% males vs. 25% females), again in a predominantly female population of instrumentalists.

There was no reported exposure to neuroleptics and no family history of dystonia. Identifiable triggers of dystonia were retrospectively noticed in more than half of the patients. This is consistent with previous reports, describing between 53% and 67% of identifiable predisposing events (2,4,7). Entrapment neuropathies, particularly ulnar nerve compression at the elbow, have been previously described as predisposing to the development of limb dystonia (15). Twenty-five of our patients had nerve conduction and electromyography (EMG) studies, mostly prior to the initial visit, with mild abnormalities in eight, leading to nerve decompression in four, none with noticeable improvement. Once present, dystonia progressed over 6 to 12 months, ending in a plateau without remission. Between 20% and 33% of patients experienced spread of dystonia to other tasks.

The clinical features in our patients with limb and embouchure dystonia were similar to other musicians with FTSD reported in the literature (4,5,7,9,12). Symptoms usually began between ages 33 and 39 years and progressed slowly over time. Remissions, fluctuations, and spread to other body regions were rare. Instrument-specific stresses on the fingers and hand seem to determine the side affected. In our series the instrument-holding hand in clarinet, oboe, and flute instrumentalists was predominantly involved. The left side of bagpipers is more likely to be affected. The reason might be that the left arm is draped over the instrument, supporting the bag (16). Previous studies also demonstrated predominant involvement of the left fingering hand in bowed string players (4,7,8).

Among our 16 string instrumentalists with hand dystonia, 25% profited from refingering exercises and another one had a very good outcome after surgical immobilization of his affected distal interphalangeal joint. The majority of string players (64%) including all musicians with bowing arm dystonia abandoned their musical careers. Four of the 18 woodwind players with limb dystonia described benefit from immobilization of their affected fingers with splints or incidental casting. In another three patients, trihexyphenidyl alone or in combination with botulinum toxin improved the symptoms to an extent that allowed them to play their instrument. Differences among the string and woodwind players in terms of treatment options might be explained with the more unidirectional movements of the fingers in woodwind players amenable to treatment with splint devices and botulinum toxin. Because of the more complex lateral movements in string players and the higher risk of excessive weakness with botulinum injections, treatment options are often restricted to refingering exercises or medication. Attempts with botulinum toxin in two musicians with bowing arm dystonia were only partially effective. In the small group of woodwind players with embouchure dystonia, two of the six woodwind players experienced good results with rebuilding their embouchure. In summary, approximately half of the string instrumentalists with hand dystonia and the woodwind players with limb or embouchure dystonia were able to continue their professional career. The outcome in string players with bowing arm dystonia seems to be even less favorable.

Although our understanding of the pathophysiology of FTSD is limited, studies support the idea of disturbed central processing of sensory information and distorted cortical representation of motor function in focal dystonia (17–20). Refingering exercises in hand dystonia and rebuilding the embouchure might influence and alleviate some of these disturbed central processes. Splint devices used while playing the instrument can exert a beneficial mechanical effect, but can also influence sensory pathways. More recently, a preliminary study demonstrated significant improvement after prolonged immobilization of the affected limb for 4 to 5 weeks in a series of seven musicians and one patient with writer's cramp (21). Long-term data in 11 professional instrumentalists treated with constraint-induced therapy, now renamed as sensory motor retuning, showed substantial benefit in six pianists and two guitarists but not in the three woodwind players (22). Data from controlled, randomized trials are needed to firmly establish benefit from these new treatment options.

REFERENCES

1. Fahn S, Marsden CD, Calne DB. Classification and investigations of dystonia. In: Marsden CD, Fahn S, eds. *Movement disorders 2*. London: Butterworths, 1987: 332–358.
2. Lederman RJ. Dystonia in musicians. *Musical Performance* 2000;2(4):45–53.
3. Hochberg FH, Leffert RD, Heller MD, et al. Hand difficulties among musicians. *JAMA* 1983;249:1869–1872.
4. Newmark J, Hochberg FH. Isolated painless manual incoordination in 57 musicians. *J Neurol Neurosurg Psychiatry* 1987;50:291–295.
5. Lederman RJ. Occupational cramp in instrumental musicians. *Med Probl Perform Art* 1988;3:45–51.
6. Lederman RJ. AAEM minimonograph #43: neuromuscular problems in the performing arts. *Muscle Nerve* 1994;17:569–577.
7. Brandfonbrener AG. Musicians with focal dystonia: a report of 58 cases seen during a ten-year period at a performing art medicine clinic. *Med Probl Perform Art* 1995;10:121–127.
8. Lederman RJ. Focal dystonia in instrumentalists: clinical features. *Med Probl Perform Art* 1991;6:132–136.
9. Frucht SJ, Fahn S, Greene PE, et al. The natural history of embouchure dystonia. *Mov Disord* 2001;16(5):899–906.
10. Lederman RJ. Treatment outcome in instrumentalists: a longterm follow-up study. *Med Probl Perform Art* 1995; 10:115–120.
11. Altenmueller E, Jabusch HC, Lim V. Therapy of musician's dystonia. *Mov Disord* 2002;17(5):1134A.
12. Brandfonbrener AG, Robson C. A review of 111 musicians with focal dystonia seen at a performing artist's clinic 1985–2002. *Mov Disord* 2002;17(5):1135A.
13. Schuele S, Lederman RJ. Focal dystonia in woodwind instrumentalists: long-term outcome. *Med Probl Perform Art* 2003;18:15–20.
14. Schuele SU, Lederman RJ. Focal dystonia in violin and viola instrumentalists. *Mov Disord* 2002;17(5):1136A.
15. Charness ME, Ross MH, Shefner JM. Ulnar neuropathy and dystonic flexion of the fourth and fifth digits: a clinical correlation in musicians. *Muscle Nerve* 1996; 19(4):431–437.
16. Lederman RJ. Piper's palsy: a focal dystonia. *Med Probl Perform Art* 1998;13:14–18.
17. Tinazzi M, Priori A, Bertolasi L, et al. Abnormal central integration of a dual somatosensory input in dystonia. Evidence for sensory overflow. *Brain* 2000;123(1): 42–50.
18. Hallett M. The neurophysiology of dystonia. *Arch Neurol* 1998;55(5):601–603.
19. Byl NN, Melnick M. The neural consequences of repetition: clinical implications of a learning hypothesis. *J Hand Ther* 1997;10:160–174.
20. Elbert T, Candia V, Altenmuller E, et al. Alteration of digital representations in somatosensory cortex in focal hand dystonia. *NeuroReport* 1998;9(16):3571–3575.
21. Priori A, Pesenti A, Cappellari A, et al. Limb immobilization for the treatment of focal occupational dystonia. *Neurology* 2001;57(3):405–409.
22. Candia V, Schafer T, Taub E, et al. Sensory motor retuning: a behavioral treatment for focal hand dystonia of pianists and guitarists. *Arch Phys Rehabil* 2002;83: 1342–1348.

Dystonia 4: Advances in Neurology, Vol. 94. Edited
by Stanley Fahn, Mark Hallett, and Mahlon R.
DeLong. Lippincott Williams & Wilkins,
Philadelphia © 2004.

37

Abnormal Sensorimotor Processing in Pianists with Focal Dystonia

*Vanessa K. Lim, †John L. Bradshaw, ‡Michael E. R. Nicholls, and
§Eckart Altenmüller

*Department of Sport and Exercise Science, The University of Auckland, Auckland, New Zealand.
†Department of Psychology, Monash University, Clayton, Australia. ‡Department of Psychology,
School of Behavioural Sciences, University of Melbourne, Melbourne, Australia.
§Institute of Music Physiology and Musicians' Medicine, University of Music and Drama,
Hanover, Germany*

Musicians perform highly complex movements that require temporospatial accuracy and auditory and tactile feedback. In some individuals a task-specific, (usually) painless cramping or incoordination of the fingers and hands may occur. This condition is referred to as focal dystonia (1), in general, and in the case of musicians this disorder may be referred to as musicians' cramp.

The prevalence of musicians' cramp is approximately 0.2% to 0.5% in professional musicians (2). Risk factors for the development of musicians' cramp include the number of practice hours, personality, genetic predisposition, and performance factors (3,4). Of particular importance is the gender and the instrument played by the patient, both of which have a significant role in the prevalence of musicians' cramp; male musicians are more likely than females to develop symptoms in keyboard, string, woodwind, and plucking instruments (3).

Although risk factors have been identified, the causes of focal dystonia have yet to be determined. Musicians' cramp affects integration of the sensorimotor system at many levels (for a review see ref. 4). Dystonia is associated with functional disturbances of the basal ganglia and according to recent studies, dystonia is also associated with deficits in sensorimotor integration (5–8).

This chapter discusses the contingent negative variation (CNV), which was recorded using electroencephalography (EEG) in patients with musicians' cramp and in musician controls. This paradigm involves a warning stimulus (S1) followed by a short delay and an imperative stimulus (S2). Typically, tones are used as the stimuli; in the current study, mechanical/tactile stimuli were employed for both S1 and S2. The early CNV (750 to 850 ms after S1) is thought to reflect stimulus processing, while the late CNV (1,900 to 2,000 ms), which occurs before the S2, is thought to reflect response preparation (9).

STUDY RATIONALE

The CNV is a relevant paradigm for musicians because it involves—as in music performance—a complex interaction among incoming sensory inputs, motor initiation, output, and personal expectations (10). Dystonia has been considered a basal ganglia disorder (11,12). Although the exact generators are unknown, the CNV is highly influenced by the basal-ganglia-thalamocortical loop (13). Additionally, the CNV has been recorded using deep electrodes in the basal ganglia and the cortex (14). Therefore, the CNV was considered a highly relevant experimental paradigm for investigations into motor and sensory changes in patients with musicians' cramp.

The first aim of this study was to investigate the cortical activity prior to a sensory event. Two conditions, with and without movement, were employed. The nonmovement condition served as a control. This was necessary because the CNV is a complex paradigm, and controlling for the movement aspect of the paradigm was important. Following previous research on patients with writers' cramp (15,16), it was expected that the CNV prior to movement (late CNV) of the patients would be significantly diminished compared to controls in the movement condition if musicians' cramp is a disorder of movement or movement preparation. In addition, group differences would not be expected in the non–movement-elicited CNV, and that the electromyography (EMG) recordings would not show differences between groups in either condition.

In addition to group differences for the cortical amplitudes, it was also expected that the reaction times of the responses to the S2 stimulus would be correlated with the electrophysiologic activity prior to movement. Typically, the faster the reaction times, the greater the CNV amplitude (9). Group differences between patients and controls may indicate possible dysfunction in producing movement or integrating sensory feedback.

METHOD

Participants

All participants were professional male pianists. Seven patients had dystonic symptoms primarily in their small finger, six of whom only displayed dystonic cramping during playing the piano (Table 37-1). The controls were matched as close as possible with respect to age (38 ± 16 years), handed-

ness, and style of music played (primarily classical).

Electrophysiology: CNV

Continuous EEG was recorded with ten scalp electrodes (Fz, CF3, CFz, CF4, C3, Cz, C4, CP3, CPz, CP4) mounted on an elastic cap (EasyCap, Germany), referenced to linked mastoids. EEG signals were amplified (Synamps amplifiers, Neuroscan Inc., USA) with a bandpass filter (DC—1,000 Hz). Additionally there were four bipolar EMG channels (extensor digitorum) recorded (bandpass filter: 30–200 Hz). Vertical electro-oculogram (VEOG) was also recorded, and was used for artifact rejection.

Stimuli

All tactile stimuli were 7 ms in duration and were placed 2 mm away from the middle of the small fingernail. The average force of each stimulus was 8.21 ± 1.51 newtons (N).

PROCEDURE

Movement Condition

There were 448 trials using an S1-S2 choice-reaction time, with a fixed interstimulus interval of 2 seconds. The interval between S2 and the next S1 varied randomly between 5 and 8 seconds (mean 6.5 seconds). After S2, the participants were required to press a button upon which the small fingers directly rested. The S1 stimulus provided information about the side on which the S2 stimulus was likely to occur (75% valid). When the S2 stimulus was presented on the same side as the S1 stimulus, the trial was designated a valid trial. When the S2 occurred on the opposite side of S1, the trial was invalid (25%).

Nonmovement Condition

This condition served as a control, and the order of presentation of the two conditions

TABLE 37-1. *Clinical profiles of the pianists with focal dystonia in this study*

Patient ID	Age	Number of years playing	Entrance into music academy	Duration of problem (years)	Handedness	Side of symptom	Symptom	Task specific	Previous medication	Family history
1	37	31	20	3	Right	Right	3, 4, 5 F	Yes	No	Father with writer's cramp
2	32	21	21	2.5	Left	Right	3, 4, 5 E	Yes	No	None
3	69	59	18	5	Right	Right	4, 5 F; 3, 4	Yes	40 U*	Son has musician's cramp
4	40	34	18	3	Right	Left	Unstable	No**	No	None
5	38	28	21	3	Right	Right	3, 4 F	Yes	80 U*	None
6	57	51	19	8	Right	Right	2, 4, 5 F; 3 E; 2,	Yes	No	None
7	32	20	22	4	Right	Right	4, 5 F	Yes	No	None

*Dysport (U: units).
**Also had problems when grasping certain instruments.
Symptomatic fingers: 3, middle; 4, ring; 5, small; F, flexion; E, extension.

was counterbalanced. This condition followed the same S1-S2 design; in 56 trials (invalid) there were "double presentations," which were 20 ms apart for S2. Participants were not required to move in this condition; instead participants counted the number of "double presentations" that they felt.

RESULTS

For the analyses, the nonmovement condition was subtracted from the movement condition; thus factors not directly related to the response preparation were minimized. Greenhouse-Geisser correction was used for all EEG and EMG analyses (17). Consistent with the thesis that musicians with dystonia and controls showed similar levels of processing of S1, there was indeed no group difference for the processing of the warning stimuli [early CNV; $F_{(1,12)} = 0.34$; nonsignificant (NS)]. In contrast, the late CNV motor component revealed a significant group difference ($F_{(1,12)} = 6.04$; p <.05). The musicians with dystonia ($-5.04\ \mu V$) had a significantly greater activation compared to the controls ($-1.34\ \mu V$). Figure 37-1 demon-

strates this increase in the motor part of the CNV with aspects unrelated to motor preparation minimized.

There were no group differences in hands (affected and unaffected) in either early or late CNV ($F_{(1,12)} = 1.23$; NS and $F_{(1,12)} = 0.54$; NS). This was also shown for the EMG analysis, which showed no significant group differences ($F_{(1,12)} = 0.82$; NS).

BEHAVIORAL AND ELECTROPHYSIOLOGIC CORRELATIONS

Controls were slower than patients in valid (339 ms and 278 ms) and invalid (414 ms and 287 ms) trials ($F_{(1,12)} = 8.52$; p <.05). Median reaction times for both hands were correlated with amplitudes of early and late CNV at Cz [r-critical for degrees of freedom $_{(1,5)} = 0.75$ at the alpha level of .05). There were no significant correlations for either hands or early or late CNVs for the patients with musicians' cramp shown. In contrast, the controls had significant correlations between the amplitude of the late CNV and reaction time, replicating the

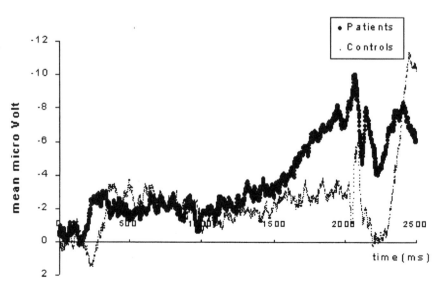

FIG. 37-1. Subtracted grand average contingent negative variation (CNV) for both hands and all trials for patients and controls over Cz (Vertex) with negative voltages up.

relationship between reaction time and electrophysiologic potentials that has been previously demonstrated (9). That is, for the controls, the faster the reaction times (both hands), the larger the late CNV amplitudes were; this was not the case for the patients. The behavioral results for the nonmovement condition demonstrated no significant group differences for the discrimination of the "double presentations" ($F_{(1,12)} = 0.60$; NS).

DISCUSSION

The results of the current study suggest that patients with musicians' cramp have an overall increase in activation or deficient inhibition prior to movement. This was demonstrated by the increase in the late CNV amplitudes of patients compared to controls. EMG signals (movement task) and the perceptual abilities (nonmovement task) of the patients were not different from controls.

Amplitude, but not distributional differences, was found prior to movement between groups. This cannot be attributed to arousal differences between groups, as the early CNV did not differ. While it is acknowledged that the patients with musician's cramp were somewhat faster than the controls, it is possible that they were merely trying to "prove" themselves. The difference does not reflect training differences, as all musicians were professional pianists and all played primarily classical music (controls and patients). Furthermore, only the reaction times of the musician controls correlated with the amplitude of the late CNV. The relation between faster reaction time and CNV amplitude is well established (9). Therefore, the increased late CNV in the patients compared to controls is not simply due to longer reaction times. This result is in fact suggestive of a further abnormality between musicians with and without dystonia. It is possible that it reflects an abnormality within the basal-ganglia-thalamo-cortical loop.

To our knowledge this is the first study investigating the CNV on patients with musicians' cramp. It is fortunate that this current study was able to examine a group of professional piano players with specific dystonic symptoms. The CNV is an appropriate paradigm for musicians, as the procedure is similar to playing an instrument. For example, reading a note is similar to the initial attention and warning stimulus (S1), and the waiting period before movement (before S2) is similar to waiting to play the notes that have been already read within a given period of time. A manipulation of the musicians' expectancy or cuing (valid and invalid trials) is not unlike playing a correct or incorrect note.

It is tempting to suggest a functional, and possibly pathophysiologic, difference in musicians with focal dystonia compared to patients with writer's cramp. That is, the results contrast previous research using the CNV paradigm (10,15,18). The direction of activation is opposite to that of other patients with focal dystonia (e.g., writer's cramp and cervical dystonia). The current study did not find diminished CNV values but rather increased values.

There are, however, several methodologic differences between this study and previous research. The current study used mechanical stimulation, which is another sensory modality that musicians rely on heavily. The previous research employed tones and may not be a sensory modality that is relevant for patients with writer's cramp. Also, expectancy of the trials was manipulated by cuing, which provided information about the upcoming event. As described earlier, the CNV is highly contextual, and the more complex the task and the more "important" the "message," the greater the negativity of the CNV (9). This is also reflected in the reaction times of the patients, which were faster than those of the controls. This paradigm may thus be more relevant to musicians who may, therefore, demonstrate greater negativity. It is unlikely, however, that the patients with writer's cramp in previous studies were in any way less motivated. Finally, while the results are inconsistent with previous studies employing EEGs, they are indeed consistent with studies employing paradigms that induced dystonic symptoms (19,20), and with transcranial magnetic stimulation (TMS) studies on patients with focal dystonia (21–26).

Although none of the patients developed overt dystonic symptoms during this task, it is a highly relevant task in a framework closely related to playing music. It is likely that the increase in motor activation prior to movement demonstrated in patients with musicians' cramp compared to controls was due to context specificity. Increased activation of the sensorimotor areas does not have to occur with dystonic symptoms; rather, an important factor appears to be the context and its relevance in which the patients are tested. This argues in favor of the basal-ganglia-thalamocortical loop as one of the main areas of dysfunction in focal dystonia.

CONCLUSION

The overactivity in the sensorimotor areas prior to movement was demonstrated in a group of professional pianists with focal dystonia. The results are consistent with an increase in sensorimotor excitability caused by dysfunctions in the basal ganglia. While this study was unable to investigate intracortical inhibition, it is possible that this is also impaired. The results are also consistent with previous research investigating focal dystonia in task-relevant paradigms (20). These results were demonstrated without inducing dystonic symptoms and suggest that contextual relevancy is important for the expression of symptoms. Therefore, it is important for future research to examine focal dystonia in task-relevant or symptom-inducing paradigms to enable a greater understanding of the disorder.

SUMMARY

Focal dystonia is a task-specific sensorimotor disorder that is characterized by sustained muscle contractions, which may cause twisting, repetitive movements, or abnormal postures. In the current study, the contingent negative variation was recorded in a group of professional pianists with focal dystonia (mu-

sicians' cramp) and compared to pianist controls. The CNV is composed of an early stimulus processing component and a later response preparation component. The CNV can be elicited in tasks that require movement and nonmovement. A subtractive analysis with a nonmovement condition was used to minimize effects of the CNV not related to response preparation. The current results revealed no group differences for the early CNV (processing of stimulus properties). In contrast, a significant group difference was found in the late CNV (movement preparation) between patients and controls, with the patients showing significantly higher activation prior to movement. The current study demonstrates an increase in overall sensorimotor activity prior to movement in patients with musicians' cramp. This overexcitation of the cortex may be the result of a dysfunction in the globus pallidus, resulting in a lack of inhibition and/or an increase in excitation.

ACKNOWLEDGMENTS

The first author is supported by the Deutscher Akademischer Austauschdienst (DAAD) Short-term Research Scholarship, the University of Melbourne Postgraduate Overseas Research Scholarship, the University of Melbourne Psychology Department Grant, and a grant from the Education and Welfare Committee (University of Melbourne).

REFERENCES

1. Fahn S, Marsden CD, Calne DB. Classification and investigation of dystonia. In: Marsden CD, Fahn S, eds. *Movement disorders 2.* London: Butterworths, 1987: 332–358.
2. Altenmüller E. Causes and cures of focal limb-dystonia in musicians. *Int Soc Study Tens Perform* 1998;9:13–17.
3. Lim VK, Altenmüller E. Musicians' cramp: instrumental and gender differences. *Med Prob Perf Artists (in press).*
4. Lim VK, Altenmüller E, Bradshaw JL. Focal dystonia: current theories. *Hum Mov Sci* 2001;20:875–914.
5. Abbruzzese G, Marchese R, Buccolieri A, et al. Abnormalities of sensorimotor integration in focal dystonia—a transcranial magnetic stimulation study. *Brain* 2001; 124:537–545.
6. Sanger TD, Merzenich MM. Computational model of the role of sensory disorganization in focal task-specific dystonia. *J Neurophysiol* 2000;84:2458–2464.

7. Schenk T, Mai N. Is writer's cramp caused by a deficit of sensorimotor integration? *Exp Brain Res* 2001;136: 321–330.

8. Serrien DJ, Burgunder JM, Wiesendanger M. Disturbed sensorimotor processing during control of precision grip in patients with writer's cramp. *Mov Disord* 2000; 15:965–972.

9. Brunia CHM. Neural aspects of anticipatory behavior. *Acta Psychol* 1999;101:213–242.

10. Kaji R, et al. Physiological study of cervical dystonia—task-specific abnormality in contingent negative variation. *Brain* 1995;118:511–522.

11. Hallett M. The neurophysiology of dystonia. *Arch Neurol* 1998;55:601–603.

12. Hallett M. Physiology of dystonia. *Adv Neurol* 1998;78: 11–18.

13. Ikeda A, et al. Dissociation between contingent negative variation and Bereitschaftspotential in a patient with cerebellar efferent lesion. *Electroencephalogr Clin Neurophysiol* 1994;90:359–364.

14. Bares M, Rektor I. Basal ganglia involvement in sensory and cognitive processing. A depth electrode CNV study in human subjects. *Clin Neurophysiol* 2001;112: 2022–2030.

15. Hamano T, et al. Abnormal contingent negative variation in writer's cramp. *Clin Neurophysiol* 1999;110:508–515.

16. Kaji R, Shibasaki H, Kimura J. Writer's cramp—a disorder of motor subroutine. *Ann Neurol* 1995;38: 837–838.

17. Greenhouse S, Geisser S. On methods in analysis of profile data. *Psychometrika* 1959;24:95–112.

18. Ikeda A, et al. Abnormal sensorimotor integration in writer's cramp: study of contingent negative variation. *Mov Disord* 1996;11:683–690.

19. Odergren T, Stone-Elander S, Ingvar M. Cerebral and cerebellar activation in correlation to the action-induced dystonia in writer's cramp. *Mov Disord* 1998;13:497–508.

20. Pujol J, et al. Brain cortical activation during guitar-induced hand dystonia studied by functional MRI. *Neuroimage* 2000;12:257–267.

21. Chen R, Wassermann EM, Hallett M. Impairment of cortical inhibition in focal dystonia. *Ann Neurol* 1996; 40:T180.

22. Ikoma K, Samii A, Mercuri B, et al. Abnormal cortical motor excitability in dystonia. *Neurology* 1996;46: 1371–1376.

23. Mavroudakis N, Caroyer JM, Brunko E, et al. Abnormal motor evoked responses to transcranial magnetic stimulation in focal dystonia. *Neurology* 1995;45:1671–1677.

24. Ridding MC, Sheean G, Rothwell JC, et al. Changes in the balance between motor cortical excitation and inhibition in focal, task specific dystonia. *J Neurol Neurosurg Psychiatry* 1995;59:493–498.

25. Rosenkranz K, Altenmüller E, Siggelkow S, et al. Alteration of sensorimotor integration in musician's cramp: impaired focusing of proprioception. *Clin Neurophysiol* 2000;111:2040–2045.

26. Siebner HR, Auer C, Conrad B. Abnormal increase in the corticomotor output to the affected hand during repetitive transcranial magnetic stimulation of the primary motor cortex in patients with writer's cramp. *Neurosci Lett* 1999;262:133–136.

Dystonia 4: Advances in Neurology, Vol. 94. Edited by Stanley Fahn, Mark Hallett, and Mahlon R. DeLong. Lippincott Williams & Wilkins, Philadelphia © 2004.

38

Dystonia: Medical Therapy and Botulinum Toxin

Joseph Jankovic

Department of Neurology, Parkinson's Disease Center and Movement Disorders Clinic, Baylor College of Medicine, Houston, Texas

The symptomatic treatment of dystonia has markedly improved, particularly since the introduction of botulinum toxin (BT) and new advances in stereotactic surgery (Table 38-1) (Fig. 38-1). This chapter discusses only medical therapy; surgical treatment of dystonia is reviewed elsewhere in this volume and is covered in other reviews (1,2). In most cases of dystonia, the treatment is merely symptomatic, designed to improve posture and function and to relieve associated pain. In rare patients, however, dystonia can be so severe that the dystonic movements may compromise respiration or cause muscle breakdown and a life-threatening hyperthermia, rhabdomyolysis, and myoglobinuria. In such cases of "dystonic storm" or "status dystonicus," proper therapeutic intervention can be lifesaving (3,4).

To objectively assess the response to various therapeutic interventions, it is critical not only to use appropriate rating scales, but also to take into account the intervention's effects on activities of daily living and quality of life. This is a particularly challenging task in dystonia, because this syndrome has different etiologies, anatomic distributions, and heterogeneous clinical manifestations, producing variable disability. A variety of instruments have been used to assess the response in patients with different forms of dystonia, most frequently for the focal dystonias such as blepharospasm (5) and cervical dystonia (Toronto Western Spasmodic Torticollis Rating Scale or TWSTRS) (6,7). In addition, various scales, such as the Burke-Fahn-Marsden Scale (BFMS) and the Unified Dystonia Rating Scale (UDRS) have been used to assess patients with generalized dystonia (8,9). Any long-term assessment of patients with dystonia must take into account the natural history of the disease, including the possibility of spontaneous, albeit often transient, remissions. Furthermore, a large placebo effect has been demonstrated in clinical trials of dystonia (10).

The selection of a particular choice of therapy is largely guided by personal clinical experience and by empirical trials (11). The age of the patient, the anatomic distribution of dystonia, and the potential risk of adverse effects are also important determinants of the choice of therapy. The identification of a specific cause of dystonia, such as drug-induced dystonias or Wilson's disease, may lead to a treatment that is targeted to the particular etiology. It is, therefore, prudent to search for identifiable causes of dystonia, particularly when some atypical features are present. It is beyond the scope of this chapter to discuss the diagnostic approaches to patients with dystonia; this topic is covered elsewhere in this volume and in other reviews (12).

TABLE 38-1. *Treatment of dystonia*

Focal dystonias
  Blepharospasm
    1. Botulinum toxin injections
    2. Clonazepam, lorazepam
    3. Trihexyphenidyl
    4. Orbicularis oculi myectomy
  Oromandibular dystonia
    1. Baclofen
    2. Trihexyphenidyl
    3. Botulinum toxin injections
  Spasmodic dysphonia
    1. Botulinum toxin injections
    2. Voice and supportive therapy
  Cervical
    1. Botulinum toxin injections
    2. Trihexyphenidyl
    3. Diazepam, lorazepam, clonazepam
    4. Tetrabenazine
    5. Cyclobenzaprine
    6. Carbamazepine
    7. Baclofen (oral)
    8. Peripheral surgical denervation
  Task-specific dystonias (e.g., writer's cramp)
    1. Benztropine, trihexyphenidyl
    2. Botulinum toxin injections
    3. Occupational therapy
Segmental and generalized dystonias
    1. Levodopa (in children and young adults)
    2. Trihexyphenidyl, benztropine
    3. Diazepam, lorazepam, clonazepam
    4. Baclofen (oral, intrathecal)
    5. Carbamazepine
    6. Tetrabenazine (with lithium)
    7. Triple therapy: tetrabenazine, fluphenazine, trihexyphenidyl
    8. Intrathecal baclofen infusion (axial dystonia)
    9. Thalamotomy (in distal dystonia or hemidystonia)
    10. Deep brain stimulation (GPi)

PHYSICAL AND SUPPORTIVE THERAPY

Before reviewing pharmacologic and surgical therapy of dystonia, it is important to emphasize the role of patient education and supportive care, as these are integral components of a comprehensive approach to patients with dystonia. Physical therapy and well-fitted braces are designed primarily to improve posture and to prevent contractures. Although braces are often poorly tolerated, particularly by children, in some cases they may be used as a substitute for a "sensory trick." For example, in some of our patients with cervical dystonia we were able to construct neck-head braces that seem to provide sensory input by touching certain portions of the neck or head in a fashion similar to the patient's own sensory trick, thus enabling the patient to maintain a desirable head position.

Various hand devices have been developed in an attempt to help patients with writer's cramp to use their hands more effectively and comfortably (13). In one small study of five professional musicians with focal dystonia, Candia et al. (14) reported success with immobilization by splints of one or more of the digits other than the dystonic finger followed by intensive repetitive exercises of the dystonic finger. It is not clear, however, whether this therapy provides lasting benefits. In another study involving eight patients with idiopathic occupational focal dystonia of the upper limb, immobilization with a splint for 4 to 5 weeks resulted in a significant improvement at a 24-week follow-up visit, based on the Arm Dystonia Disability Scale (0 = normal; 3 = marked difficulty in playing) and the Tubiana and Chamagne Score (0 = unable to play, 5 = returns to concert performances), and was considered marked in four, moderate in three, and the initial improvement disappeared in one (15). The splint was applied for 24 hours every day except for 10 minutes; once a week it was removed for brief local hygiene. Immediately upon removal of the splint, all patients reported marked clumsiness and weakness, which resolved in 4 weeks. There was also some local subcutaneous and joint edema and pain in the immobilized joint, and nail growth stopped; none developed contractures. Although the mechanisms of action of immobilization is unknown, the authors have postulated that removing all motor and sensory input to a limb may allow the cortical map to "reset" to the previous normal topography.

One major concern about immobilization of a limb, particularly a dystonic limb, is that such immobilization can actually increase the risk of exacerbating or even precipitating dystonia, as has been well demonstrated in dystonia following casting or other peripheral causes of dystonia (16). A variation of the immobilization therapy, the so-called constraint-

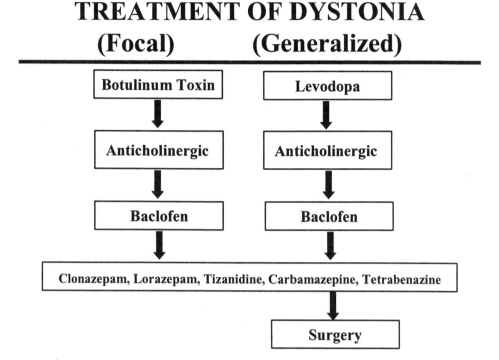

FIG. 38-1. Algorithm for the treatment of dystonia.

induced movement therapy, has been used successfully in rehabilitation of patients after stroke and other brain insults, and the observed benefit has been attributed to cortical reorganization (17,18). Some patients find various muscle relaxation techniques and sensory feedback therapy useful adjuncts to medical or surgical treatments. Because some patients with dystonia have impaired sensory perception, it has been postulated that sensory training may relieve dystonia. In a study of ten patients with focal hand dystonia, Zeuner et al. (19) showed that reading Braille for 30 to 60 minutes daily for 8 weeks improved spatial acuity and dystonia. Sensory training, to restore sensory representation of the hand along with mirror imagery and mental practice techniques, also has been reported to be useful in the treatment of focal hand dystonia (20).

Using repetitive transcranial magnetic stimulation (rTMS) delivered at low frequencies (≤1 Hz) for 20 minutes, Siebner et al. (21) showed that handwriting impaired by dystonic writer's cramp improved for at least 3 hours, presumably by increasing inhibition (and thus reducing excitability) of the underlying cortex. Finally, long-term neck muscle vibration of the contracting muscle may have a therapeutic value in patients with cervical dystonia. This is suggested by transient (minutes) improvement in head position in one patient treated for 15 minutes with muscle vibration (22). Such observation is consistent with the notion that proprioceptive sensory input affects cervical dystonia.

DOPAMINERGIC THERAPY

Unlike Parkinson's disease, in which therapy with levodopa replacement is based on the finding of depletion of dopamine in the brains of parkinsonian animals and humans, our knowledge of biochemical alterations in idiopathic dystonia is very limited (Table 38-2).

TABLE 38-2. *Therapeutic options for patients with dystonia*

Generic name	Trade name	Daily dosage (*)	Mechanism of action
Trihexyphenidyl	Artane	6–100	Anticholinergic
Benztropine	Cogentin	4–15	Anticholinergic
Orphenadrine	Norflex	200–800	Anticholinergic
Clonazepam	Klonopin	1–12	Serotonergic; relaxant
Lorazepam	Ativan	1–16	Relaxant
Diazepam	Valium	10–100	Relaxant
Cyclobenzaprine	Flexeril	20–60	Relaxant
Chlordiazepoxide	Librium	10–100	Relaxant
Baclofen	Lioresal	40–120	Antispastic; GABA agonist; substance P antagonist
Baclofen intrathecal infusion	Lioresal	200–1,500 µg/day	
Primidone	Mysoline	50–800	Antiepileptic; antitremor
Valproate	Depakote	500–1,500	Antiepileptic; GABA-T inhibitor
Carbamazepine	Tegretol	1,600	Antiepileptic
Levodopa/carbidopa	Sinemet (CR)	75/300–200/2,000	Dopamine precursor
Lithium	Lithobid	600–1,800	Antidopaminergic
Tetrabenazine	Xenazine 25	50–300	Monoamine depleter
Botulinum toxin A	BOTOX	5–400 Mouse units	Blocks Ach release at the neuromuscular junction by cleaving SNAP-25
Botulinum toxin B	MYOBLOC	100–15,000 Mouse units	Blocks Ach release at the neuromuscular junction by cleaving synaptobrevin (VAMP)
Surgery—peripheral denervation, myectomy, thalamotomy, pallidotomy, pallidal deep brain stimulation			

*Dose in mg unless otherwise specified.
GABA, γ-aminobutyric acid; VAMP, vesicle-associated membrane potential.

One exception is the dopa-responsive dystonia (DRD), in which the biochemical and genetic mechanisms have been elucidated by studies of postmortem brains and by molecular DNA and biochemical studies. Decreased neuromelanin in the substantia nigra with otherwise normal nigral cell count and morphology and normal tyrosine hydroxylase immunoreactivity were found in one brain of a patient with classic DRD (23). There was a marked reduction in dopamine in the substantia nigra and in striatum. These findings suggested that in DRD the primary abnormality was a defect in dopamine synthesis. This proposal is supported by the finding of a mutation in the guanosine triphosphate (GTP) cyclohydrolase I gene on chromosome 14q, which indirectly regulates the production of tetrahydrobiopterin, a cofactor for tyrosine hydroxylase, the rate-limiting enzyme in the synthesis of dopamine (24,25). The combination of levodopa-responsive dystonia and parkinsonism, inherited in an autosomal-dominant pattern, was also reported in a family characterized by

rapidly evolving dystonia (over a period of days to weeks) starting between ages 14 and 45 (26).

Most patients with DRD improve dramatically even with small doses of levodopa (100 mg of levodopa with 25 mg of decarboxylase inhibitor), but some may require doses of levodopa as high as 1,000 mg per day. In contrast to patients with juvenile Parkinson's disease, DRD patients usually do not develop levodopa-induced fluctuations or dyskinesias. If no clinically evident improvement is noted after 3 months of therapy, the diagnosis of DRD is probably in error and levodopa can be discontinued. In addition to levodopa, patients with DRD also improve with dopamine agonists, anticholinergic drugs, and carbamazepine (27). The take-home message from these reports is that a therapeutic trial of levodopa should be considered in all patients with childhood-onset dystonia, whether they have classic features of DRD or not. Since up to 25% of patients with adult-onset primary and secondary dystonia benefit at least partially from levodopa, some investigators have proposed that all patients with dystonia should be given at least a brief trial of levodopa. Apomorphine, perhaps by decreasing dopamine as well as serotonin release, may also ameliorate dystonia (28).

ANTIDOPAMINERGIC THERAPY

Paradoxically, some patients with dystonia benefit not from dopaminergic but from antidopaminergic therapy. Most clinical trials, however, have produced mixed results with dopamine receptor blocking drugs. Because of the poor response and the possibility of undesirable side effects, particularly sedation, parkinsonism, and tardive dyskinesia, the use of dopamine receptor blocking drugs (typical neuroleptics) in the treatment of dystonia should be discouraged (29). Although antidopaminergic drugs have been reported to be beneficial in the treatment of dystonia, the potential clinical benefit is usually limited by the development of side effects. Dopamine-depleting drugs, however, such as tetrabenazine, have been found useful in some patients with dystonia, particularly in those with tardive dystonia (30). Tetrabenazine has the advantage over other antidopaminergic drugs in that it does not cause tardive dyskinesia, although it may cause transient acute dystonic reaction (30). The drug is not readily available in the United States, but it is dispensed by prescription under the trade name Nitoman or Xenazine 25 in other countries, including the United Kingdom and Canada.

It is possible that some of the new atypical neuroleptic drugs will be useful not only as antipsychotics, but also in the treatment of hyperkinetic movement disorders. Clozapine, an atypical neuroleptic, has been reported in a small, open trial to be moderately effective in the treatment of segmental and generalized dystonia, but its usefulness was limited by potential side effects (31). Risperidone, a D_2 dopamine receptor blocking drug with a high affinity for 5-hydroxytryptamine (5-HT$_2$) receptors, has been reported to be useful in a 4-week trial of five patients with various forms

of dystonia (28). The treatment of tardive dystonia and other tardive syndromes is discussed elsewhere in this volume and in other reviews (29).

ANTICHOLINERGIC THERAPY

Anticholinergic medications such as trihexyphenidyl have been found to be most useful in the treatment of generalized and segmental dystonia (32). In the experience of Greene et al. (33), patients with blepharospasm, generalized dystonia, tonic (in contrast to clonic) dystonia, and onset of dystonia earlier than the age of 19 seemed to respond better to anticholinergic drugs than other subgroups, but this difference did not reach statistical significance. Except for short duration of symptoms before onset of therapy, there was no other variable, such as gender or severity, that reliably predicted a favorable response. This therapy is generally well tolerated when the dose is increased slowly. We recommend starting with a 2-mg preparation, half a tablet at bedtime, and advancing up to 12 mg per day over the next 4 to 6 weeks. Some patients require up to 60 to 100 mg/day, but may experience dose-related drowsiness, confusion, memory difficulty, blurring of vision, bladder retention, and hallucinations. In one study of 20 cognitively intact patients with dystonia, only 12 of whom could tolerate 15 to 74 of daily trihexyphenidyl, drug-induced impairments of recall and slowing of mentation was noted particularly in the older patients (34).

Diphenhydramine, an anticholinergic with histamine H_1 antagonist properties, has been reported to have an antidystonic effect in three of five patients (35). The drug, however, was not effective in ten other patients with cervical dystonia, and it was associated with sedation and other anticholinergic side effects in most patients. Pyridostigmine, peripherally acting anticholinesterase, and eye drops of pilocarpine (a muscarinic agonist) often ameliorate at least some of the peripheral side effects such as urinary retention and blurred vision. Pilocarpine (Salagen) 5 mg four times per day, cevimeline (Evoxac) 30 mg three times per day, and synthetic saliva (Salagen, Salivart, Salix) have been found effective in the treatment of dry mouth.

OTHER PHARMACOLOGIC THERAPIES

Many patients with dystonia require a combination of several medications and treatments (Table 38-2) (36). Benzodiazepines (diazepam, lorazepam, or clonazepam) may provide additional benefit for patients whose response to anticholinergic drugs is unsatisfactory. Clonazepam may be particularly useful in patients with blepharospasm and with myoclonic dystonia. Tizanidine hydrochloride (Zanaflex) has been approved for the treatment of spasticity, but it is not yet known whether the drug also will be useful in the treatment of dystonia (37). A centrally acting α_2-adrenergic agonist, its postulated mechanism of action involves increased presynaptic inhibition of motor neurons. Other muscle relaxants useful in the treatment of dystonia include cyclobenzaprine (Flexeril, 30 to 40 mg/day), metaxalone (Skelaxin, 800 mg two to three times per day), carisoprodol (Soma), orphenadrine (Norflex), and chlorzoxazone (Parafon forte). Structurally and pharmacologically similar to amitriptyline, cyclobenzaprine has been found at doses 30 to 40 mg/day to be superior to placebo but equal to diazepam.

Oral baclofen may be occasionally helpful, particularly in the treatment of oromandibular dystonia. This γ-aminobutyric acid (GABA)$_B$ autoreceptor agonist has been found to produce substantial and sustained improvement in 29% of children at a mean dose of 92 mg per day (range: 40–180) (38). Although initially effective in 28 of 60 (47%) of adults with cranial dystonia, only 18% continued baclofen at a mean dose of 105 mg/day after a mean of 30.6 months. Narayan et al. (39) first suggested that intrathecal baclofen (ITB) may be effective in the treatment of dystonia in a 1991 report of an 18-year-old man with severe cervical and truncal dystonic spasms, who was refractory to all forms of oral therapy and to large doses of paraspinal BT injections. Muscle-paralyzing agents were necessary to relieve these spasms, which compromised his respiration. Within a few hours after the institution of ITB infusion the patient's dystonia markedly improved and he was able to be discharged from the intensive care unit within 1 to 2 days. Our long-term experience with ITB has confirmed that this form of therapy is particularly useful in patients with spastic dystonia or dystonia affecting predominantly the trunk and legs (40). This has been also suggested by others (41,42).

In a study involving 86 patients, ages 3 to 42 (mean 13 years), with generalized dystonia (secondary to cerebral palsy in 71% of patients), external infusion or bolus-dose screening was positive in approximately 90% of patients (43). Programmable pumps were implanted in 77 patients. Infusion began at 200 µg/day, and increased by 10% to 20% per day until the best dose was achieved. Median-duration ITB therapy was 26 months. Mean dose increased over time, from 395 µg at 3 months, to 610 µg at 24 months, to 960 µg at 36 months. Quality of life and ease of care were rated by patients and caregivers as improved in approximately 85% of patients. Seven patients, including four with cerebral palsy, lost their response to ITB during the study, usually during the first year. The most common side effects were increased constipation (19%), decreased neck/trunk control, and drowsiness. Surgical and device complications occurred in 38% of patients, including infections and catheter breakage and disconnection. Complication rates decreased over time. In a long-term (6 years) follow-up of 14 patients, five were found to have improvement in their rating scale scores, although only two had sustained "clear clinical benefit" (44).

Continuous ITB has been found to be safe and effective in some patients with reflex sympathetic dystrophy (RSD) and dystonia (45). It is not yet clear whether ITB can induce lasting remissions in patients with dystonia. The American Academy for Cerebral Palsy and Developmental Medicine has published a systematic review of the use of ITB for spastic and dystonic cerebral palsy (46). The limited published data show that ITB reduced spasticity and dystonia, particularly in the lower extremities.

Other medications are used in the treatment of dystonia. For example, slow-release morphine sulfate has been shown to reduce not only pain but also dystonic movement in some patients with primary and tardive dystonia (47). In addition to clonazepam, γ-hydroxybutyrate (GHB), used in the treatment of alcohol abuse, has been found beneficial in the treatment of myoclonus-dystonia syndrome (48). It is not known whether acamprosate, another drug used in the treatment of alcohol abuse, is useful in the treatment of myoclonus-dystonia.

Peripheral deafferentiation with anesthetic was previously reported to improve tremor, but this approach also may be useful in the treatment of focal dystonia such as writer's cramp (49) or oromandibular dystonia (50), unresponsive to other pharmacologic therapy. An injection of 5 to 10 mL of 0.5% lidocaine into the target muscle improved focal dystonia for up to 24 hours. This short effect can be extended for up to several weeks if ethanol is injected simultaneously. The observation that the blocking of muscle spindle afferents reduces dystonia suggests that somatosensory input is important in the pathogenesis of dystonia. Mexiletine, an oral derivative of lidocaine, has been found effective in the treatment of cervical dystonia at doses ranging from 450 to 1,200 mg/day (51). Two thirds of the patients, however, experienced adverse effects such as heartburn, drowsiness, ataxia, tremor, and other side effects. Based on a review and a rating of videotapes by a "blind" rater, Lucetti et al. (52) reported a significant improvement in six patients with cervical dystonia treated with mexiletine.

Local electromyographic (EMG)-guided injection of phenol is currently being investigated as a potential treatment of cervical dystonia, but the results have not been very encouraging because of pain associated with the procedure and unpredictable response (53). Chemomyectomy with muscle necrotizing drugs, such as doxorubicin, has been tried in some patients with blepharospasm and hemifacial spasm (54), but because of severe local irritation it is doubtful that this approach will be adopted into clinical practice.

Attacks of kinesigenic paroxysmal dystonia may be controlled with anticonvulsants (e.g., carbamazepine, phenytoin). The nonkinesigenic forms of paroxysmal dystonia are less responsive to pharmacologic therapy, although clonazepam and acetazolamide may be beneficial. Treatment of paroxysmal dyskinesias is covered in other chapters in this volume and in other reviews (55).

BOTULINUM TOXIN

The introduction of BT into clinical practice in the late 1980s revolutionized treatment of dystonia. The most potent biologic toxin, BT has become a powerful therapeutic tool in the treatment of a variety of neurologic, ophthalmic, and other disorders manifested by abnormal, excessive, or inappropriate muscle contractions (56). In December 1989, after extensive laboratory and clinical testing, the Food and Drug Administration (FDA) approved this biologic (BT-A or Botox) as a therapeutic agent for patients with strabismus, blepharospasm, and other facial nerve disorders, including hemifacial spasm. In December 2000, the FDA approved Botox and BT-B (Myobloc) as treatments for cervical dystonia. Although its widest application is still in the treatment of disorders manifested by abnormal, excessive, or inappropriate muscle contractions, the use of BT is rapidly expanding to include treatment of a variety of ophthalmologic, gastrointestinal, urologic, orthopedic, dermatologic, secretory, painful, and cosmetic disorders (57,58).

Few therapeutic agents have been better understood in terms of their mechanism of action before their clinical application or have had greater impact on patient's functioning than BT (56). The therapeutic value of BT is a result of its ability to cause chemodenervation and to produce local paralysis when injected into a muscle. There are seven immunologically distinct toxins that share structurally homologous subunits. Synthesized as single-chain polypeptides (molecular weight of 150 kd), these toxin molecules have relatively little potency until they are cleaved by trypsin or bacterial enzymes into a heavy chain (100 kd) and light chain (50 kd). The 150-kd protein, the active portion of the molecule, complexes with one or more nontoxin proteins that support its structure and protect it from degradation (Table 38-3).

BT-A has been studied most intensely and used most widely, but the clinical applications of other types of toxins, including B and F, are also expanding (56,59). Although the efficacy and duration of benefits of BT-B or Myobloc, formerly NeuroBloc (Elan), are thought to be generally comparable to BT-A (Botox and Dysport), no head-to-head comparisons of the various products have been performed. An *in vivo* study using injections into the extensor digitorum brevis (EDB) of healthy volunteers suggested that the muscle paralysis from BT-B was not as complete or long-lasting as that from BT-A (60). Whether M-wave amplitude is a reliable measure of clinical response and whether the doses of BT-A (7.5–10 U) and BT-B (320–480 U), with a B-A ratio of about 45:1, are comparable is, however, debatable. The apparent longer duration of action of BT-A as compared to BT-B may be possibly explained by the observation that vesicle-associated membrane protein (VAMP) cleaved by BT-B cannot form a stable soluble NSF (N-ethylmaleimide) attachment protein receptor

(SNARE) complex and it turns over to form new VAMP, whereas SNAP-25, the substrate for BT-A, forms a truncated $SNAP-25_A$, which prevents degradation of SNARE, as a result of which the inhibition of exocytosis persists for 40 to 60 days. This correlates well with the reappearance of the original terminals (61).

A small percentage of patients receiving repeated injections develop antibodies against BT, causing the patients to be completely resistant to the effects of subsequent BT injections (62). In addition to the need for high and frequent dosages, young age may be a potential risk factor for the development of immunoresistance to BT-A (63). The original preparation of Botox contained 25 ng of neurotoxin complex protein per 100 units, but in 1997 the FDA approved a new preparation that contains only 5 ng per 100 units, which presumably should have lower antigenicity. In a 3-year follow-up of patients treated with the current Botox we have found no evidence of blocking antibodies as compared to 9.4% frequency of blocking antibodies in patients treated with the original Botox for the same period (64).

Blepharospasm

The effectiveness of BT in blepharospasm was first demonstrated in a double-blind, placebo-controlled trial in 1987 (5). In subsequent reports, moderate or marked improvement has been noted in 94% of blepharospasm patients. The average latency from the time of the injection to the onset of improvement was 4.2 days, the average duration of maximum benefit was 12.4 weeks, but the total benefit lasted considerably longer, averaging 15.7 weeks. Although 41% of all treatment sessions were followed by some side effects (ptosis, blurring of vision or diplopia, tearing, and local hematoma), only 2% of these side effects affected patient's functioning. Complications usually improved spontaneously in less than 2 weeks. In addition to idiopathic blepharospasm, BT injections have been used effectively in the treatment of blepharospasm in-

TABLE 38-3. *Botulinum neurotoxins*

Neurotoxin	Substrate	Localization
BT—A, E	SNAP-25	Presynaptic plasma membrane
BT—B, D, F	VAMP/ synaptobrevin	Synaptic vesicle membrane
BT—C	Syntaxin	Presynaptic plasma membrane

BT, botulinum toxin; VAMP, vesicle-associated membrane protein.

duced by drugs (e.g., levodopa in parkinsonian patients or neuroleptics in patients with tardive dystonia), dystonic eyelid and facial tics in patients with Tourette's syndrome, and in patients in whom blepharospasm was associated with apraxia of the eyelid opening (65).

Oromandibular Dystonia

Oromandibular dystonia is among the most challenging forms of focal dystonia to treat with BT; it rarely improves with medications, there are no surgical treatments, and BT therapy can be complicated by swallowing problems. The masseter muscles are usually injected in patients with jaw-closure dystonia, and in patients with jaw-opening dystonia either the submental muscle complex or the lateral pterygoid muscles are injected. A meaningful reduction in the oromandibular-lingual spasms and an improvement in chewing and speech can be achieved in more than 70% of all patients. BT can provide lasting improvement not only in patients with primary (idiopathic) dystonia but also in orolingual-mandibular tardive dystonia. Clenching and bruxism are frequent manifestations of oromandibular dystonia, although nocturnal and diurnal bruxism can occur even without evident dystonia (66,67).

Laryngeal Dystonia (Spasmodic Dysphonia)

Several studies have established the efficacy and safety of BT in the treatment of laryngeal dystonia, and this approach is considered by most to be the treatment of choice for spasmodic dysphonia (68). There are three approaches currently used in the BT treatment of spasmodic dysphonia: (a) unilateral EMG-guided injection of 5 to 30 U (69); (b) bilateral approach, injecting with EMG guidance 1.25 U to 4 U in each vocal fold; and (c) an injection via indirect laryngoscopy without EMG. Irrespective of the technique, most investigators report about 75% to 95% improvement in voice symptoms. Adverse experiences include transient breathy hypophonia,

hoarseness, and rare dysphagia with aspiration. Outcome assessments clearly show that BT injections for spasmodic dysphonia produce measurable improvements in the quality of life of patients with this disorder (70).

Cervical Dystonia

The efficacy and safety of BT in the treatment of cervical dystonia has been demonstrated in several controlled and open trials (71). Most trials report that about 90% of patients experience improvement in function and control of the head and neck and in pain. The average latency between injection and the onset of improvement (and muscle atrophy) is 1 week, and the average duration of maximum improvement is 3 to 4 months. On average, the injections are repeated every 4 to 6 months. Patients with long-duration dystonia have been found to respond less well than those treated relatively early, possibly because prolonged dystonia produced contractures. Complications, such as dysphagia and neck weakness, are probably related to local spread of biologic activity into adjacent muscles. Most complications resolve spontaneously, usually within 2 weeks. Lindeboom et al. (72) found that neurologic impairment and pain usually improve following BT injections, but only functional status measures differentiate patients who improve from those who have an insufficient response. There have been only a few long-term studies of BT treatment in cervical dystonia (73,74). Brashear et al. (74) showed that two thirds of patients who received BT reported the injections always helped.

Results similar to those obtained with BT-A have been obtained in patients treated for cervical dystonia with BT-B (59). Using the TWSTRS, 77% of the patients were found to respond at week 4. Other studies have subsequently confirmed the efficacy of BT-B (75), even in patients who are resistant to BT-A (76). In a 16-week, randomized, multicenter, double-blind, placebo-controlled trial of BT-B, 109 patients, who previously responded well to BT-A, were randomized into one of the following treatment groups: placebo,

5,000 U, and 10,000 U administered into two to four cervical muscles (75). At week 4, the total TWSTRS score improved by 4.3, 9.3 (p = .01), and 11.7 (p = .0004), respectively, when compared to baseline, and this was accompanied by significant improvements in pain, disability, and severity. The estimated median time until the total TWSTRS score returned to baseline was 63, 114, and 111 days, respectively. The most frequent side effects associated with BT-B included dysphagia and dry mouth. An identical design was used in another study of BT-B in cervical dystonia with one exception: the patients were resistant to BT-A as determined by the fluorescent treponemal antibody test (FTAT) (56). A total of 77 patients were randomized to receive placebo or 10,000 U of BT-B. At week 4, the total TWSTRS scores improved by 2 (placebo) and 11 (10,000 U) (p = .0001). There was also significant improvement in secondary and tertiary outcome measures including global assessments and pain visual analog scores as well as other measures of pain, disability, and severity. The estimated duration of effect, based on Kaplan-Meier survival analysis, was 112 days (12–16 weeks). Subsequent studies have suggested that dosages as high as 45,000 U of BT-B (Myobloc) per session may be effective and safe in patients with cervical dystonia. The most important determinants of a favorable response to BT treatments are a proper selection of the involved muscles and an appropriate dosage (Table 38-2). The general consensus among most BT users is that EMG is not needed in the vast majority of patients, except in rare instances when the muscles cannot be adequately palpated or the patient does not obtain adequate relief of symptoms with a conventional approach (77).

Writer's Cramp and Other Limb Dystonias

Treatments of writer's cramp with muscle relaxation techniques, physical and occupational therapy, and medical and surgical therapies, have been disappointing. Several trials

have concluded that BT injections into selected hand and forearm muscles probably provide the most effective relief in patients with these task-specific occupational dystonias. In some studies, fine-wire electrodes were used to localize bursts of muscle activation during the task and the toxin was injected through a hollow EMG needle into the belly of the most active muscle (78). Similar beneficial results, however, were obtained in other studies without complex EMG studies (79). Several lines of evidence support the notion that an intramuscular injection of BT into the forearm muscles corrects the abnormal reciprocal inhibition (80). Although one study showed that only 14 of 38 (37%) of needle placement attempts reached the proper hand muscles in the absence of EMG guidance, this does not mean that placement with EMG guidance correlates with better results, since the selection of the muscle involved in the hand dystonia is based on clinical examination and not on EMG (81). One study showed that voluntary activity of the hand immediately after the treatment for 30 minutes enhanced the weakness produced by the injection (82).

REFERENCES

1. Krack P, Vercueil L. Review of the functional surgical treatment of dystonia. *Eur J Neurol* 2001;8:389–399.
2. Bereznai B, Steude U, Seelos K, et al. Chronic high-frequency globus pallidus internus stimulation in different types of dystonia: a clinical, video, and MRI report of six patients presenting with segmental, cervical, and generalized dystonia. *Mov Disord* 2002;17:138–144.
3. Manji H, Howard RS, Miller DH, et al. Status dystonicus: the syndrome and its management. *Brain* 1998; 121:243–252.
4. Opal P, Tintner R, Jankovic J, et al. Intrafamilial phenotypic variability of the DYT1 dystonia: from asymptomatic TOR1A gene carrier status to dystonic storm. *Mov Disord* 2002;17:339–345.
5. Jankovic J, Orman J. Botulinum A toxin for cranial-cervical dystonia: a double-blind, placebo-controlled study. *Neurology* 1987;37:616–623.
6. Consky ES, Lang AE. Clinical assessments of patients with cervical dystonia. In: Jankovic J, Hallett M, eds. *Therapy with botulinum toxin.* New York: Marcel Dekker, 1994:211–237.
7. Comella CL, Stebbins GT, Goetz CG, et al. Teaching tape for the motor section of the Toronto Western Spasmodic Torticollis Scale. *Mov Disord* 1997;12:570–575.
8. Burke RE, Fahn S, Marsden CD. Torsion dystonia: a double-blind, prospective trial of high-dosage trihexyphenidyl. *Neurology* 1986;36:160–164.

9. Ondo WG, Desaloms M, Jankovic J, et al. Surgical pallidotomy for the treatment of generalized dystonia. *Mov Disord* 1998;13:693–698.

10. Lindeboom R, de Haan RJ, Brans JWM, et al. Treatment outcomes in cervical dystonia: a clinimetric study. *Mov Disord* 1996;11:371–376.

11. Brin MF, Hallett M, Jankovic J. Scientific and Therapeutic Aspects of Botulinum Toxin. Lippincott Williams & Wilkins, Philadelphia, PA, 2002:1–507.

12. Jankovic J, Fahn S. Dystonic disorders. In: Jankovic J, Tolosa E, eds. Parkinson's Disease and Movement Disorders, 4th ed. Philadelphia: Lippincott Williams & Wilkins, 2002:331–357.

13. Tas N, Karatas K, Sepici V. Hand orthosis as a writing aid in writer's cramp. *Mov Disord* 2001;16:1185–1189.

14. Candia V, Elbert T, Altenmüller E, et al. Constraint-induced movement therapy for focal hand dystonia in musicians. *Lancet* 1999;53:42.

15. Priori A, Pesenti A, Cappellari A, et al. Limb immobilization for the treatment of focal occupational dystonia. *Neurology* 2001;57:405–409.

16. Jankovic J. Can peripheral trauma induce dystonia and other movement disorders? Yes! *Mov Disord* 2001;16:7–12.

17. Levy CE, Nichols DS, Schmalbrock PM, et al. Functional MRI evidence of cortical reorganization in upper-limb stroke hemiplegia treated with constraint-induced movement therapy. *Am J Phys Med Rehabil* 2001;80:4–12.

18. Taub E, Uswatte G, Elbert T. New treatments in neurorehabilitation founded on basic research. *Nature Rev* 2002;3:226–236.

19. Zeuner KE, Bara-Jimenez W, Noguchi PS, et al. Sensory training for patients with focal hand dystonia. *Ann Neurol* 2002;51:593–598.

20. Byl NN, McKenzie A. Treatment effectiveness for patients with a history of repetitive hand use and focal hand dystonia: a planned, prospective follow-up study. *J Hand Ther* 2000;13:289–301.

21. Siebner HR, Tormos JM, Ceballos-Baumann AO, et al. Low-frequency repetitive transcranial magnetic stimulation of the motor cortex in writer's cramp. *Neurology* 1999;52:529–537.

22. Karnath H-O, Konczak J, Dichgans J. Effect of prolonged neck muscle vibration on lateral head tilt in severe spasmodic torticollis. *J Neurol Neurosurg Psychiatry* 2000;69:658–660.

23. Rajput AH, Gibb WRG, Zhong XH, et al. DOPA-responsive dystonia—pathological and biochemical observations in a case. *Ann Neurol* 1994;35:396–402.

24. Ichinose H, Ohye T, Takahi E, et al. Hereditary progressive dystonia with marked diurnal fluctuation caused by mutations in the GTP cyclohydrolase I gene. *Nature Gen* 1994;8:236–242.

25. Steinberger D, Korinthenber R, Topka H, et al. Dopa-responsive dystonia: mutation analysis of GCH1 and analysis of therapeutic doses of L-dopa. *Neurology* 2000;55:1735–1737.

26. Brashear A, Farlow MR, Butler IJ, et al. Variable phenotype of rapid-onset dystonia-parkinsonism. *Mov Disord* 1996;11:151–156.

27. Nygaard TG, Marsden CD, Fahn S. Dopa-responsive dystonia: Long-term treatment response and prognosis. *Neurology* 1991;41:174–181.

28. Zudas A, Cianchetti C. Efficacy of risperidone in idiopathic segmental dystonia. *Lancet* 1996;347:127–128.

29. Jankovic J. Tardive syndromes and other drug-induced movement disorders. *Clin Neuropharmacol* 1995;18:197–214.

30. Jankovic J, Beach J. Long-term effects of tetrabenazine in hyperkinetic movement disorders. *Neurology* 1997;48:358–362.

31. Karp BI, Goldstein SR, Chen R, et al. An open trial of clozapine for dystonia. *Mov Disord* 1999;14:652–657.

32. Hoon AH Jr, Freese PO, Reinhardt EM, et al. Age-dependent effects of trihexyphenidyl in extrapyramidal cerebral palsy. *Pediatr Neurol* 2001;25:55–58.

33. Greene P, Shale H, Fahn S. Analysis of open-label trials in torsion dystonia using high dosage of anticholinergics and other drugs. *Mov Disord* 1988;3:46–60.

34. Taylor AE, Lang AE, Saint-Cyr JA, et al. Cognitive processes in idiopathic dystonia treated with high-dose anticholinergic therapy: implications for treatment strategies. *Clin Neuropharmacol* 1991;14:62–77.

35. Truong DD, Sandromi P, van der Noort S, et al. Diphenhydramine is effective in the treatment of idiopathic dystonia. *Arch Neurol* 1995;52:405–407.

36. Jankovic J. Dystonia: medical therapy and botulinum toxin in dystonia. In: Fahn S, Marsden CD, DeLong DR, eds. *Dystonia 3, advances in neurology,* vol 78. Philadelphia: Lippincott-Raven, 1998:169–184.

37. Nance PW, Bugaresti J, Shellenberger K, et al. Efficacy and safety of tizanidine in the treatment of spasticity in patients with spinal cord injury. *Neurology* 1994;44 (suppl 9):S44–S52.

38. Greene P. Baclofen in the treatment of dystonia. *Clin Neuropharmacol* 1992;15:276–288.

39. Narayan RK, Loubser PG, Jankovic J, et al. Intrathecal baclofen for intractable axial dystonia. *Neurology* 1991;41:1141–1142.

40. Hou JG, Ondo W, Jankovic J. Intrathecal baclofen for dystonia. *Mov Disord* 2001;16:1201–1202.

41. van Hilten JJ, Hoff JI, Thang MC, et al. Clinimetric issues of screening for responsiveness to intrathecal baclofen in dystonia. *J Neural Transm* 1999;106:931–941.

42. Ford B, Greene PE, Louis ED, et al. Intrathecal baclofen in the treatment of dystonia. *Adv Neurol* 1998;78:199–210.

43. Albright AL, Barry MJ, Shafron DH, et al. Intrathecal baclofen for generalized dystonia. *Dev Med Child Neurol* 2001;43:652–657.

44. Walker RH, Danisi FO, Swope DM, et al. Intrathecal baclofen for dystonia: benefits and complications during six years of experience. *Mov Disord* 2000;15:1242–1247.

45. van Hilten BJ, van de Beek WJ, Hoff JI, et al. Intrathecal baclofen for the treatment of dystonia in patients with reflex sympathetic dystrophy. *N Engl J Med* 2000;343:625–630.

46. Butler C, Campbell S, AACPDM Treatment Outcomes Committee Review Panel. Evidence of the effects of intrathecal baclofen for spastic and dystonic cerebral palsy. *Dev Med Child Neurol* 2000;42:634–645.

47. Berg D, Becker G, Naumann M, et al. Morphine in tardive and idiopathic dystonia. *J Neural Transm* 2001;108:1035–1041.

48. Priori A, Bertolasi L, Pesenti A, et al. Gamma-hydroxybutyric acid for alcohol-sensitive myoclonus in dystonia. *Neurology* 2000;54:1706.

49. Kaji R, Kohara N, Katayama M, et al. Muscle afferent block by intramuscular injection of lidocaine for the treatment of writer's cramp. *Muscle Nerve* 1995;18:234–235.

50. Yoshida K, Kaji R, Kubori T, et al. Muscle afferent block for the treatment of oromandibular dystonia. *Mov Disord* 1998;13:699–705.

51. Ohara S, Hayashi R, Momoi H, et al. Mexiletine in the treatment of spasmodic torticollis. *Mov Disord* 1998; 13:934–940.

52. Lucetti C, Nuti A, Gambaccini G, et al. Mexiletine in the treatment of torticollis and generalized dystonia. *Clin Neuropharmacol* 2000;23:186–189.

53. Massey JM. EMG-guided chemodenervation with phenol in cervical dystonia (spasmodic torticollis). In: Brin MF, Hallett M, Jankovic J, eds. *Scientific and therapeutic aspects of botulinum toxin.* Philadelphia: Lippincott Williams & Wilkins, 2002:459–462.

54. Wirtschafter JD, McLoon LK. Long-term efficacy of local doxorubicin chemomyectomy in patients with blepharospasm and hemifacial spasm. *Ophthalmology* 1998;105:342–346.

55. Jankovic J, Demirkiran M. Classification of paroxysmal dyskinesias and ataxias. In: Frucht S, Fahn S, eds. *Myoclonus and paroxysmal dyskinesias, advances in neurology.* Philadelphia: Lippincott Williams & Wilkins, 2002:387–400.

56. Thant ZS, Tan EK. Emerging therapeutic applications of botulinum toxin. *Med Sci Monit* 2003;9:40–48.

57. Tintner R, Jankovic J. Focal dystonia: the role of botulinum toxin. *Curr Neurol Neurosci* 2001;1:337–345.

58. Jankovic J, Brin M. Botulinum toxin: Historical perspective and potential new indications. In: Mayer NH, Simpson DM, eds. Spasticity: Etiology, Evaluation, Management and the role of Botulinum Toxin; WE-MOVE, New York, NY, 2002:100–109.

59. Figgitt DP, Noble S. Botulinum toxin B. A review of its therapeutic potential in the management of cervical dystonia. *Drugs* 2002;62:705–755.

60. Sloop RR, Cole BA, Escutin RO. Human response to botulinum toxin injection: type B compared with type A. *Neurology* 1997;49:189–194.

61. de Paiva A, Meunier FA, Molgó J, et al. Functional repair of motor endplates after botulinum neurotoxin A poisoning: Bi-phasic switch of synaptic activity between nerve sprouts and their parent terminals. *Proc Natl Acad Sci USA* 1999;96:3200–3205.

62. Jankovic J. Botulinum toxin: clinical implications of antigenicity and immunoresistance. In: Brin MF, Hallett M, Jankovic J, eds. *Scientific and therapeutic aspects of botulinum toxin.* Philadelphia: Lippincott Williams & Wilkins, 2002:409–416.

63. Hanna PA, Jankovic J, Vincent A. Comparison of mouse bioassay and immunoprecipitation assay for botulinum toxin antibodies. *J Neurol Neurosurg Psychiatry* 1999; 66:612–616.

64. Jankovic J, Vuong KD, Ahsan J. Comparison of efficacy and immunogenicity of original versus current botulinum toxin in cervical dystonia. *Neurology* 2003;60:1186–1188.

65. Forget R, Tozlovanu V, Iancu A, et al. Botulinum toxin improves lid opening in blepharospasm-associated apraxia of lid opening. *Neurology* 2002;58:1843–1846.

66. Tan E-K, Jankovic J. Botulinum toxin A in patients with oromandibular dystonia: long-term follow-up. *Neurology* 1999;53:2102–2105.

67. Tan E-K, Jankovic J. Treating severe bruxism with botulinum toxin. *J Am Dent Assoc* 2000;131:211–216a.

68. Blitzer A, Zalvan C, Gonzalez-Yanez O, et al. Botulinum toxin type A injections for the management of the hyperfunctional larynx. In: Brin MF, Hallett M, Jankovic J, eds. *Scientific and therapeutic aspects of botulinum toxin.* Philadelphia: Lippincott Williams & Wilkins, 2002:207–216.

69. Jankovic J, Schwartz K, Donovan DT. Botulinum toxin treatment of cranial-cervical dystonia, spasmodic dysphonia, other focal dystonias and hemifacial spasm. *J Neurol Neurosurg Psychiatry* 1990;53:633–639.

70. Courey MS, Garrett CG, Billante CR, et al. Outcomes assessment following treatment of spasmodic dysphonia with botulinum toxin. *Ann Otol Rhinol Laryngol* 2000;109:819–822.

71. Jankovic J. Treatment of cervical dystonia. In: Brin MF, Comella C, Jankovic J, eds. *Dystonia.* Philadelphia: Lippincott Williams & Wilkins, 2003 *(in press).*

72. Lindeboom R, Brans JWM, Aramideh M, et al. Treatment of cervical dystonia: a comparison of measures for outcome assessment. *Mov Disord* 1998;13:706–712.

73. Jankovic J, Schwartz K. Longitudinal experience with botulinum toxin injections for treatment of blepharospasm and cervical dystonia. *Neurology* 1993;43: 834–836.

74. Brashear A, Bergan K, Wojcieszek J, et al. Patients' perception of stopping or continuing treatment of cervical dystonia with botulinum toxin type A. *Mov Disord* 2000;15:150–153.

75. Brashear A, Lew MF, Dykstra DD, et al. Safety and efficacy of Neurobloc (botulinum toxin type B) in type A-responsive cervical dystonia. *Neurology* 1999;53: 1439–1446.

76. Brin MF, Lew MF, Adler CH, et al. Safety and efficacy of NeuroBloc (botulinum toxin type B) in type A-resistant cervical dystonia. *Neurology* 1999;53:1431–1438.

77. Jankovic J. Needle EMG guidance is rarely required. *Muscle Nerve* 2001;24:1568–1570.

78. Cole R, Hallett M, Cohen LG. Double-blind trial of botulinum toxin for treatment of focal hand dystonia. *Mov Disord* 1995;10:466–471.

79. Rivest J, Lees AJ, Marsden CD. Writer's cramp: treatment with botulinum toxin injections. *Mov Disord* 1990;6:55–59.

80. Priori A, Berardelli A, Mercuri B, et al. Physiological effects produced by botulinum toxin treatment of upper limb dystonia. Changes in reciprocal inhibition between forearm muscles. *Brain* 1995;118:801–807.

81. Molloy FM, Shill HA, Kaelin-Lang A, et al. Accuracy of muscle localization without EMG: implications of limb dystonia. *Neurology* 2002;58:805–807.

82. Chen R, Karp BI, Goldstein SR, et al. Effect of muscle activity immediately after botulinum toxin injection for writer's cramp. *Mov Disord* 1999;14:307–312.

Dystonia 4: Advances in Neurology, Vol. 94. Edited by Stanley Fahn, Mark Hallett, and Mahlon R. DeLong. Lippincott Williams & Wilkins, Philadelphia © 2004.

39

Pallidotomy for Generalized Dystonia

Blair Ford

Neurological Institute, Columbia University, New York, New York

Dystonia is a syndrome of sustained muscle contractions causing twisting movements and postures (1). With the exception of dopa-responsive dystonia, the pathophysiology of dystonia remains unknown, and the treatment empiric. Surgically based approaches for severe, generalized dystonia have been undertaken since the early 1940s. Innovative surgeons placed lesions in different parts of the basal ganglia, including thalamus, globus pallidus, caudate, and putamen. In the 1990s, driven by successful results in treating Parkinson's disease, advances in neuroimaging, refinements in neurosurgical technique, and a deeper understanding of motor physiology, improved surgical treatments for dystonia were developed. Based on several case reports and small series, posteroventral medial pallidotomy, a surgical lesion created in the sensorimotor portion of the globus pallidus interna (GPi), emerged as the most effective ablative technique for the treatment of dystonia. Despite documentation of dramatic benefit in selected patients, pallidotomy remains incompletely studied as a treatment for dystonia, even as it is being replaced by deep brain stimulation.

HISTORICAL DEVELOPMENT

Meyers (2,3) was the first neurosurgeon to treat movement disorders by creating lesions in selected regions of the basal ganglia. Meyers made the seminal observation that lesions of the basal ganglia could abolish abnormal involuntary movements without producing weakness. By using newly developed localization and ablative techniques, he treated patients with Parkinson's disease, dystonia, hemiballism, and choreoathetoid cerebral palsy by extirpating the head of caudate, oral putamen, or oral globus pallidus; by sectioning the anterior limb of the internal capsule; or by interrupting pallidofugal fibers. The complication rate of this work was unacceptably high, with a mortality approaching 15%, but several patients experienced a reduction in their involuntary movements. Meyers proposed a schematic of basal ganglia circuitry that anticipated by several decades the current model of brain motor networks (Fig. 39-1). Meyers' model consisted of two parallel pathways that oppose and regulate each: a kinetic "K" circuit, the seat of dyskinetic movements, and a suppressor "S" circuit that modulated excessive activity in the K pathways. The entire system was a feedback loop, and the S circuit included the inhibitory pallidothalamic output that is the centerpiece of the current model of basal ganglia physiology.

Meyers' approach was quickly replicated by contemporary surgeons, who improved greatly on the safety of stereotactic lesion surgery (4–10). Lesions were placed in a variety of deep brain regions, sometimes in combination, targeting many different thalamic nuclei and the internal capsule, cerebral peduncle, subthalamic nucleus, dentate nucleus, globus pallidus, and ansa lenticularis. Lesions were created using injections of procaine and

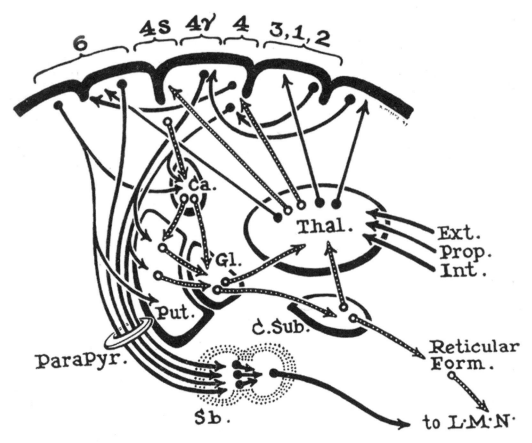

FIG. 39-1. Meyers' reverberating circuit theory of hemiballistic neural function. The kinetic "K" circuit is represented by *solid black lines* and the suppressor "S" circuit by *black lines* with *white dots.* The circuit input derives from exteroceptive (Ext), proprioceptive (Prop), and interoceptive (Int) sources converging on the thalamus. c.sub, corpus subthalamicus (subthalamic nucleus); ca, caudate; Gl, globus pallidus; LMN, lower motor neuron pool; ParaPyr, parapyramidal fibers; Put, putamen; Sb, subcortical nuclei; Thal, thalamus. (From Meyers R. The role of surgery in the abnormal movements of patients with cerebral palsy. *Q Rev Pediatr* 1951;6:157–173, with permission.)

alcohol (11), liquid nitrogen delivered by cannula (12), and electrical coagulation (13). It was not possible for these workers to know whether they achieved their target, and there was no ability to correlate clinical outcome with lesion size or location.

The early pallidotomy was a lesion in the anterodorsal part of the globus pallidus, a target for treating Parkinson's disease, dystonia, and various hyperkinetic disorders (14). Medial pallidal lesions were avoided because of proximity to the corticospinal tract, and perhaps due to Meyers' (2) observation that pal-

lidofugal section alone was inadequate. Between 1960 and 1990, reports of pallidotomy as a treatment for dystonia, using the anterodorsal target, produced variably poor results (6,9,15).

In treating patients with Parkinson's disease beginning in 1958, Leksell noted improved outcomes as he gradually moved the pallidal target posteroventrally to the site from which the ansa lenticularis emerges (16). Leksell's posteroventral medial pallidotomy led to strikingly reduced levodopa-induced dyskinesias in Parkinson patients, a finding overlooked until the early 1990s, when this palli-dal site became the primary target for dysto-nia.

ANATOMIC CONSIDERATIONS

The modern pallidotomy, as established by Leksell and reemphasized by Laitenen et al. (16), creates a lesion that is more posterior, ventral, and medial than the pallidotomy tar-gets of old. The modern posteroventral medial pallidotomy targets the sensorimotor projec-tion to the thalamus (Fig. 39-2). A lesion at this site interrupts the abnormal neuronal sig-naling in the pallido-thalamocortical pathway that is the putative anatomic substrate for dys-tonia and other hyperkinetic disorders. Fibers emerging from the medial pallidal segment project to the thalamus via the ansa lenticu-laris and the lenticular fasciculus. These fiber tracts merge as the thalamic fasciculus, and terminate in the ventral anterior (VA) and ventral lateral (VL) thalamic nuclei, giving off collaterals that terminate in the centrome-

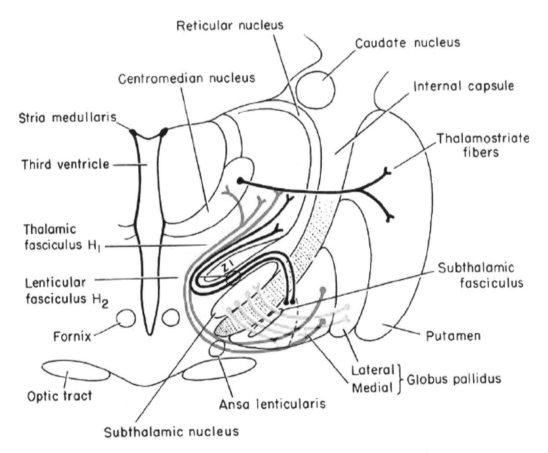

FIG. 39-2. Anatomy of the globus pallidus. This schematic illustrates the efferent fibers of the globus pallidus. The ansa lenticularis *(light)* arises from the outer portion of the medial pallidal segment and winds around the internal capsule to enter the prerubral field. The lenticular fasciculus *(dark)* crosses the posterior limb of the internal capsule, and merges with the ansa lenticularis. The subthalamic fas-ciculus consists of reciprocal pathways between the lateral globus pallidus and subthalamic nucleus. (From Carpenter MB. *Core text of neuroanatomy,* 3rd ed. Baltimore: Williams & Wilkins, 1985, with permission.)

dian (CM) nucleus. Reductions in dystonia following isolated lesions of the ansa lenticularis, which issues from the most lateral portion of the medial pallidal segment, suggest that a medially placed lesion is important in creating an effective pallidotomy.

ELECTROPHYSIOLOGIC MODEL OF DYSTONIA

The current model of basal ganglia electrophysiology is relevant to lesion surgery, and derives in part from intracellular recordings performed during pallidotomy for dystonia and Parkinson's disease. The electrophysiologic data include neuronal firing rates in different parts of the basal ganglia, patterns of neuronal activity, and somatosensory responsiveness of neurons in the globus pallidus. The pathophysiology of dystonia is not understood, and the model of basal ganglia circuitry partly assumes that dystonia and other hyperkinetic disorders are the inverse counterparts of Parkinson's disease.

Single neuron recordings obtained in patients with dystonia undergoing pallidotomy reveal two main findings: decreased mean neuronal firing rates in the GPi and globus pallidus externa (GPe) (Table 39-1), and abnormal patterns of firing, containing irregularly grouped discharges with intermittent pauses (17,18) (Fig. 39-3). The mean discharge rate of GPi neurons in dystonia is in the range of 20 to 40 Hz, as compared to a firing rate of 70 Hz in normal nonhuman primates, or 80 to 85 Hz in patients with Parkinson's disease (17–19). In dystonia, lower rates of GPi neuronal firing correlate with greater dystonia severity on the opposite body side (19).

The physiologic model of dystonia proposes that a decrease in the tonic inhibitory output from the globus pallidus allows abnormal excessive activity in centromedian and ventral lateral thalamic nuclei. Hyperactive thalamic neurons, in turn, excite the cerebral cortex in an excessive and unregulated manner, leading to abnormal, excessive, and uncontrolled movement (Fig. 39-4). This electrophysiologic model is supported by fluorodeoxyglucose (FDG) positron emission tomographic (PET) studies showing increased glucose metabolism in the lentiform nucleus, cerebellum, thalamus, and supplementary motor cortex (20,21). However, a model based solely on neuronal firing rate does not explain why lesioning the globus pallidus, which further reduces pallidal output, may improve dystonia. Many other characteristics of the electrophysiologic changes in dystonia appear relevant, including the finding of expanded, reorganized receptive fields in pallidal neurons in patients with dystonia (17). Supporting the idea that the pattern of discharge plays a key role in dystonia, a hamster model of paroxysmal dystonia shows increased irregularity of entopeduncular neuronal firing in proportion to dystonia severity (22).

Lesions of the globus pallidus have been shown to restore GPi neuronal activity toward

TABLE 39-1. *Electrophysiologic recordings in patients with dystonia*

Reference	Dystonia etiology	GPi firing rate	GPi somatosensory response	GPe firing rate
Lozano et al., 1997 (19)	Primary (1 pt)	Decreased	—	—
Lenz et al., 1998 (17)	Primary (1)	Decreased and irregular	Widened receptive fields	Decreased
Vitek et al., 1999 (18)	Primary (2) Tardive (1)	Decreased and irregular	Widened receptive fields	Decreased
Kumar et al., 1999 (23)	Primary (1)	Decreased	—	—
Hashimoto 2000 (51)	Parkinsonian off dystonia (1)	Decreased and irregular	—	Decreased
Cubo et al., 2000 (41)	Huntington's disease (1)	Decreased: 29 Hz	—	—

Adapted from Hashimoto (51). GPe, globus pallidus externa; GPi, globus pallidus interna.

FIG. 39-3. Single electrode recordings from the globus pallidus interna (GPi), showing irregularly grouped discharges at low firing frequency. (From Lenz FA, Suarez JI, Verhagen Metman L, et al. Pallidal activity during dystonia: somatosensory reorganization and changes with severity. *J Neurol Neurosurg Psychiatry* 1998;65:767–770, with permission.)

normal (18), and correct abnormalities of glucose metabolism present in the brains of patients with dystonia (23). Interrupting pallidal output may reduce dystonia by recalibrating abnormal discharge patterns of neuronal firing (19), but measurements of electrophysiologic changes following pallidotomy have never been reported. The clinical results of pallidotomy are not acute. It is further proposed that gradual improvements occurring in some patients may result from widespread compensatory network effects that evolve over months (24).

SURGICAL TECHNIQUE

The accuracy, safety, and clinical outcome of pallidotomy all depend critically on brain mapping. The operative technique varies between medical centers, and has been reviewed in detail (25,26). Patients are placed into a stereotactic head frame and undergo preoper-

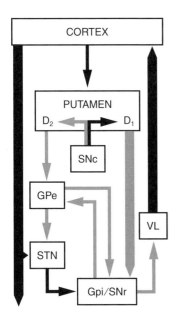

FIG. 39-4. Current model of basal ganglia electrophysiology in dystonia. A schematic of the basal ganglia illustrates inhibitory *(white)* and excitatory *(black)* projections. SNc, substantia nigra pars compacta; STN, subthalamic nucleus; GPi, globus pallidus interna; GPe, globus pallidus externa; SNr, substantia nigra pars reticulata; VL, ventrolateral thalamus. (Modified from Vitek JL, Giroux M. Physiology of hypokinetic and hyperkinetic movement disorders: model for dystonia. *Ann Neurol* 2000;47:S131–S140.)

ative magnetic resonance imaging (MRI) or computed tomography (CT) for direct visualization of the pallidal target, and indirect calculation of the target location, based on its relationship to the anterior (AC) and posterior commissures (PC). The typical location, according to Leksell, is 19 to 21 mm lateral to midline, 3 to 5 mm below the AC-PC line, and 2 to 3 mm anterior to the midcommissural point (Figs. 39-5 and 39-6).

Centers with the largest experience perform intraoperative single neuron recordings for basal ganglia surgery. Lesion placement within the globus pallidus may be inaccurate if based solely on neuroimaging data (25). In the absence of electrophysiologic mapping, discrepancies between expected target and actual lesion location have led to surgical complications. Electrophysiologic mapping pro-

vides an important confirmation of target site, although it does not guarantee optimal placement of a thermal lesion because the recording electrode must be replaced by the lesioning electrode.

The patient is taken to the operating room and positioned on the operating table. For a unilateral pallidotomy, a paramedian incision is made at the level of coronal suture. The operation can be accomplished under local anesthesia, but for children or adults with severe dystonia, general anesthesia or intravenous sedation is used. A burr hole is created, the dura is opened, and a recording microelectrode is driven toward the GPi site. The discharge frequency and patterns of individual neurons at deep brain sites provide accurate identification of neuronal structures. Microelectrode recordings can identify the GPe, the

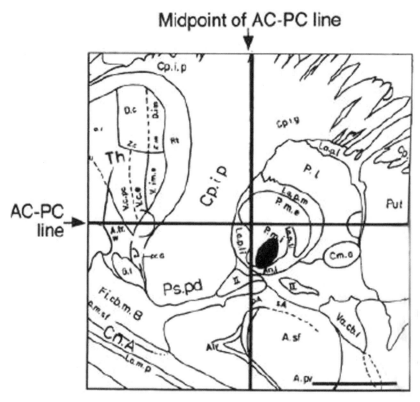

FIG. 39-5. Schematic of pallidotomy lesion target. (From Yoshor D, Hamilton WJ, Ondo W, et al. Comparison of thalamotomy and pallidotomy for the treatment of dystonia. *Neurosurgery* 2001;48:818–826, with permission.)

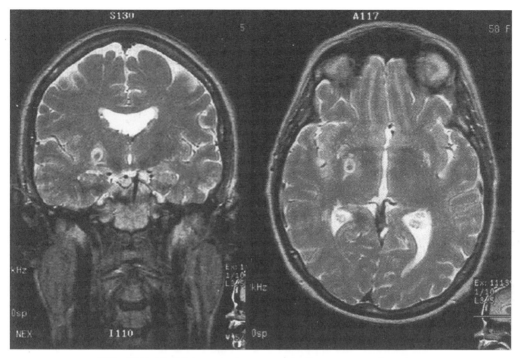

FIG. 39-6. Pallidotomy lesion on magnetic resonance imaging.

lamina between GPe and GPi, GPi neurons, the internal capsule, and the optic tract (25). GPi neurons are examined for receptive field properties. Cells of the sensorimotor GPi fire in response to active and passive movements of the limbs and trunk. The number of needle passes using the recording electrode may vary but is usually two or three.

Two potential complications of pallidotomy are hemiparesis and visual field deficit. As such it is especially important to identify the site of the internal capsule, located posteriorly and medially to GPi, and the optic tract, located 2 or 3 mm ventral to GPi. The optic tract is identified by a flash-evoked action potential in the optic tract, and by contralateral phosphenes in response to stimulation using the microelectrode (25,27).

Once the GPi target is located, the recording microelectrode is removed, and replaced by a lesioning electrode. A radiofrequency lesion is created by a thermistor-coupled electrode that heats the tissue to 60° to 90°C for 60 to 90 seconds. In some centers, several small lesions are created along a vertical axis to produce the pallidotomy lesion. The lesion must destroy a volume of 40 to 200 mm^3 of brain tissue to be effective (28).

OUTCOME OF TREATMENT

Most of the literature over six decades of surgical treatment for generalized dystonia consists of open-label, retrospective series. Most studies did not use control or comparison groups, rating scales or functional outcome measures, confirmation of lesion location, or adequate follow-up. Surgical technique and lesion location have varied considerably over the decades, and no surgical series is readily comparable to any other.

Early Series

The early surgical series included hundreds of patients with dystonia, and targeted multiple sites within the basal ganglia. Although the largest series consisted of thalamotomy procedures (7,10,29), no single target lesion was ever compared to any other, or shown to be superior. By contrast, the modern pallidotomy reports and series involve fewer patients, perhaps 75 individuals, but focused almost exclusively on a single lesion site, the posteroventral GPi.

The thalamotomy series consisted of patients who underwent combined lesions in the ventrolateral thalamus as well as the centromedian nucleus, pulvinar, and globus pallidus. The largest series is that of Cooper (10), who performed up to seven operations, creating up to 13 lesion sites, in a single patient. In all, he performed 504 operations on 226 patients. Follow-up information was obtained on 208 patients at a mean postoperative interval of 8 years. Using a global rating assessment, 70% patients were markedly or moderately improved. Other large thalamotomy series gave similar results (7,29,30). Patients with primary or familial dystonia tended to have a superior prognosis in most but not all (29) series, as compared to those with secondary dystonia. Patients whose symptoms were progressing at the time of surgery fared worse (10). A major complication of bilateral thalamotomy was severe dysarthria, approaching 60% in one series (31).

Modern Series

After 1990, investigators with previous experience using thalamotomy immediately recognized the superiority of the posteroventral medial pallidotomy, both in terms of efficacy and safety. Bilateral procedures were remarkably well tolerated. Severe dysarthria resulting from bilateral thalamotomy did not occur. Neuropsychiatric complications of bilateral pallidotomy in patients with Parkinson's disease, including speech dysfluency, visuospatial processing deficits, and abulia (32), did not occur in dystonia patients.

Several initial case reports described dramatic reductions in dystonia (Table 39-2). Iacono et al. (33) performed bilateral pallidoansotomy lesions in a 17-year-old, wheelchairbound boy with incapacitating, generalized dystonia; at the 12-month interval, the patient had reacquired the ability to use his hands and could ambulate independently. Lozano et al. (19) described a 9-year-old boy with severe generalized DYT1 dystonia, wheelchair-bound and with severe axial involvement. After bilateral pallidotomy, beginning 3 days after surgery, the patient's dystonia progressively improved. At 10 days, he could ambulate, and after 3 months was completely independent. However, after 2 years, his symptoms recurred.

Vitek described three individuals with severe generalized dystonia (18), including one with tardive dystonia. All patients underwent unilateral pallidotomy on the brain side opposite the most severe clinical symptoms. Dystonia severity ratings were reduced by 53% at the 7- to 14-month follow-up point, using the Burke-Fahn-Marsden dystonia rating scale (34). However, one individual with predominantly axial involvement had recurrence of symptoms over the following year, and underwent implantation of a GPi stimulator opposite the pallidotomy, with subsequent sustained improvement over 4 years (35).

Several larger series, with more complete follow-up and quantitative evaluations were reported. Ondo et al. (36) described a series of eight patients with severe generalized or hemidystonia who underwent pallidotomy, five bilaterally and three unilaterally. After a mean follow-up interval of 17.5 weeks, the unblinded dystonia severity ratings (34) improved by 61.2%. Medication intake was reduced postoperatively, and patients' average weight increased by 9%. Complications included mild hemiparesis in one patient related to lesion placement near the internal capsule. In a follow-up report (37), extending the series to 12 patients, the authors noted that the most effective reduction of dystonia occurred in the hands and arms, with modest benefit in leg function and gait, and little improvement in midline and cranial structures.

The largest modern series is that of Lin et al. (38), published as a letter, consisting of 18 patients who underwent bilateral pallidotomy for intractable dystonia. All of these individuals had secondary dystonia: cerebral palsy

TABLE 39-2. *Pallidotomy for dystonia: summary of recently reported cases*

Reference	n	Dystonia etiology	Age[a] (yrs)	Outcome	Follow-up (mo)	Remarks
Kwon and Whang, 1995 (42)	1	Postinfectious L. hemidystonia	37	Improved	—	Gamma knife pallidotomy; complicated by hemianopsia
Iacono et al., 1996 (33)	1	Idiopathic	17	Marked improvements in dystonia and functional capacity	12	Progressive improvement postoperatively
Lozano et al., 1997 (19)	1	Idiopathic	9	Marked improvements in dystonia and functional capacity, reduction in B-F-M[b] dystonia scale 75 to 16	3	Progressive improvement postoperatively
Weetman 1997 (52)	1	Tardive	31	Improvements in dystonia and functional capacity, reduction in B-F-M dystonia scale score 76 to 21	8	
Vitek et al., 1998 (48)	3	Idiopathic (2), tardive (1)	—	Improvements in dystonia and functional capacity, reduction in B-F-M dystonia scale scores by 72%–80%	—	
Lin et al., 1998 (46)	1	Hypotensive shock	36	Improvement in B-F-M dystonia scale scores from 74 to 28, 55% improvement in ADL capacity	9	Progressive improvement
Bhatia 1998 (53)	1	Paroxysmal dystonia	47	Paroxysmal dystonia completely resolved, patient discontinued meds	6	Unilateral
Iacono 1998 (54)	6	2 pts. generalized dystonia (idiopathic, cerebral palsy): 4 pts. focal or segmental	17–71	5 pts. underwent pallidotomy or ansa-pallidotomy, 3 unilaterally; 1 underwent thalamotomy; improvements in two patients with generalized dystonia; improvements in torticollis, craniofacial, and leg dystonia but not in dysphonia	6–24	
Ondo et al., 1998 (36)	8	Primary dystonia (4), secondary (4): CNS trauma (2), peripheral trauma (1), anoxia (1)	9–56	59% reduction in B-F-M scores	17.5 weeks	3 unilateral 5 bilateral
Lai 1999 (55)	1	Idiopathic	14	Improvements in dystonia and functional capacity	—	
Lin et al., 1999 (38)	1	Perinatal asphyxia	29	30% improvement over baseline dystonia	12	
Lin et al., 1999 (47)[c]	8	Cerebral palsy (8 patients), hypoxia (6), carbon monoxide poisoning (2), encephalitis (1) and post-infectious (1)	14–36	13% reduction in B-F-M dystonia severity scores	12	
Justesen et al., 1999 (40)	1	Hallervorden-Spatz	10	Reduction in dystonia and painful dystonic spasms, improvements in ADL capacity	6	
Ford et al., 2000 (39)	6	Idiopathic (5) and tardive (1)	15–34	30% reduction in B-F-M dystonia scale score (mean score 59.2 to 49.3)[d]	8–42	4 bilateral 2 unilateral
Cubo et al., 2000 (41)	1	Huntington disease (Westphal variant)	13	Minimal improvement; B-F-M score reduced from 56 to 49	3	
Teive, 2001 (56)	5	Idiopathic (4), posttraumatic (1)	28–40	52.3% reduction in B-F-M dystonia severity scale at 6 month follow-up	6	
Yoshor et al., 2001 (43)[e]	1	Primary (8)	8–57	Improvement marked in 7 pts and moderate in 2; 5 pts no functional benefit	12	10 bilateral
	4	Secondary (6)		1 pt experienced persistent dysarthria and hypophonia	12	4 unilateral

[a]Age at time of operation.
[b]Burke-Fahn-Marsden (B-F-M) dystonia rating scale (Burke 1985).
[c]Includes the patients reported in Lin 1998 and Lin 1999.
[d]Bilaterally operated patients.
[e]Includes the patients previously reported in Ondo 1998.
ADL, activity of daily living.

(eight patients), hypoxia (six), carbon monoxide poisoning (two), encephalitis (one), and postinfectious (one). Improvement in dystonia was delayed, peaking at 6 months, with some diminution thereafter. At the 1-year follow-up point, the overall outcome was a 13% reduction in dystonia severity ($p = .0017$), with the greatest effect on neck dystonia. Complications in this series included visual field deficits in two patients and hemiparesis in two others.

An objective measure of pallidotomy outcome, using videotaped examinations rated by a shielded observer, was performed in a series of six patients with severe generalized dystonia (39). The series included one patient with *DYT1* dystonia, four with non-*DYT1* primary dystonia, and one with tardive dystonia. Three individuals underwent unilateral pallidotomy. After a mean follow-up interval of 20 months, there was a 29% reduction in dystonia severity ratings, with improvements in limb, trunk, and neck dystonia, but not speech. Disability scores improved by 18%, mainly due to improved ambulation. The best outcome occurred in the individual with tardive dystonia. In subsequent follow-up, one patient developed severe dysarthria 1 year after the procedure due to spread of dystonia into cranial structures, and underwent bilateral GPi deep brain stimulator implantation.

Patients with symptomatic dystonia due to progressive neurodegenerative disorders have undergone pallidotomy to palliate intractable dystonic spasms. A 10-year-old boy with Hallervorden-Spatz disease underwent a left pallidotomy, which greatly reduced his painful right-sided dystonia, and enabled useful hand function (40). A 13-year-old girl with juvenile Huntington's disease underwent bilateral pallidotomy but showed minimal reduction in her dystonia, and died 4 months postoperatively (41).

The only report of gamma knife pallidotomy describes a radiofrequency lesion created in the right GPi of a 37-year-old woman with left hemidystonia (42). The cause was an infarct of the right basal ganglia due to tuberculous meningitis during childhood. The

surgery was complicated by a homonymous hemianopsia, but at 16 months postoperatively the patient had an 80% improvement in left hand function.

Pallidotomy and Thalamotomy

As noted, the most frequently performed operation for generalized dystonia, thalamotomy, has never been systematically or directly compared to pallidotomy. A recent report describes 14 patients who underwent bilateral pallidotomy between 1996 and 1999, comparing the results to those from a group of 18 patients treated using bilateral thalamotomy at the same institution between 1981 and 1996 (43). Approximately half the patients in each group had secondary dystonia. Ten patients underwent bilateral pallidotomy and four unilateral; two of the unilateral procedures were performed contralaterally to a previous thalamotomy. Seven patients (50%) experienced marked improvement, according to a global outcome scale, while two others were moderately improved, after a mean follow-up interval of 1 year. Of the seven with the greatest improvement, five had idiopathic dystonia and two had symptomatic dystonia. By contrast, only two of 18 patients in the thalamotomy group showed marked improvement at a mean follow-up interval of 42.9 months (43).

Pallidotomy for Cervical Dystonia

In addition to generalized dystonia, pallidotomy has been performed in patients with cervical dystonia and segmental dystonia (44). Between 1960 and 1980, approximately 300 patients underwent lesion surgery targeting mainly thalamic nuclei but also the GPi, zona incerta, Forel's fields H1 and H2, and the interstitial nucleus of Cajal. As with the generalized dystonia series, limited outcome measures and duration of follow-up preclude an accurate appraisal of these approaches. Improvement was reported in 50% to 70% of patients, and the incidence of postoperative dysarthria following bilateral thalamic lesions was in the range of 15%. By the 1990s, lesion-based surgery for torticollis declined, becoming replaced by deep brain stimulation in the GPi (45).

General Observations

Pallidotomy is associated with marked reduction in severe, medication-refractory dystonia in selected patients. Bilateral pallidotomy is generally required for bilateral or axial symptoms. According to several recent case reports and series, bilateral pallidotomy can reduce symptoms of dystonia by 30% to 80% when measured by dystonia severity rating scale scores. In several reports, this reduction in dystonic spasms has translated into important gains in functional capacity. Improvement following a unilateral pallidotomy is maximal in the contralateral limbs; bilateral pallidotomy can reduce axial dystonia, including torticollis. Primary dystonia appears to respond better than secondary dystonia. In patients with dystonia, unlike those with Parkinson's disease, bilateral pallidotomy can be accomplished without obvious neurologic, cognitive, or psychiatric morbidity.

Several reports describe a delay in the onset of benefit after pallidotomy (19,36,46,47), with progressive improvement over many months following surgery that cannot be attributed to changes in edema at the operative site. In these instances, it is suggested that the surgical lesion induces a gradual restoration of signaling in the motor control networks. The literature contains few descriptions of long-term outcome, but several patients had recurrence or spread of symptoms after initial benefit (35,36,39), including the patients described in the initial reports (19,48). Several of these patients subsequently underwent implantation of deep brain stimulators in the GPi.

CONCLUSION

Pallidotomy, a procedure developed in the 1930s, remains a promising approach for severe medication-refractory generalized dystonia. The technique has never been compared to any other approach in a prospective randomized clinical trial, and long-term, detailed follow-up is lacking. The recent literature describes clinical outcomes, ranging from 3 to 42 months, in approximately 75 patients. Clinical experience indicates that GPi pallidotomy is the most effective lesion-based treatment for dystonia. Pallidotomy can reduce axial dystonia and improve gait when performed bilaterally. Patients with primary or idiopathic dystonia as well as those with tardive dystonia appear to have a better surgical prognosis than those with pathologic lesions involving the basal ganglia. The identification of the posteroventral medial GPi site as an effective target for dystonia has provided the direction for current and future interventions using deep brain stimulation.

Perhaps the most important drawback to pallidotomy is the unpredictability of the long-term outcome. Every published series includes individuals who derived excellent and sustained benefit. But each series also contains patients who experienced only temporary benefit, or subsequent progression of dystonia, even with optimally placed lesions. In contrast to thalamotomy for refractory tremor, or pallidotomy for dyskinesias in Parkinson's disease, pallidotomy has proven far less predictable in its effect on dystonia. Therefore, despite its advantages over all previous lesion-based approaches for dystonia, pallidotomy seems destined to be replaced by GPi deep brain stimulation, a technique that in its earliest application already appears to be more effective and safer (23,49,50).

REFERENCES

1. Fahn S. Concept and classification of dystonia. *Adv Neurol* 1988;50:1–8.
2. Meyers R. The present state of neurosurgical procedures directed against the extrapyramidal diseases. *NY State J Med* 1942;42:317–325.
3. Meyers R. The role of surgery in the abnormal movements of patients with cerebral palsy. *Q Rev Pediatr* 1951;6:157–173.
4. Talairach MMJ, Paillas JE, David M. Dyskinesie de type hemiballiqu traitee par cortectomie frontale limitee, puis par coagulation de l'anse lenticulaire et de la portion interne du globus pallidus. Amelioration importante depuis un an. *Rev Neurol* 1950;83:440–451.

5. Guiot G, Brion S. Traitement neuro-chirugical de syn-dromes choreo-athetosique et parkinsonien. *Semin Hop Paris* 1952;49:2095–2099.
6. Hassler R, Reichert T, Mundinger F, et al. Physiological observations in stereotactic operations in extrapyrami-dal motor disturbances. *Brain* 1960;83:337–350.
7. Riechert T. Long term follow-up of results of stereo-taxic treatment in extrapyramidal disorders. *Confin Neurol* 1962;22:356–363.
8. Markham CH, Rand RW. Physiological and anatomical influences on dystonia. *Trans Am Med Assoc* 1961;86: 135–137.
9. Gros C, Frerebeau PH, Perez-Dominguez E, et al. Long-term results of stereotaxic surgery for infantile dystonia and dyskinesia. *Neurochirugica* 1976;19: 171–178.
10. Cooper IS. 20-year follow-up study of the neurosurgical treatment of dystonia musculorum deformans. *Adv Neurol* 1976;14:423–452.
11. Cooper IS. Intracerebral injection of procaine into the globus pallidus in hyperkinetic disorders. *Science* 1954; 119:417–418.
12. Cooper IS, Gioino G, Terry R. The cryogenic lesion. *Confin Neurol* 1965;26:161–177.
13. Spiegel AE, Wycis HT. Pallidothalamotomy in chorea. *Arch Neurol Psychiatry* 1950;64:295–296.
14. Guiot G, Brion S. Traitement des mouvements anor-maux par la coagulation pallidale. Technique et resul-tants. *Rev Neurol* 1953;89:578–580.
15. Burzaco J. Stereotactic pallidotomy in extrapyramidal disorders. *Appl Neurophysiol* 1985;48:283–287.
16. Laitenen LV, Bergenheim AT, Hariz MI. Leksell's pos-teroventral pallidotomy in the treatment of Parkinson's disease. *J Neurosurg* 1992;76:53–61.
17. Lenz FA, Suarez JI, Verhagen Metman L, et al. Pallidal activity during dystonia: somatosensory reorganization and changes with severity. *J Neurol Neurosurg Psychi-atry* 1998;65:767–770.
18. Vitek JL, Chockkan V, Zhang J-Y, et al. Neuronal ac-tivity in the basal ganglia in patients with generalized dystonia and hemiballismus. *Ann Neurol* 1999;46: 222–235.
19. Lozano AM, Kumar R, Gross RE, et al. Globus pallidus internus pallidotomy for generalized dystonia. *Mov Dis-ord* 1997;12:865–870.
20. Ceballos-Bauman AO, Passingham RE, Warner T, et al. Overactive prefrontal and underactive motor cortical ar-eas in idiopathic dystonia. *Ann Neurol* 1995;37:636–372.
21. Eidelberg D, Moeller JR, Antonini A, et al. Functional brain networks in DYT1 dystonia. *Ann Neurol* 1998;44: 303–312.
22. Gernert M, Bennay M, Fedrowitz M, et al. Altered dis-charge pattern of basal ganglia output neurons in an an-imal model of idiopathic dystonia. *J Neurosci* 2002;22: 7244–7253.
23. Kumar R, Dagher A, Hutchison WD, et al. Globus pal-lidus deep brain stimulation for generalized dystonia: clinical and PET investigation. *Neurology* 1999;53: 871–874.
24. Vitek JL, Giroux M. Physiology of hypokinetic and hy-perkinetic movement disorders: model for dystonia. *Ann Neurol* 2000;47:S131–S140.
25. Lozano A, Hutchison W, Kiss Z, et al. Methods for mi-croelectrode-guided posteroventral pallidotomy. *J Neu-rosurg* 1996;84:194–202.

26. Vitek J, Bakay RAE, Hashimoto T, et al. Microelec-trode-guided pallidotomy: technical approach and its application in medically intractable Parkinson's disease. *J Neurosurg* 1998a;88:1027–1043.
27. Lozano AM, Hutchison WD. Microelectrode recordings in the pallidum. *Mov Disord* 2002;17(suppl 3): S150–S154.
28. Hirai T, Miyazaki M, Nakajima H, et al. The correla-tion between tremor characteristics and the predicted volume of effective lesions in stereotaxic nucleus ventralis intermedius thalamotomy. *Brain* 1983;106: 1001–1018.
29. Tasker RR, Doorly T, Yamashiro K. Thalamotomy in generalized dystonia. *Adv Neurol* 1988;50:615–631.
30. Andrew J, Rice Edwards JM, Rudolf N de, M. Place-ment of stereotaxic lesions for involuntary movements other than in Parkinson's disease. *Acta Neurochir Suppl* 1974;Suppl.21:39–47.
31. Andrew J, Fowler CL, Harrison MJG. Stereotaxic thal-amotomy in 55 cases of dystonia. *Brain* 1983;106: 981–1000.
32. Ghika J, Ghika-Schmid F, Fankhauser H. Bilateral contemporaneous posteroventral pallidotomy for the treatment of Parkinson's disease: neuropsychological and neurological side-effects. *J Neurosurg* 1999;91:313–321.
33. Iacono R, Kuniyoshi S, Lonser R, et al. Simultaneous bilateral pallidoansotomy for idiopathic dystonia mus-culorum deformans. *Pediatr Neurol* 1996;14:145–148.
34. Burke RE, Fahn S, Marsden CD, et al. Validity and reli-ability of a rating scale for the primary torsion dysto-nias. *Neurology* 1985;35:73–77.
35. Abosch A, Vitek JL, Lozano AM. Pallidotomy and pal-lidal deep brain stimulation for dystonia. In: Tarsy D, Vitek JL, Lozano AM, eds. *Surgical treatment of Parkinson's disease and other movement disorders.* To-towa, NJ: Humana Press, 2003;265–274.
36. Ondo WG, Desaloms JM, Jankovic J, et al. Pallido-tomy for generalized dystonia. *Mov Disord* 1998;13: 693–698.
37. Ondo WG, Desaloms M, Krauss JK, et al. Pallidotomy and thalamotomy for dystonia. In: Krauss JK, Jankovic J, Grossman RG, eds. *Surgery for Parkinson's disease and movement disorders.* Philadelphia: Lippincott Williams & Wilkins, 2001;299–306.
38. Lin J-J, Lin G-Y, Shih C, et al. Benefit of bilateral pal-lidotomy in the treatment of generalized dystonia. *J Neurosurg* 1999;90:974–976.
39. Ford B, Winfield L, Frucht S, et al. Treatment of severe generalized dystonia using stereotactic pallidotomy. *Neurology* 2000;54:(suppl 3):A219.
40. Justesen CR, Penn RD, Kroin JS, et al. Stereotactic pal-lidotomy in a child with Hallervorden-Spatz disease. *J Neurosurg* 1999;90:551–554.
41. Cubo E, Shannon K, Penn RD, et al. Internal globus pal-lidotomy in dystonia secondary to Huntington's disease. *Mov Disord* 2000;15:1248–1251.
42. Kwon Y, Whang CJ. Stereotactic gamma knife radio-surgery for the treatment of dystonia. *Stereotact Funct Neurosurg* 1995;64(suppl):222–227.
43. Yoshor D, Hamilton WJ, Ondo W, et al. Comparison of thalamotomy and pallidotomy for the treatment of dys-tonia. *Neurosurgery* 2001;48:818–826.
44. Krauss JK, Pohle T, Stibal A, et al. Functional stereo-tactic surgery for the treatment of cervical dystonia. In: Krauss JK, Jankovic J, Grossman RG, eds. *Surgery for*

Parkinson's disease and movement disorders. Philadelphia: Lippincott Williams & Wilkins, 2001;343–349.

45. Krauss JK, Pohle T, Weber S. Bilateral stimulation of the globus pallidus internus for treatment of cervical dystonia. *Lancet* 1999;13(suppl 2):134.

46. Lin J-J, Lin S-Z, Lin G-Y, et al. Application of bilateral sequential pallidotomy to treat a patient with generalized dystonia. *Eur Neurol* 1998;40:108–110.

47. Lin J-J, Lin S-Z, Chang D-C. Pallidotomy and generalized dystonia. *Mov Disord* 1999;14:1057–1059.

48. Vitek JL, Zhang J, Evatt M, et al. GPi pallidotomy for dystonia: clinical outcome and neuronal activity. *Adv Neurol* 1998;78:211–219.

49. Coubes P, Echenne B, Roubertie A, et al. Traitment de la dystonie generalise a debut precoce par stimulation chronique bilaterale des globus pallidus internes. *Neurochirugie* 1999;45:139–144.

50. Loher TJ, Hasdemir MG, Burgunder J-M, et al. Long-term follow-up study of chronic globus pallidus internus stimulation for post-traumatic hemidystonia. *J Neurosurg* 2000;92:457–460.

51. Hashimoto T. Neuronal activity in the globus pallidus in primary dystonia. *J Neurol* 2000;247(Suppl.5): V49–V52.

52. Weetman J, Anderson IM, Gregory RP, Gill SS. Bilateral posteroventral pallidotomy for severe antipsychotic induced tardive dyskinesia and dystonia. *J Neurol Neurosurg Psychiatry* 1997 Oct;63(4):554–556.

53. Bhatia KP, Marsden CD, Thomas DG. Posteroventral pallidotomy can ameliorate attacks of paroxysmal dystonia induced by exercise. *J Neurol Neurosurg Psychiatry* 1998 Oct;65(4):604–605.

54. Iacono RP, Kuniyoshi SM, Schoonenberg T. Experience with stereotactics for dystonia: case examples. *Adv Neurol* 1998;78:221–226.

55. Lai T, Lai JM, Grossman RG. Functional recovery after bilateral pallidotomy for the treatment of early-onset primary generalized dystonia. *Arch Phys Med Rehabil* 1999 Oct;80(10):1340–1342.

56. Teive HA, Sa DS, Grande CV, Antoniuk A, Werneck LC. Bilateral pallidotomy for genrallized dystonia. *Arq Neuropsiquiatr* 2001 Jun;59(2-B):353–357.

Dystonia 4: Advances in Neurology, Vol. 94. Edited by Stanley Fahn, Mark Hallett, and Mahlon R. DeLong. Lippincott Williams & Wilkins, Philadelphia © 2004.

40

Pallidal Stimulation for Dystonia

Andres M. Lozano and Aviva Abosch

Division of Neurosurgery, Toronto Western Hospital, Toronto, Ontario, Canada

The dystonias are a varied group of disorders characterized by striking disruptions in motor function. They can be classified according to their etiology, distribution, age of onset, or severity. Of particular interest is the occurrence of severe abnormalities in the function of the motor system in the face of what is sometimes little or no obvious structural or chemical abnormality in the brain in the so-called idiopathic dystonias. This emphasizes that changes in neuronal activity play a crucial role in the pathogenesis of dystonia. The changes in cellular activity and network properties leading to these abnormalities are incompletely understood, but recent laboratory-based experiments and observations in humans are beginning to make an impact.

Neurosurgeons have sought to disrupt the abnormalities in brain function leading to dystonia through intervention directed at various components of the motor system or neural networks including the cerebellum, internal capsule, spinal cord, thalamus, and pallidum (1–10). These procedures have for the most part been empirical, based on improvements seen with neurosurgical interventions for other disorders including chorea or Parkinson's disease (PD).

RATIONALE FOR PALLIDAL INTERVENTIONS IN DYSTONIA

There have been a number of historical and more recent advances that now provide a strong rationale and justification for a re-appraisal of pallidal procedures in the treatment of dystonia.

The first large experience with pallidal procedures in dystonia comes from the work of Irving Cooper. Although Cooper had extensive experience with thalamic procedures in treating dystonia, he also utilized the globus pallidus as a surgical target with varying degrees of effectiveness (11,12).

More recently, pallidotomy and pallidal stimulation have been shown to have profound effects on the "off-period" dystonia— the dystonia associated with levodopa-induced dyskinesias in patients with PD (13,14). In addition, new pathophysiologic data derived from functional imaging studies show abnormal activation of premotor areas in patients with dystonia (15–17). These cortical fields are targets of globus pallidus interna (GPi) outflow (18) and can thus be influenced by interventions at the level of the globus pallidus.

It is interesting that these abnormalities in cortical function persist even in patients without overt manifestations of dystonia or in patients in whom the dystonia is ameliorated by peripheral interventions. Indeed the abnormalities in the activity of cortical motor networks seen with functional imaging are also seen in nonmanifesting carriers of the *DYT1* mutation (16) and in patients with writer's cramp treated with botulinum toxin (19,20). These observations suggest that the cortical motor network abnormality, under the influence of pathologic basal ganglia outflow, may play a primary and causal role in the pathogenesis of dystonia.

While the pallidum is now being considered, it is clear that there is more experience with the thalamus as a surgical target for the treatment of dystonia. The relative attributes and benefits of each of these targets are far from settled. On theoretical grounds, GPi has certain advantages. GPi outflow neurons have a dual output to the thalamus and to locomotor areas of the brainstem (21). Neurons in the motor thalamus project predominantly to the cortex. Pallidal interventions have the possibility of direct access to the brainstem as well as to cortical fields. This may be an important advantage.

The success of functional neurosurgery for PD, the lack of adequate pharmacotherapy for many patients, and the development of resistance to botulinum toxins are factors in the reevaluation of stereotactic surgery for dystonia. Recent preliminary observations of striking clinical benefit with pallidal interventions in certain patients with dystonia, and the description of disrupted pallidal activity in GPi in dystonia provide further rationale to reappraise the role of GPi in the pathogenesis and treatment of dystonia.

UNILATERAL AND BILATERAL PALLIDOTOMY AND PALLIDAL DEEP BRAIN STIMULATION

Patient Selection

The indications for surgery are evolving. Only patients who continue to have significant disability despite adequate trials of pharmacotherapy that may, in some cases, also include botulinum toxin injections and intrathecal baclofen are considered for surgery. The indications for pallidal stimulation are the same as for pallidotomy, with the added potential benefits of avoiding a lesion and of a procedure that is both reversible and modifiable. These characteristics may be desirable in younger patients, such as those with juvenile-onset dystonia or in patients with secondary dystonia in whom the structural lesions may contribute to unexpected side effects.

A number of dystonia syndromes have been treated with pallidotomy and a lesser number with pallidal deep brain stimulation (DBS) with a varying degree of effectiveness. These include primary generalized dystonia, segmental dystonia, off-period dystonia of Parkinson's disease, dystonia associated with cerebral palsy (22,23), Huntington's (24), and Hallervorden-Spatz disease (25), and dystonia associated with trauma and structural lesions (26). It is unclear whether pallidal lesions differ from pallidal DBS in their clinical effects on patients with dystonia. For this reason, clinical outcomes in both pallidal lesion and stimulation surgery will be considered together.

Intraoperative and Postoperative Issues

The technical details of surgery are covered elsewhere (27,28). If possible, surgery is performed under local anesthesia. For children and patients with a severe movement disorder, the procedure can be performed with general anesthesia or with intravenous sedation. Physiologic localization with microelectrode recording data is important to target identification, particularly in patients under general anesthesia. Reliance solely on magnetic resonance imaging (MRI)-based anatomic localization is problematic given the frequent discrepancies between the expected location based on MRI data and the actual location based on physiology.

The pattern of discharge of GPi neurons in dystonia patients has been reported to differ from that in PD patients. Generally, pallidal neurons in dystonia discharge at slower rates (20–50 Hz) (29,30) than those in PD patients (80–85 Hz) (28,31). Somatosensory responses of GPi neurons in dystonia patients reported so far appear to be similar to those reported for PD, with neurons responding to multiple directions about multiple joints, often in more than one limb (30). The recording techniques and states of consciousness may have influenced some of these findings, particularly the data on discharge rates. For example, intravenous propofol has been shown to decrease neuronal firing rates in locus ceruleus and neocortical neurons (32,33), confounding assessments of neuronal firing rate in the dystonic pallidum in patients receiving certain anesthetics. As yet, no reports have been published that correlate the characteristics of neuronal activity, i.e., neuronal firing rates and patterns, with surgical outcome.

An important goal of intraoperative mapping is to identify the sensorimotor territory of the GPi, that region populated by neurons that respond to active and passive movements of the body and limbs. Other structures to be identified and to be avoided with lesioning or DBS are the optic tract that lies ventral to GPi and the fibers of the internal capsule apposed to the medial and posterior borders of the GPi. Once the desired location within the GPi has been identified, the microelectrodes are removed and either a lesioning probe or DBS electrodes are inserted into the target. The precise location

within the GPi to be targeted is still unresolved. From the experience in PD, it is likely that different regions in the GPi will have differential clinical effects on motor function. This may be related to the multiple segregated motor output channels in the GPi (18), or which neural elements including adjacent white matter tracts are affected by lesions or activated with stimulation (34). The usual radiofrequency lesions in GPi are approximately 6 mm in diameter (28). The technique for placement of DBS electrodes has been described elsewhere (35). In programming DBS stimulators for certain dystonia patients, a much longer pulse width (> 210 μs) is generally required to achieve an effect than that typically used for PD patients (60–90 μs) (27). The optimal parameters for rate, pulse width, and amplitude of stimulation for each patient have to be derived empirically. The appearance of bilateral GPi DBS electrodes is shown in Fig. 40-1.

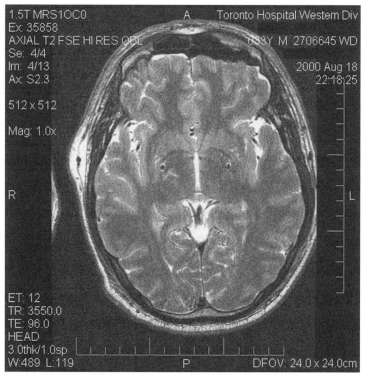

FIG. 40-1. Axial magnetic resonance imaging of patient with cervical dystonia treated with bilateral globus pallidus interna deep brain stimulation.

Results

Pallidotomy and Pallidal DBS in Dystonia

A number of small series have documented the clinical response to pallidotomy and pallidal DBS in various types of dystonia (Tables 40-1 and 40-2). Because there are no clear differences in outcomes between lesion and stimulation surgery at this stage, they are considered together.

An overview of these cases suggests that patients with idiopathic generalized dystonia show a greater response to pallidal surgery than patients with secondary dystonia (36,37). The improvements in patients with *DYT1* dystonia are particularly striking. Improvement on the Burke-Fahn-Marsden Dystonia Rating Scale for Movement (BFMDRS-M) and Disability (BFMDRS-D) scales can reach very high levels, with *DYT1* dystonia patients experiencing improvements of up to 80% or 90% with either pallidal lesions or stimulation (29,38–41). In patients with generalized dystonia treated with unilateral surgery, Vitek et al. (30) found lasting (7 to 14 months) contralateral limb dystonia improvement but unsustained axial improvement. Subsequent implantation on the nonoperated side of a deep brain stimulator in the GPi led to dramatic improvement in axial symptoms

with an overall improvement in the BFM-DRS-M of 82%, which has remained over the 4-year period of follow-up (Vitek, personal communication).

Although there can be some immediate improvement in the dystonia with surgery, in many cases, the response is delayed and there can be progressive improvement. For example, in a child with *DYT1* dystonia undergoing bilateral pallidotomy, there was no immediate improvement. By 5 days, however, the BFM-DRS score improved by 31%, and by 3 months by 79% (29). The gradual improvement in symptoms seen following surgery for dystonia, requiring weeks to months, might be a consequence of a gradual normalization of physiologic disruptions that occurred in structures downstream to the pallidum, relearning of tasks, or plasticity of the nervous system.

The issue of the surgical response of various primary and secondary forms of dystonia is slowly being resolved. The group from Baylor University (42,43) reported four patients with primary and four with secondary dystonia undergoing bilateral or unilateral pallidotomy. The mean score on the BFM-DRS improved by 61.2 ± 13.6% (p <.01), with a mean follow-up of 17.5 weeks (Table 40-2). The authors noted that the typical time-course of symptom amelioration was moder-

TABLE 40-1. *Pallidotomy for dystonia*

Study	Diagnosis	Procedure	n	Length of follow-up	Improvement (scale)
Lin et al., 1999 (22)	2° generalized	Bilat. pallidotomy	1	12 months	34% (BFMDRS)
Lin et al., 1999 (23)	2° generalized	Bilat. pallidotomy	18	12 months	13% (BFMDRS)
Vitek et al., 1999 (30)	1° generalized	Unilat. pallidotomy	3	14, 11, and 7 months	Mean = 56% (BFMDRS)
Ondo et al., 1998 (37)	1° and 2° generalized and hemidystonia	5 bilat. pallidotomy Unilat. pallidotomy	5 3	Mean = 17.5 weeks	Mean = 61% (BFMDRS)
Lozano et al., 1997 (29)	Generalized	Bilat. GPi pallidotomy	1	3 months	79% (BFMDRS)
Iacono et al., 1996 (36)	1° generalized	Bilat. pallidoansotomy	1	12 months	100% (no evidence of dystonia)
Kwon and Whang, 1995 (6)	2° hemidystonia	Unilat. pallidotomy gamma knife	1	16 months	"Improved"

BFMDRS, Burke-Fahn-Marsden Dystonia Rating Scale; GPi, globus pallidus interna.

TABLE 40-2. *Deep brain stimulation for dystonia*

Study	Diagnosis	Procedure	n	Length of follow-up	Mean improvement (scale)
Krauss et al., 1999 (45)	Cervical dystonia	Bilateral GPi DBS	3	6–15 months	49–80% TWSTRS
Islekel, et al., 1999 (46)	Cervical dystonia	Unilateral GPi DBS	1	3 weeks	Improved
Kulisevsky et al., 2000 (47)	Cervical dystonia	Bilateral GPi DBS	2	17–24 weeks	Improved pain scores but little improvement in severity
Parkin et al., 2001 (48)	Cervical dystonia	Bilateral GPi DBS	3	2–6 months	Improved
Andaluz et al., 2001 (49)	Cervical dystonia	Bilateral GPi DBS	1	8 months	50% TWSTRS
Coubes et al., 2000 (39)	1° (DYT1) generalized	Bilateral GPi DBS	7	12 months	90% (BFMDRS)
Tronnier and Fogel, 2000 (44)	1° and 2° generalized	Bilateral GPi DBS	3	6 months	59%, 14%, 34% (BFMDRS)
Loher et al., 2000 (26)	2° hemidystonia	R GPi DBS and thalamotomy	1	4 years	Improved
Kumar et al., 1999 (27)	1° generalized	Bilateral GPi DBS	1	12 months	67% (BFMDRS)
Sellal et al., 1993 (50)	2° hemidystonia	L-VPL thalamic DBS	1	8 months	Improved

BFMDRS, Burke-Fahn-Marsden Dystonia Ratying Scale; GPi, globus pallidus interna; DBS, deep brain stimulation; TWSTRS, Toronto Western Spasmodic Torticollis Rating Scale.

ate in the immediate postoperative period, with continued improvements over the subsequent 1 to 3 months. The authors noted that the patient receiving the least postoperative benefit had a diagnosis of posttraumatic dystonia. They noted that one patient who underwent a staged bilateral pallidotomy derived predominantly contralateral benefits following the first procedure, and axial and bilateral improvement following the second procedure. These observations are consistent with the suggestion that axial symptoms respond to a greater degree, and more consistently following bilateral than unilateral procedures. In another series, Lin and colleagues (22,23) reported the results of their treatment of 18 patients with secondary generalized dystonia of a variety of different etiologies, by bilateral posteroventral pallidotomy. These investigators noted only a 13% improvement in BFM-DRS scores at 12 months after surgery. This highlights the heterogeneous nature of the dystonias, and serves as a cautionary note in

the attempt to apply broadly the findings of any of the individual studies listed.

The striking benefit obtained with bilateral pallidotomy in patients with generalized dystonia led to the placement of bilateral GPi DBS electrodes (27) by our group in Toronto. Our first GPi DBS patient with idiopathic generalized dystonia noted significant improvements (67% BFM scores) in all aspects of her dystonia (Table 40-2). This same patient underwent positron emission tomographic (PET) imaging during a motor task 1 year postoperatively, with and without GPi stimulation. In this double-blinded PET imaging study, GPi stimulation was found to reverse the abnormal excessive activation in motor cortical areas, including primary motor, lateral premotor, supplementary motor, anterior cingulate, and prefrontal areas, which is characteristic of dystonia. Because the GPi is known to modulate primary and association motor cortex activity, and excessive activation of these areas is present in primary and secondary dystonia, these authors proposed that the mechanism of GPi stimulation might be one of directly suppressing excess motor area activation.

Several other series of GPi DBS in dystonia have now been reported (Table 40-2). As with pallidotomy, the most striking improvements are in patients with *DYT1* dystonia. Coubes and colleagues (39) reported bilateral GPi stimulation in seven patients with *DYT1* generalized dystonia. The patients included six children and one adult, with a mean preoperative BFMDRS score of 62 (out of 120). All surgeries were carried out under general anesthesia, using MRI-based stereotactic localization of the posteroventral portion of the GPi, and without microelectrode recordings. Improvements were noted to occur gradually over the course of 3 months, with a 90% improvement in BFMDRS scores at 1 year after surgery.

Patients with secondary dystonias can also benefit from pallidal DBS but usually not to the same extent (44). Loher and colleagues (26) reported their long-term results in a 24-year-old man with posttraumatic left-sided hemidystonia, pain, and tremor following a head injury at the age of 15 who underwent chronic GPi stimulation. A previous right-sided thalamotomy improved his tremor, but only transiently ameliorated the dystonic symptoms. Unilateral GPi stimulation with parameters set initially at amplitude 0.75 V, pulse width 180 µs, and frequency 130 Hz, resulted in early postoperative improvements in both the patient's pain and dystonia. The improvements in the patient's dystonia were sustained at 4 years of follow-up.

Cervical Dystonia

The use of pallidal DBS is also showing some promise in the treatment of cervical dystonia. Several small series with a total of ten patients have shown improvements of approximately 50% to 80% in the Toronto Western Spasmodic Torticollis Rating Scale (TW-STRS) and relief of associated pain with pallidal DBS (Table 40-2). This procedure

could prove useful in primary and secondary nonresponders to botulinum toxin.

CONCLUSION

The accumulated reports indicate that pallidotomy and pallidal stimulation can each be safe and effective treatments for dystonia. However, determination of the optimal surgical treatment for dystonia is difficult given the variability in techniques, targets, underlying pathophysiologic mechanisms, the length and nature of follow-up, the small numbers of patients per study, and the lack of blinded, prospective trials. It appears that patients with idiopathic generalized dystonia, particularly those with *DYT1*, respond best to pallidal interventions. The response in secondary dystonias is more variable and reflects the heterogeneity in the extent of the lesion and distribution of involvement of neural structures and the accompanying neurologic deficits.

SUMMARY

The net output of the basal ganglia is tightly regulated by the activity and balance of driving and inhibitory circuitry. In pathologic states, disrupted activity in the main outflow nucleus, the globus pallidus interna (GPi), is relayed to the motor areas of the thalamus and brainstem. The behavior of these targets receiving this disrupted outflow is consequently also disrupted, which in turn produces the profound disturbances in motor function that are characteristic of parkinsonian states and certain forms of dystonia. Therapeutic efforts are directed at reversing or canceling the pathologic basal ganglia output. When drugs are ineffective or have shortcomings, surgical approaches can be considered. It is interesting and paradoxical that elimination of this abnormal activity with destruction of the motor GPi is usually well tolerated and produces little in the way of overt motor deficit. Indeed having no motor pallidum appears to be preferable to having a pallidum generating and transmitting pathologic inputs to downstream targets. This observation brings into question the mysterious role of the GPi in normal motor function. Nevertheless, bilateral pallidal lesions can be associated with significant adverse effects including speech difficulties and cognitive disturbances. It is for this reason that neurosurgeons have sought to develop surgical procedures that offer the efficacy of selective pallidal lesions but have a better index of safety. With the introduction of DBS to treat first chronic pain and then PD, it became logical to apply DBS to treat dystonia. There is now increasing experience in the use of DBS to treat various forms of dystonia. The initial results suggest that certain primary dystonias can show a strong improvement with GPi DBS.

REFERENCES

1. Andrew J, Fowler CL, Harrison MJG. Stereotaxic thalamotomy in 55 cases of dystonia. *Brain* 1983;106:981–1000.
2. Cooper IS. 20-year follow-up study of the neurosurgical treatment of dystonia musculorum deformans. *Adv Neurol* 1976;14:423–452.
3. Cooper IS, Upton AR, Amin I. Reversibility of chronic neurologic deficits. Some effects of electrical stimulation of the thalamus and internal capsule in man. *Appl Neurophysiol* 1980;43:244–258.
4. Fahn S. Lack of benefit from cervical cord stimulation for dystonia. *NEJM* 1985;313:1229.
5. Gildenberg PL. Treatment of spasmodic torticollis by dorsal column stimulation. *Appl Neurophysiol* 1978; 41:113–121.
6. Kwon Y, Whang CJ. Stereotactic Gamma Knife radiosurgery for the treatment of dystonia. *Stereotact Funct Neurosurg* 1995;64:222–227.
7. Lang AE. Surgical treatment of dystonia. *Adv Neurol* 1998;78:185–198.
8. Manrique M, Oya S, Vaquero J, et al. Chronic paleocerebellar stimulation for the treatment of neuromuscular disorders. Four case reports. *Appl Neurophysiol* 1978;41:237–247.
9. Tasker RR, Doorly T, Yamashiro K. Thalamotomy in generalized dystonia. *Adv Neurol* 1988;50:615–631.
10. Zervas NT. Long-term review of dentatectomy in dystonia musculorum deformans and cerebral palsy. *Acta Neurochir (Wien)* 1977;suppl:49–51.
11. Cooper IS. Dystonia: surgical approaches to treatment and physiological implications. In: Yahr MD, ed. *The basal ganglia: research publications. Association for Research in Nervous and Mental Disease.* New York: Raven Press, 1976:369–384.
12. Cooper IS, Cullinan T, Riklan M. The natural history of dystonia. *Adv Neurol* 1976;14:156–169.
13. Fine J, Duff J, Chen R, et al. Long-term follow-up of unilateral pallidotomy in advanced Parkinson's disease. *N Engl J Med* 2000;342:1708–1714.
14. Lozano AM, Lang AE, Galvez-Jimenez N, et al. Effect of GPi pallidotomy on motor function in Parkinson's disease (see comments) (published erratum appears in *Lancet* 1996;348:1108). *Lancet* 1995;346:1383–1387.
15. Eidelberg D. Abnormal brain networks in DYT1 dystonia. *Adv Neurol* 1998;78:127–133.
16. Eidelberg D, Moeller JR, Antonini A, et al. Functional brain networks in DYT1 dystonia. *Ann Neurol* 1998;44:303–312.
17. Eidelberg D, Moeller JR, Ishikawa T, et al. The metabolic topography of idiopathic torsion dystonia. *Brain* 1995;118:1473–1484.
18. Hoover JE, Strick PL. Multiple output channels in the basal ganglia. *Science* 1993;259:819–821.
19. Ceballos-Baumann AO, Brooks DJ. Activation positron emission tomography scanning in dystonia. *Adv Neurol* 1998;78:135–152.
20. Ceballos-Baumann AO, Sheean G, Passingham RE, et al. Botulinum toxin does not reverse the cortical dysfunction associated with writer's cramp. A PET study. *Brain* 1997;120:571–582.
21. Pahapill PA, Lozano AM. The pedunculopontine nucleus and Parkinson's disease. *Brain* 2000;123:1767–1783.
22. Lin JJ, Lin GY, Shih C, et al. Benefit of bilateral pallidotomy in the treatment of generalized dystonia. Case report. *J Neurosurg* 1999;90:974–976.
23. Lin JJ, Lin SZ, Chang DC. Pallidotomy and generalized dystonia. *Mov Disord* 1999;14:1057–1059.
24. Cubo E, Shannon KM, Penn RD, et al. Internal globus pallidotomy in dystonia secondary to Huntington's disease. *Mov Disord* 2000;15:1248–1251.
25. Justesen CR, Penn RD, Kroin JS, et al. Stereotactic pallidotomy in a child with Hallervorden-Spatz disease. Case report. *J Neurosurg* 1999;90:551–554.
26. Loher TJ, Hasdemir MG, Burgunder JM, et al. Long-term follow-up study of chronic globus pallidus internus stimulation for posttraumatic hemidystonia. *J Neurosurg* 2000;92:457–460.
27. Kumar R, Dagher A, Hutchison WD, et al. Globus pallidus deep brain stimulation for generalized dystonia: clinical and PET investigation. *Neurology* 1999;53: 871–874.
28. Lozano AM, Hutchison WD, Kiss Z, et al. Methods for microelectrode-guided posteroventral pallidotomy. *J Neurosurg* 1996;84:194–202.
29. Lozano AM, Kumar R, Gross RE, et al. Globus pallidus internus pallidotomy for generalized dystonia. *Mov Disord* 1997;12:865–870.
30. Vitek JL, Chockkan V, Zhang JY, et al. Neuronal activity in the basal ganglia in patients with generalized dystonia and hemiballismus. *Ann Neurol* 1999;46:22–35.
31. Hutchison WD, Lozano AM, Davis KD, et al. Differential neuronal activity in segments of globus pallidus in Parkinson's disease. *NeuroReport* 1994;5:1533–1537.
32. Antkowiak B. Different actions of general anesthetics on the firing patterns of neocortical neurons mediated by the GABA(A) receptor. *Anesthesiology* 1999;91:500–511.
33. Chen CL, Yang YR, Chiu TH. Activation of rat locus coeruleus neuron GABA(A) receptors by propofol and its potentiation by pentobarbital or alphaxalone. *Eur J Pharmacol* 1999;386:201–210.
34. Ranck JB Jr. Which elements are excited in electrical stimulation of mammalian central nervous system: a review. *Brain Res* 1975;98:417–440.
35. Galvez-Jimenez N, Lozano A, Tasker R, et al. Pallidal

stimulation in Parkinson's disease patients with a prior unilateral pallidotomy. *Can J Neurol Sci* 1998;25: 300–305.

36. Iacono RP, Kuniyoshi SM, Lonser RR, et al. Simultaneous bilateral pallidoansotomy for idiopathic dystonia musculorum deformans. *Pediatr Neurol* 1996;14:145–148.

37. Ondo WG, Desaloms JM, Jankovic J, et al. Pallidotomy for generalized dystonia. *Mov Disord* 1998;13: 693–698.

38. Coubes P, Echenne B, Roubertie A, et al. Treatment of early-onset generalized dystonia by chronic bilateral stimulation of the internal globus pallidus. Apropos of a case. *Neurochirurgie* 1999;45:139–144.

39. Coubes P, Roubertie A, Vayssiere N, et al. Treatment of DYT1-generalised dystonia by stimulation of the internal globus pallidus. *Lancet* 2000;355:2220–2221.

40. Roubertie A, Echenne B, Cif L, et al. Treatment of early-onset dystonia: update and a new perspective. *Childs Nerv Syst* 2000;16:334–340.

41. Vayssiere N, Hemm S, Zanca M, et al. Magnetic resonance imaging stereotactic target localization for deep brain stimulation in dystonic children. *J Neurosurg* 2000;93:784–790.

42. Ondo WG, Desaloms JM, Jankovic J, et al. Pallidotomy for generalized dystonia. *Mov Disord* 1998;13: 693–698.

43. Yoshor D, Hamilton WJ, Ondo W, et al. Comparison of thalamotomy and pallidotomy for the treatment of dystonia. *Neurosurgery* 2001;48:818–824; discussion 824–826.

44. Tronnier VM, Fogel W. Pallidal stimulation for generalized dystonia. Report of three cases. *J Neurosurg* 2000; 92:453–456.

45. Krauss JK, Pohle T, Weber S, Ozdoba C, Burgunder JM. Bilateral stimulation of globus pallidus internus for treatment of cervical dystonia. *Lancet* 1999 Sep 4;354 (9181):837–838.

46. Islekel S, Zileli M, Zileli B. R Unilateral pallidal stimulation in cervical dystonia. *Stereotact Funct Neurosurg* 1999;72(2–4):248–252.

47. Kulisevsky J, Lleo A, Gironell A, Molet J, Pascual-Sedano B, Pares P. Related Articles Links Bilateral pallidal stimulation for cervical dystonia: dissociated pain and motor improvement. *Neurology* 2000 Dec 12; 55(11):1754–1755.

48. Parkin S, Aziz T, Gregory R, Bain P. Bilateral internal globus pallidus stimulation for the treatment of spasmodic torticollis. *Mov Disord* 2001 May;16(3):489–493.

49. Andaluz N, Taha JM, Dalvi A. Bilateral pallidal deep brain stimulation for cervical and truncal dystonia. *Neurology* 2001 Aug 14;57(3):557–558.

50. Sellal F, Hirsch E, Barth P, Blond S, Marescaux C. A case of symptomatic hemidystonia improved by ventroposterolateral thalamic electrostimulation. *Mov Disord* 1993 Oct;8(4):515–518.

Dystonia 4: Advances in Neurology, Vol. 94. Edited by Stanley Fahn, Mark Hallett, and Mahlon R. DeLong. Lippincott Williams & Wilkins, Philadelphia © 2004.

41

Off-Period Dystonia in Parkinson's Disease but Not Generalized Dystonia Is Improved By High-Frequency Stimulation of the Subthalamic Nucleus

Olivier Detante, Laurent Vercueil, Paul Krack, Stéphan Chabardes, Alim-Louis Benabid, and Pierre Pollak

Department of Biological and Clinical Neurosciences, Grenoble, France; INSERM, Joseph Fourier University, Grenoble, France; and Department of Neurology, CHU Grenoble, Grenoble, France

Off-period dystonia in idiopathic Parkinson's disease (IPD) and generalized dystonia share the same clinical definition of dystonia, namely abnormal postures or repetitive twisting movements induced by involuntary muscle contractions (1). However, identifiable clinical differences between the two exist. Segmental fixed postures are mostly characteristic of off-period dystonia, whereas repetitive twisting movements are commonly observed in primary generalized dystonia. However, fixed postures can also be noted in the late stage of primary generalized dystonia or can be associated with specific etiologies, especially in secondary dystonia. Since both parkinsonism and dystonia can lead to debilitating states and medical treatment efficacy is limited, they are amenable to functional brain surgery. Historically, brain surgery for dystonia followed the development of surgery for IPD and the observation of an improvement of dystonic symptoms in parkinsonian subjects (2). The ablative procedures, especially thalamotomy, were used for generalized dystonia and produced a substantial benefit (3). More recently, with the renewal of posteroventral pallidotomy in IPD (4–6), pallido-

tomy was also rediscovered as the treatment for generalized dystonia, producing marked improvement in dystonic movements and motor function (7,8). The introduction of deep brain stimulation (DBS) of the thalamic Vim nucleus for the treatment of tremors (9,10) was followed by the application of the same procedure to the subthalamic nucleus (STN) (11–13) and to the globus pallidus interna (GPi) (14). The improvement of off-period dystonia with STN stimulation (15) suggested that DBS could constitute a first-line surgical treatment for generalized dystonia (2). Moreover, unlike ablative surgery, DBS is reversible and adjustable.

At present, the STN is the commonly preferred target for high-frequency stimulation (HFS) for IPD (11–13). Given the increasing number of clinical reports showing obvious efficacy of pallidal stimulation in generalized dystonia (16–18), the rationale to choose STN as a target in generalized dystonia is as follows: (a) when dystonia is associated with pallidal lesions as in Hallervorden-Spatz disease, it is logically assumed that this pallidal lesion will prevent the DBS from this site being effective; (b) when dystonia is associated with bradykinesia and rigidity, the STN could be proposed as a means of dramatically improving such clinical signs by using HFS (11–13); (c) the significant benefit from STN stimulation in off-period dystonia in IPD (15) could be transposed to dystonia from other causes; (d) according to some authors, the STN could be involved in the pathophysiology of generalized dystonia (19).

The aim of our retrospective study was to compare the efficacy of STN-HFS in IPD patients with off-period dystonia with that in patients with generalized dystonia.

PATIENTS AND METHODS

Methods

To evaluate the dystonia severity in both disorders (IPD and generalized dystonia), we used a Dystonia Severity Score (DSS) developed by our group to score off-period dystonia in IPD patients (Table 41-1) (15). On the basis of videotape recordings, the same examiner scored each limb in the preoperative period and 3 months after surgery in two conditions of stimulation: on-stimulation and off-stimulation. The on-stimulation condition was defined by parameters providing the best clinical improvement. The off-stimulation condition was defined by switching the stimulator off for more than 20 minutes before scoring. The DSS was obtained for each hemibody corresponding with each electrode (two per patient).

We used the Wilcoxon signed rank test to compare the DSS in the preoperative period with that at 3 months after surgery for each

TABLE 41-1. *Dystonia Severity Score (DSS) rated for each limb (maximum = 16) in preoperative period and 3 months after stimulation*

0 = absent
1 = minimal dystonia or abnormal posture
2 = moderate dystonia
3 = severe dystonia (moderate interference with movement)
4 = severe dystonia (intense interference with movement)

TABLE 41-2. *General characteristics of four patients with high-frequency stimulation (HFS) of the subthalamic nucleus (STN) for severe generalized dystonia*

Patient	Sex	Diagnosis	Age at onset	Age at surgery (HFS)
1	F	HSD	16	29
2	M	HSD	7	10
3	M	Primary dystonia	44	60
4	M	HSD	12	26

HSD, Hallervorden-Spatz disease.

group independently. A *p* value of <.05 was considered significant.

Patients

Of the complete series of patients with IPD treated in our center by STN stimulation (*n* = 185), 22 patients exhibited severe preoperative off-period dystonia rated ≥3 (DSS) in at least one limb. For generalized dystonia, we reported four cases with bilateral STN-HFS, including three cases of Hallervorden-Spatz disease and one case of late-onset primary dystonia. In addition to abnormal postures, these patients suffered from mobile repetitive dystonic movements of the four limbs and the spine; however, we did not take into account axial dystonia for the purpose of comparison with IPD patients. The clinical characteristics of these four patients are shown in Table 41-2. Electrical variables are shown in Table 41-3 for both groups.

RESULTS

High-Frequency Stimulation of the Subthalamic Nucleus in Off-Period Dystonia of Idiopathic Parkinson's Disease

In IPD, bilateral STN-HFS reduced the severity of off-period dystonia by 70%. The preoperative mean value of the DSS was 2.03 ± 1.49 per limb, whereas the postoperative DSS was 0.6 ± 0.78 for the on-stimulation condition associated with the best clinical ef-

TABLE 41-3. *Electrical variables of high-frequency stimulation (HFS) of the subthalamic nucleus (STN): four patients with generalized dystonia and 22 patients with idiopathic Parkinson's disease (IPD) and severe off-period dystonia*

	Voltage (V) [range (mean)]	Pulse width (µs)	Frequency (Hz)
IPD—off-period dystonia	1.1–3.6 (2.7)	60–90	130–185
Generalized dystonia	2.2–3.6 (2.8)	60–120	130

fect. As shown in Fig. 41-1, we also noted a significant improvement of dystonia severity in the off-stimulation condition, 3 months after surgery (p <.0001). Moreover, an additional benefit was present due to the direct effect of DBS as proved by the significant difference between on- and off-stimulation conditions (p <.05) during the postoperative period.

High-Frequency Stimulation of the Subthalamic Nucleus in Generalized Dystonia

Bilateral STN-HFS had no effect on the severity of generalized dystonia. The preoperative mean DSS was 3.25 ± 0.77 per limb and the postoperative mean DSS was 3.12 ± 0.62 in the on-stimulation condition. We did not observe any significant differences between preoperative and postoperative periods or between the on- and off-stimulation conditions (Fig. 41-2).

DISCUSSION

Although we were not able to perform between-group comparisons due to the difference in the samples sizes ($n = 4$ for generalized dystonia; $n = 22$ for IPD), our findings suggest that preoperative severity of dystonia was more important in generalized dystonia (DSS = 3.25 ± 0.77) than in off-period dystonia (DSS = 2.03 ± 1.49). It is important to distinguish the different clinical forms of dystonia. We would like to point out that within the same clinical definition of dystonia, off-period dystonia in IPD is characterized by fixed postures, whereas the dystonia of the four non-IPD patients is characterized by repetitive movements, most accurately described by

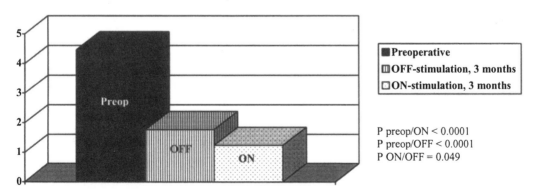

Preoperative
OFF-stimulation, 3 months
ON-stimulation, 3 months

P preop/ON < 0.0001
P preop/OFF < 0.0001
P ON/OFF = 0.049

FIG. 41-1. Improvement of off-period dystonia severity in 22 idiopathic Parkinson's disease (IPD) patients by high-frequency stimulation (HFS) of the subthalamic nucleus (STN) evaluated with the Dystonia Severity Score (DSS).

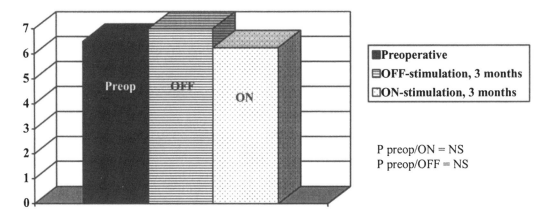

FIG. 41-2. No effect of high-frequency stimulation (HFS) of the subthalamic nucleus (STN) on generalized dystonia severity in four patients, evaluated with the Dystonia Severity Score (DSS). NS, nonsignificant.

the term mobile dystonia. These clinical differences may account for different pathophysiologic mechanisms, especially regarding the putative involvement of the STN.

Improvement of Off-Period Dystonia in Idiopathic Parkinson's Disease by High-Frequency Stimulation of the Subthalamic Nucleus

STN-HFS has been shown to improve parkinsonian signs and symptoms (11–13). Moreover, in a previous study, it was shown that bilateral STN-HFS reduced the severity of off-period dystonia in eight patients by 90% when the stimulator was switched on (15). We confirmed this dramatic improvement in our 22 cases. To explain this beneficial effect, studies related a normalization of force excess related to off-period dystonia and other forms of dyskinesia in IPD, suggesting a direct effect of chronic STN-HFS on force regulation and dyskinesias (20,21). In addition, all types of dyskinesias are indirectly improved by a decrease in dopaminergic treatment. Although the exact mechanism of the effect of DBS remains unknown, STN-HFS might induce a functional inhibition of the glutamatergic neuronal hyperactivity of the STN in IPD given a similarity to the effect induced by STN lesions (22).

No Effect of High-Frequency Stimulation of the Subthalamic Nucleus in Generalized Dystonia

We observed that STN-HFS had no effect on generalized dystonia in contrast to the dramatic improvement of off-period dystonia in IPD. However, our study included only a few heterogeneous cases of generalized dystonia ($n = 4$), including generalized dystonia of rare causes: Hallervorden-Spatz disease and late-onset primary dystonia. It is important to note that this study does not include any cases of *DYT1* dystonia. Moreover, because of the absence of acute benefit, STN-HFS was stopped after a few days for these four patients. So this study cannot predict a potential effect of chronic stimulation. As predicted by clinical differences and the poor effect of STN-HFS in generalized dystonia, we suggest that the pathophysiologic mechanism for generalized dystonia is different from that for the off-period dystonia in IPD. Assuming the hypothesis that HFS creates a functional inhibition of local neuronal activity, our findings suggest that there is no hyperactivity of the STN in generalized dystonia. This hypothesis contrasts with the model suggesting an increased activity of the STN in dystonia (19). It is also probable that the different forms of generalized dystonia with distinct clinical presentations implicate different pathophysiologic mechanisms. For example, in symptomatic dystonia due to putaminal lesion, the absence of neuronal inhibitory projections from the putamen would lead to overactivity of the globus pallidus externa (GPe) that would inhibit the STN via γ-aminobutyric acid (GABA)ergic inhibitory projections.

Regarding the poor clinical effects of STN-HFS, we suggest that the posterolateral GPi is a better target for HFS in generalized dystonia. Indeed, highly irregular activity of the GPi with grouped discharges separated by periods of pauses was observed in this disorder (23), and the first studies about the therapeutic effects of GPi-HFS in generalized dystonia showed a substantial clinical benefit (16–18).

CONCLUSION

In spite of some clinical similarities between off-period dystonia in IPD and generalized dystonia, the effect of chronic bilateral STN-HFS was clearly different between the two. STN-HFS was highly effective in off-period dystonia of IPD, whereas it did not improve various types of generalized dystonia. Pathophysiologic mechanisms underlying the different forms of dystonia are still poorly understood. Assuming that STN-HFS inhibits local neuronal activity, our findings suggest that the pathophysiology of these disorders is variable, especially regarding the STN neuronal activity.

SUMMARY

STN-HFS is well known to improve patients with IPD. Because off-period dystonia mimics focal or generalized dystonia of other causes, we proposed bilateral STN-HFS to some patients with generalized dystonia. The aim of this study was to compare the efficacy of STN stimulation on off-period dystonia and generalized dystonia. From a larger series of patients with IPD, we selected 22 patients based on the presence of severe preoperative off-period dystonia rated ≥3 in at least one limb on a severity score ranging from 0 to 4.

Four patients with generalized dystonia (Hallervorden-Spatz disease, $n = 3$; primary, $n = 1$) underwent bilateral STN-HFS. Dystonia of the four limbs was rated on video recordings in all patients before surgery and 3 months after surgery. In IPD, bilateral STN stimulation reduced the severity of off-period dystonia by 70% on the four limbs (preoperative mean severity score = 2.03 ± 1.49; postoperative mean severity score = 0.60 ± 0.78). In contrast, bilateral STN-HFS had no effect on generalized dystonia (preoperative mean severity score = 3.25 ± 0.77; postoperative mean severity score = 3.12 ± 0.62).

Despite clinical similarities between off-period dystonia in Parkinson's disease and generalized dystonia in certain cases, the effect of chronic bilateral STN-HFS differs. STN stimulation is highly effective in off-period dystonia of IPD, whereas it does not improve generalized dystonia. The pathophysiologic mechanisms underlying dystonia in these two disorders are still unknown. Assuming that the mechanism of action of STN-HFS is similar regardless of the cause of dystonia, our findings suggest that the STN is not similarly involved in off-period dystonia of IPD and others dystonias.

ACKNOWLEDGMENTS

We wish to thank Bradley Wallace for his helpful comments on the manuscript.

REFERENCES

1. Fahn S, Bressmann SB, Marsden CD. Classification of dystonia. *Adv Neurol* 1998;78:1–10.
2. Krack P, Vercueil L. Review of the functional surgical treatment of dystonia. *Eur J Neurol* 2001;8:389–399.
3. Cooper IS. 20 year follow-up study on the neurosurgical treatment of dystonia musculorum deformans. *Adv Neurol* 1976;14:423–452.
4. Fine J, Duff J, Chen R, et al. Long-term follow-up of unilateral pallidotomy in advanced Parkinson's disease. *N Engl J Med* 2000;342:1708–1714.
5. Lang AE, Lozano AM, Montgomery EB, et al. Posteroventral medial pallidotomy in advanced Parkinson's disease. *N Engl J Med* 1997;337:1036–1042.
6. Lozano AM, Lang AE, Galvez-Jimenez N, et al. Effect of GPi pallidotomy on motor function in Parkinson's disease. *Lancet* 1995;346:1383–1387.
7. Lozano AM, Kumar R, Gross RE, et al. Globus pallidus

internus pallidotomy for generalized dystonia. *Mov Disord* 1997;12:865–870.

8. Ondo WG, Desaloms M, Jankovic J, et al. Pallidotomy for generalized dystonia. *Mov Disord* 1998;13:693–698.

9. Benabid AL, Pollak P, Gervason C, et al. Long-term suppression of tremor by chronic stimulation of the ventral intermediate thalamic nucleus. *Lancet* 1991;337: 403–406.

10. Limousin P, Speelman JD, Gielen F, et al., and the study collaborators. Multicenter European study of thalamic stimulation in parkinsonian and essential tremor. *J Neurol Neurosurg Psychiatry* 1999;66:289–296.

11. Limousin P, Krack P, Pollak P, et al. Electrical stimulation of the subthalamic nucleus in advanced Parkinson's disease. *N Engl J Med* 1998;339:1105–1111.

12. Limousin P, Pollak P, Benazzouz A, et al. Effect on parkinsonian signs and symptoms of bilateral subthalamic nucleus stimulation. *Lancet* 1995;345:91–95.

13. Pollak P, Benabid AL, Gross C, et al. Effet de la stimulation du noyau sous-thalamique dans la maladie de Parkinson. *Rev Neurol (Paris)* 1993;149:175–176.

14. Siegfried J, Lippitz B. Bilateral chronic electrostimulation of ventroposterolateral pallidum: a new therapeutic approach for alleviating all parkinsonian symptoms. *Neurosurgery* 1994;35:1126–1130.

15. Krack P, Pollak P, Limousin P, et al. From off-period dystonia to peak-dose chorea: the clinical spectrum of varying subthalamic nucleus activity. *Brain* 1999;122: 1133–1146.

16. Coubes P, Echenne B, Roubertie A, et al. Traitement de la dystonie généralisée à début précoce par stimulation chronique bilatérale des globus pallidus internes. A propos d'un cas. *Neurochirurgie* 1999;45:139–144.

17. Coubes P, Roubertie A, Vayssière N, et al. Treatment of DYT1-generalised dystonia by stimulation of the internal globus pallidus. *Lancet* 2000;355:2220–2221.

18. Vercueil L, Pollak P, Fraix V, et al. Deep brain stimulation in the treatment of severe dystonia. *J Neurol* 2001; 248:695–700.

19. Vitek JL. Pathophysiology of dystonia: a neuronal model. *Mov Disord* 2002;17(suppl 3):S49–S62.

20. Wenzelburger R, Zhang B, Poepping M, et al. Dyskinesias and grip control in Parkinson's disease are normalized by chronic stimulation of the subthalamic nucleus. *Ann Neurol* 2002;52:240–243.

21. Wenzelburger R, Zhang B, Pohle S, et al. Force overflow and levodopa-induced dyskinesias in Parkinson's disease. *Brain* 2002;125:871–879.

22. Bergman H, Wichmann T, DeLong M. Reversal of experimental parkinsonism by lesions of the subthalamic nucleus. *Science* 1990;249:1436–1438.

23. Vitek JL, Chockkan V, Zhang JY, et al. Neuronal activity in the basal ganglia in patients with generalized dystonia and hemiballismus. *Ann Neurol* 1999;46:22–35.

Dystonia 4: Advances in Neurology, Vol. 94. Edited by Stanley Fahn, Mark Hallett, and Mahlon R. DeLong. Lippincott Williams & Wilkins, Philadelphia © 2004.

42

Autonomic Side Effects of Botulinum Toxin Type B Therapy

Dirk Dressler and Reiner Benecke

Department of Neurology, Rostock University, Rostock, Germany

For some time now, botulinum toxin type A (BT-A) has been used with great success to treat muscle hyperactivity syndromes and exocrine gland hyperfunction (1,2). Botulinum toxin type B (BT-B) was introduced as a new compound for treatment of muscle hyperactivity in cervical dystonia (3,4). When we started clinical use of BT-B we noticed side effects not seen with BT-A.

METHODS

Patients

Altogether 30 consecutive patients were studied, 13 female and 17 male. Their age was 48.1 ± 15.4 years. As summarized in Table 42-1, 24 patients suffered from idiopathic cervical dystonia (CD), nine female and 15 male. Their age was 52.4 ± 13.2 years and the duration of their CD was 11.6 ± 8.0 years. Fifteen of the CD patients (six female and nine male) had received BT-A therapy before with initially adequate improvement, but had developed therapy failure in the further course of their treatment. All of those patients presented with functionally significant antibody titers against BT-A as tested by the mouse diaphragm assay (5). After other causes for BT-A therapy failure (6) were excluded, the patients were classified as suffering from antibody-induced therapy failure (CD antibody patients). Their age was 53.4 ± 14.3 years and the duration of their CD was 14.8 ±

7.5 years. Nine of the CD patients (three female, six male) were treated with BT for the first time (CD de novo patients). Their age was 50.8 ± 11.6 years and the duration of their CD was 6.3 ± 6.1 years.

As summarized in Table 42-2, six patients (four female, two male) presented with hyperhidrosis (HH). Their mean age ±SD was 30.7 ± 11.3 years and the duration of their HH was 19.2 ± 10.5 years. Two had bilateral palmar HH, two bilateral axillary HH, one bilateral plantar, and one bilateral palmar and axillary HH. Two HH patients had received BT-A before, and four received botulinum toxin therapy for the first time. In none of the HH patients was there any indication of botulinum toxin therapy failure.

None of the CD patients and none of the HH patients were currently being treated with anticholinergics.

Botulinum Toxin Therapy

Botulinum toxin therapy was performed with BT-B or with a combination of BT-B and BT-A. BT-B therapy was performed with NeuroBloc/MyoBloc (Elan Pharmaceuticals, Shannon, Ireland). For treatment of CD, NeuroBloc/MyoBloc was used in its original dilution of 5,000 MU/ml, for treatment of HH in a dilution of 1,000 MU/ml. BT-A therapy was performed with Botox (Allergan, Irvine, CA) in a concentration of 20 MU/ml. All CD pa-

TABLE 42-1. *Therapeutic effects and side effects of botulinum toxin type B in 24 consecutive patients with cervical dystonia (CD)*

		Total	CD de novo patients	CD antibody patients
Number	[n]	24	9	15
Gender (females/males)	[n]	9/15	3/6	6/9
Age at time of study (mean ± standard deviation)	[n] [years]	52.4 ± 13.2	50.8 ± 11.6	53.4 ± 14.3
Duration of dystonia at time of study (mean ± standard deviation)	[years]	11.6 ± 8.0	6.3 ± 6.1	14.8 ± 7.5
BT-B dosage (mean ± standard deviation)	[MU NeuroBloc]	11,310 ± 2,616	10,436 ± 3,320	11,835 ± 2,039
TWSTRS-B (mean ± standard deviation)	[n]	19.7 ± 4.4	18.4 ± 5.4	20.5 ± 3.6
TWSTRS-A (mean ± standard deviation)	[n]	11.6 ± 5.4	9.2 ± 4.8	13.1 ± 5.4
TWSTRS-I (mean ± standard deviation)	[n]	8.0 ± 4.0	9.1 ± 3.8	7.4 ± 4.2
Dryness of mouth: total	[n]	21	7	14
Severe	[n]	10	2	8
Moderate	[n]	7	3	4
Mild	[n]	4	2	2
Accommodation difficulties	[n]	7	2	5
Conjunctival irritation	[n]	5	1	4
Reduced sweating	[n]	4	1	3
Swallowing difficulties	[n]	3	1	2
Heart burn	[n]	3	0	3
Constipation	[n]	3	0	3
Bladder voiding difficulties	[n]	2	1	1
Head instability	[n]	1	1	0
Dryness of nasal mucosa	[n]	1	1	0
Soor	[n]	1	0	1

BT-A; botulinum toxin type A; BT-B; botulinum toxin type B; TWSTRS-B, Toronto Western Spasmodic Torticollis Rating Scale, before BT-B therapy; TWSTRS-A, Toronto Western Spasmodic Torticollis Rating Scale, after BT-B therapy; TWSTRS-I, Toronto Western Spasmodic Torticollis Rating Scale, improvement after BT-B therapy; CD de novo patients, patients with cervical dystonia without previous exposure to BT-A or BT-B; CD antibody patients, patients with cervical dystonia and antibody-induced failure of BT-A therapy.

tients received BT-B only. Target muscle selection was based on routine clinical standards. BT-B dosages were chosen by multiplying standard BT-A dosages by a factor of 40. As summarized in Table 42-2, patients with axillary and palmar HH received 4,000 MU of BT-B each on one side and 100 MU of BT-A each on the corresponding contralateral body side. The one patient with axillary and palmar HH received 8,000 MU of BT-B in his axilla and his palm on one side and 200 MU of BT-A in his axilla and his palm on the corresponding contralateral body side. The one patient with plantar HH received a total of 10,000 MU of BT-B bilaterally. All botulinum toxin injections were placed intracutaneously at a distance of approximately 2 cm from each other. Therapeutic efficacy was evaluated with a clinical examination and the Toronto

Western Spasmodic Torticollis Rating Scale (TWSTRS) (7) for CD patients before treatment and 2 to 3 weeks thereafter. For HH patients a clinical examination and a subjective rating for the best BT-B effect (0 = none, 1 = moderate, 2 = good, 3 = excellent) were used.

Statistics

All group values are given as mean ± standard deviation. Applied statistical tests are described together with their results.

RESULTS

Cervical Dystonia Patients

As summarized in Table 42-1, the BT-B dosage used in the 24 CD patients was 11,310 ± 2,616 MU with 11,835 ± 2,039 MU used in

TABLE 42-2. *Therapeutic effects and side effects of botulinum toxin type A and of botulinum toxin type B in six consecutive patients with hyperhidrosis*

		Axillary hyperhidrosis	Palmar hyperhidrosis	Axillary and palmar hyperhidrosis	Plantar hyperhidrosis
Number	[n]	2	2	1	1
BT-B dosage per patient	[MU NeuroBloc]	4,000	4,000	8,000	10,000
BT-A dosage per patient	[MU Botox]	100	100	200	0
Maximal BT-B therapy effect (mean)	[0 = none, 1 = moderate, 2 = good, 3 = excellent]	3	3	3	3
Maximal BT-A therapy effect (mean)	[0 = none, 1 = moderate, 2 = good, 3 = excellent]	3	2	3 (ax) 2 (pal)	n/a
Duration of BT-B therapy effect (mean ± standard deviation)	[weeks]	12.7 ± 2.3	11.7 ± 3.1	10 (ax) 9 (pal)	15
Duration of BT-A therapy effect (mean ± standard deviation)	[weeks]	11.7 ± 1.5	9.3 ± 1.5	10 (ax) 8 (pal)	n/a
Accommodation difficulties	[n]	1	1	1	1
Dryness of mouth	[n]	1	0	0	1
Conjunctival irritation	[n]	1	0	0	0

ax, axilla; pal, palma; BT-A; botulinum toxin type A; BT-B; botulinum toxin type B.

the 15 CD antibody patients and 10,436 ± 3,320 MU in the nine BT de novo patients. TWSTRS score before BT-B therapy was 19.7 ± 4.4 in CD patients, with 20.5 ± 3.6 in CD antibody patients and 18.4 ± 5.4 in CD de novo patients. TWSTRS score after BT-B therapy was 11.6 ± 5.4 in CD patients, with 9.2 ± 4.8 in CD de novo patients and 13.1 ± 5.4 in CD antibody patients. Resulting TWSTRS score improvement was 8.0 ± 4.0 in CD patients with 7.4 ± 4.2 in CD antibody patients and 9.1 ± 3.8 in CD de novo patients.

The most frequent side effect in CD patients was dryness of mouth, which occurred in 21 (88%) patients. In ten (48%) patients it was severe, in seven (33%) moderate, and in four (19%) mild. Its duration was 4.4 ± 2.0 weeks. In CD de novo patients, dryness of mouth occurred in seven (78%) patients. In two patients it was severe, in three moderate, and in two mild. Its duration was 3.6 ± 1.6 weeks. In CD antibody patients, dryness of mouth occurred in 14 (93%). In eight (57%) patients it was severe, in four (29%) moderate, and in two mild. Its duration was 4.8 ± 2.1 weeks. Accommodation difficulties were the

second most common side effect. It occurred in seven (29%) CD patients, in five (33%) CD antibody patients, and in two CD de novo patients. Conjunctival irritation occurred in five (21%) CD patients; reduced sweating, either focal or generalized; in four (17%), heartburn in three (13%); constipation in three (13%), swallowing difficulties in three (13%); bladder voiding difficulties in two; and head instability, dryness of nasal mucosa, and oral and vaginal soor in one CD patient each. In one CD patient preexisting diabetes mellitus was exacerbated at the time of the study so that insulin substitution had to be introduced. Excessive pain at the injection site was not reported.

Hyperhidrosis Patients

As summarized in Table 42-2, all six HH patients reported an excellent effect from the BT-B therapy, lasting 10.7 ± 4.4 weeks. Of the five HH patients with additional BT-A therapy, three patients with axillary HH reported excellent effect and three patients with palmar HH reported a good effect from BT-A therapy.

The duration of the BT-A effect was 9.3 ± 3.6 weeks. Accommodation difficulties occurred in four HH patients, and dryness of mouth and conjunctival irritation in one each. Reduced sweating in skin areas other than the site of injection, swallowing difficulties, heartburn, constipation, head instability, bladder voiding difficulties, dryness of nasal mucosa, soor, and excessive pain at the injection site did not occur.

Dosage Dependency of Autonomic Side Effects

In CD patients receiving from 5,600 to 10,000 MU, the number of autonomic side effects was 1.54 ± 1.56, and in patients receiving more than 10,000 and up to 15,600 MU it was 2.29 ± 1.54 (Mann-Whitney U test, p = .235). Figure 42-1 shows the correlation between the severity of dryness of mouth and the BT-B dosage administered. The linear correlation was $y = 1,118.9x + 9,079.6$ (p = .041). Patients without dryness of mouth received a BT-B dosage of 9,067 ± 3,029 MU, and those with dryness of mouth 11,631 ± 2,468 MU (Mann-Whitney U test, p = .271). Patients with mild, moderate, and severe dryness of mouth had not received different BT-B dosages (Kruskal-Wallis test, p = 0.271).

DISCUSSION

BT has long been infamous for causing botulism. Some of its earliest and still some of its best clinical descriptions (8–10) highlight not only paresis but also autonomic dysfunction, especially accommodation problems, reduced sweating, high skin temperature, and reduced cerumen production as some of botulism's cardinal features. When intramuscular BT-A injections were first used to reduce

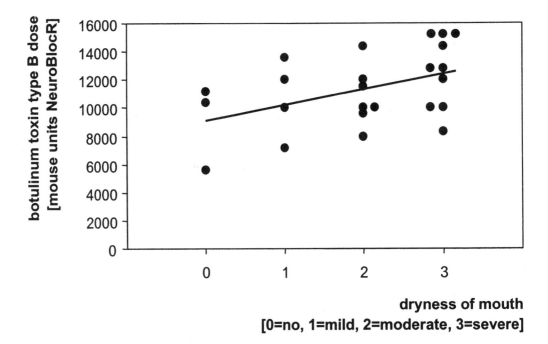

FIG. 42-1. Correlation between dryness of mouth and botulinum toxin type B dosage in 24 consecutive patients with cervical dystonia. The line shows the linear correlation [$y = 1,118.9x + 9,079.6$ (p = .041)].

muscle hyperactivity disorders, their effect was strictly local and no autonomic dysfunction was observed (11). It was believed that lack of systemic spread was due to a specific and robust BT-A binding to glycoprotein "acceptors" (12,13). Later, with the use of higher BT-A dosages, jitter examinations revealed some systemic motor side effects (14) and examination of residual urine volumes (15) and of heart rate variability (16,17) suggested possible systemic autonomic dysfunction. None of these findings, however, was noticed by the patient or became clinically relevant.

We are reporting 24 consecutive patients who received BT-B in dosages from 5,600 to 15,200 MU for DC; 92% of patients experienced at least one side effect, most often dryness of mouth, and less frequently, accommodation difficulties, conjunctival irritation, reduced sweating, swallowing difficulties, heartburn, constipation, head instability, bladder voiding difficulties, dryness of nasal mucosa, and soor. Particularly dryness of mouth was clinically relevant and frequently caused considerable distress to patients. Apart from head instability occurring in one patient only, all of the reported side effects reflect, directly or indirectly, autonomic dysfunction due to parasympathetic blockade caused by BT-B's anticholinergic action. Distribution of autonomic side effects indicates clinically relevant systemic BT-B spread. Frequency of motor side effects after BT-B application was in the same range as after BT-A application. Excessive pain at the injection site was not reported by our patients. Although there was a trend for higher BT-B dosages to produce more autonomic side effects, this trend was not statistically significant. Similarly, although the BT-B dosages and the severity of dryness of mouth showed a statistically significant linear correlation, and, although there was a trend for more severe dryness of mouth to be caused by higher BT-B dosages, BT-B dosages causing different degrees of dryness of mouth did not show a statistically significant difference. BT-B dosage reduction, therefore, may not necessarily be a promising strategy to avoid autonomic side effects, especially with BT-B dosages between 8,000 and 12,000 MU, which is, unfortunately, the most interesting dosage range to treat CD patients.

As a novel indication we used BT-B in dosages from 4,000 to 10,000 MU for treatment of focal hyperhidrosis. All of the HH patients experienced excellent reduction of sweating for 10.7 ± 4.4 weeks with BT-B. Effect of BT-A given in the corresponding contralateral body side produced the same effectiveness for a similar duration in axillary HH and a slightly weaker and shorter effect in palmar HH. Again, systemic autonomic side effects occurred. With substantially higher BT-A dosages only extremely rarely producing systemic autonomic side effects, those side effects are likely due to the BT-B application rather than to the BT-A application. Additive effects between BT-A and BT-B, however, cannot entirely be excluded.

BT-B and BT-A have clearly different affinities to neuromuscular and to autonomic synapses. Whether BT-B has a particularly low affinity for neuromuscular synapses, thus requiring BT-B dosages of around 10,000 MU to relax overactive muscles, or whether BT-B has a particularly high affinity for autonomic synapses, cannot be decided yet.

Despite its side-effect profile, BT-B is the treatment of choice for patients with BT-A antibodies. For CD de novo patients and CD patients currently under successful BT-A therapy, however, use of BT-B bears the risk of systemic autonomic side effects without, so far, offering advantages over BT-A. For indications where low BT-B dosages might be sufficient, its side-effect profile might be less relevant. Trials on BT-B for treatment of spasticity, where particularly high BT-B dosages will be necessary, should be planned and monitored carefully. Special attention should be paid when BT-B is given to patients with preexistent autonomic dysfunction, additional anticholinergic treatment, and in conditions where anticholinergics are contraindicated. Attention to those precautions should be advised in the official product information and in physicians' prescription manuals.

With its potentially high affinity for autonomic nerve endings, BT-B might have advantages over BT-A for treatment of autonomic disorders, such as hyperhidrosis, hypersalivation, and hyperlacrimation, where it might be used in lower relative dosages with less motor side effects.

ACKNOWLEDGMENT

The statistical analyses of Guenther Kundt, Institute of Medical Informatics and Biometrics, Rostock University, were greatly appreciated.

REFERENCES

1. Jankovic J, Hallett M, eds. *Therapy with botulinum toxin.* New York, Basel, Hong Kong: Marcel Dekker, 1994:267–278.
2. Dressler D. *Botulinum toxin therapy.* Stuttgart: Thieme Verlag, 2000.
3. Brashear A, Lew MF, Dykstra DD, et al. Safety and efficacy of NeuroBloc (botulinum toxin type B) in type A-responsive cervical dystonia. *Neurology* 1999;53:1439–1446.
4. Brin MF, Lew MF, Adler CH, et al. Safety and efficacy of NeuroBloc (botulinum toxin type B) in type A-resistant cervical dystonia. *Neurology* 1999;53:1431–1438.
5. Goschel H, Wohlfarth K, Frevert J, et al. Botulinum A toxin: neutralizing and nonneutralizing antibodies—therapeutic consequences. *Exp Neurol* 1997;147:96–102.
6. Dressler D. Botulinum toxin therapy failure: causes, evaluation procedures and management strategies. *Eur J Neurol* 1997;4(suppl 2):S67–S70.
7. Consky ES, Basinski A, Belle L, et al. The Toronto Western Spasmodic Torticollis Rating Scale (TW-STRS): assessment of validity and inter-rater reliability. *Neurology* 1990;40(suppl 1):445.
8. Kerner J. Vergiftung durch verdorbene Würste. *Tübinger Blätter f Naturwissensch u Arzneykunde* 1817;3:1–25.
9. Kerner J. *Neue Beobachtungen über die in Würthemberg so häufig vorfallenden tödlichen Vergiftungen durch den Genuß geräucherter Würste.* Tübingen: G F Osiander, 1820.
10. Kerner J. *Das Fettgift und die Fettsäure und ihre Wirkungen auf den thierischen Organismus. Ein Beytrag zur Untersuchung des in verdorbenen Würsten giftig wirkenden Stoffes.* Stuttgart, Tübingen: Cotta-Verlag, 1822.
11. Poewe W, Wissel J. Experience with botulinum toxin in cervical dystonia. In: Jankovic J, Hallett M, eds. *Therapy with botulinum toxin.* New York, Basel, Hong Kong: Marcel Dekker, 1994:267–278.
12. Black JD, Dolly JO. Interaction of ^{125}I-labeled botulinum neurotoxins with nerve terminals. II. Autoradiographic evidence for its uptake into motor nerves by acceptor-mediated endocytosis. *J Cell Biol* 1986;103:535–544.
13. Daniels-Holgate PU, Dolly JO. Productive and non-productive binding of botulinum neurotoxin A to motor nerve endings are distinguished by its heavy chain. *J Neurosci Res* 1996;44:263–271.
14. Garner CG, Straube A, Witt TN, et al. Time course of distant effects of local injections of botulinum toxin. *Mov Disord* 1993;8:33–37.
15. Schnider P, Berger T, Schmied M, et al. (Increased residual urine volume after local injection of botulinum A toxin) [in German]. *Nervenarzt* 1995;66:465–467.
16. Claus D, Druschky A, Erbguth F. Botulinum toxin: influence on respiratory heart rate variation. *Mov Disord* 1995;10:574–579.
17. Nebe A, Schelosky L, Wissel J, et al. No effects on heart-rate variability and cardiovascular reflex tests after botulinum toxin treatment of cervical dystonia. *Mov Disord* 1996;11:337–339.

Dystonia 4: Advances in Neurology, Vol. 94. Edited by Stanley Fahn, Mark Hallett, and Mahlon R. DeLong. Lippincott Williams & Wilkins, Philadelphia © 2004.

43

Dystonia and Headaches: Clinical Features and Response to Botulinum Toxin Therapy

*Nestor Galvez-Jimenez, †Cristina Lampuri, *Rosa Patiño-Picirrillo, *Melanie J. A. Hargreave, and *Maurice R. Hanson

*Movement Disorders, Department of Neurology, The Cleveland Clinic Florida, Weston, Florida. †State University of New York at Buffalo School of Medicine and Biomedical Sciences, Buffalo, New York

Headache is an uncommon feature of cervical spondylosis and herniated disc disease (1), yet neck pain is present in approximately 68% to 91% of patients with cervical dystonia (CD) and may be a major source of disability (2–5). Among all the dystonic conditions, CD has a high incidence of pain that distinguishes CD from other forms of focal dystonia (6). Jankovic et al. (7) reported that approximately 32% of patients with CD might have symptoms and signs associated with a concomitant cervical radiculopathy.

It has been our clinical observation that many patients with craniocervical dystonia complain of suboccipital pain, generalized head pain, "band-like pain," frontal pain or tightness, or bitemporal pain as part of their symptom complex when evaluated or treated for their craniocervical dystonia.

We found no reports describing cervicogenic headaches or headaches of neck origin in patients with CD. Similarly, we found no reports of other forms of headaches in patients suffering from blepharospasm or oromandibular dystonia except for the description of retroorbital discomfort (sand-like sensation) in patients with blepharospasm or jaw pain in some patients with oromandibular dystonia.

This chapter examines the prevalence and clinical features of the different types of facial pain and headaches, their relationship to the different types of craniocervical dystonias, and their response to botulinum toxin (BT) therapy.

METHODS

The dystonia database of the Movement Disorders Program of The Cleveland Clinic Florida was queried, and those patients with all types of dystonia of the head and neck were identified. Only active patients currently receiving BT therapy were included. Patients were examined during their routine BT therapy visit, and a history was obtained and a neurologic examination was performed to confirm the type of headache or facial pain if present, and to confirm the type of craniocervical dystonia. A questionnaire specifically developed for this study was used to prospectively assess patients' symptoms before and after BT therapy. The patients rated themselves by using a visual analog scale (VAS) where 0 represented no pain and 10 represented the worst pain. In addition to the VAS, pain severity was assessed using the Toronto Western Spasmodic Torticollis Rating Scale (TWSTRS). Headache or pain location, quality, severity, relationship to dystonia, onset, frequency, trigger factors, and associated symptoms were assessed. In addition, the questionnaire included:

1. Demographics (age, sex, ethnic origin)
2. Family history of headaches
3. Type of dystonia (CD, blepharospasm, oromandibular dystonia)
4. Types of headaches (in patient's own words)
5. Onset and frequency of headaches
6. Relationship to their dystonia (i.e., headache or facial pain present with dystonia)
7. How often the headache occurs in relationship to the dystonia
8. Location of symptoms or pain
9. Duration of symptoms
10. Character and description of symptoms or pain
11. Associated symptoms (e.g., nausea, vomiting, photophobia, phonophobia)
12. Signs of impending headache including auras
13. Trigger factors for headaches or pain
14. Sleeping difficulties
15. Menstrual relationship to the headaches
16. Seasonal relationship to the headaches/pain
17. Personality/emotional state
18. Relevant medical-surgical history
19. Prior physicians' visits for headaches
20. Prior hospital visits or admissions for headaches
21. Visual analog scale (10 = worst headache or pain; 0 = no headache)

The headaches were classified using the currently accepted classification scheme of the International Headache Society (IHS) (8).

RESULTS

Of the 234 patients treated with BT between 1996 and 2001, 70 patients were included in the study. Seventeen patients had blepharospasm, eight had oromandibular dystonia, and 45 had CD. The mean age of the patients was 57.19 years [standard deviation (SD) 13.67]. Forty-one patients (58.6%) had the following types of headaches: 34 tension type headaches, 19 cervicogenic headaches, five migraine headaches without auras, one migraine headache with auras, and one atypical facial pain. Some patients have more than one type of headache or facial pain. The average dose of botulinum toxin type A used was 175 units (range 25–325 units).

Patients reported their pain located in the following areas: 65.8% in the frontal area, 48.7% in the cervical region, 12.1% in the shoulder area, 34% at the top of the head, 73% in the temporal region, 46.3% in the occipital area, 7.3% in the masseter region, and 4.8% in the jaw.

Using a VAS, pain was reported as 7.4 before BT therapy and 1.79 after BT therapy for a 75% improvement rate; 92% of patients described their headache as a dull pressure, 46.5% as sharp stabbing, 22% as radiating from the cervical region, and 9.7% as band-like pressure.

Patients described themselves as anxious (61%), stressed (44%), depressed (17%), perfectionist (10%), and content/happy (27%).

Oromandibular Group

Only patients with jaw closure or jaw deviation dystonia were included. Those with jaw opening dystonia were excluded, as this particular group of patients does not receive BT routinely in our program. There were a total of eight patients with a mean age of 60.8 years (range 58–72). Four patients (50%) had headaches. All (100%) had features in keeping with the IHS criteria for tension-type headache (TTH) (Table 43-1, 43-2), and one patient had, in addition, features of atypical facial pain.

TABLE 43-1. *International Headache Society (IHS) definition of chronic tension type headache 8*

Average frequency of attacks 15 days/month
At least two of the following pain characteristics:
Pressing/tightening quality
Mild or moderate severity
Bilateral location
No aggravation by physical activity
No vomiting
No more than one of the following: nausea, photophobia, phonophobia
Normal neurologic and physical examination

The headaches began at onset of dystonia in all patients with a mean age at onset of headache and dystonia of 53 years (range 42–60). The headache was found to be worst when the dystonia was at its worst (usually prior to the BT therapy) (Table 43-2).

The headaches were daily in most patients 2 to 3 weeks before treatment, and were relieved 1 to 7 days (average 4) after BT therapy. In two patients (50%) the headache frequency changed from more than 15 per month to less than four per month. Using a VAS, patients rated pain to be 7 before and 1.5 after BT therapy for a differential improvement of 78% (Fig. 43-1). Warning signs of impending return

TABLE 43-2. *Headache or facial pain associated with disorder of cranium, neck, eyes, ears, nose, sinuses, teeth, mouth or other facial or cranial structures (IHS) 8*

Diagnostic criteria
  A. Clinical and/or laboratory evidence of disorders in cranium, neck, etc. (specify)
  B. Headache located to the affected facial or cranial structure and radiating to surroundings; pain may or may not be referred to more distant areas of the head
  C. Headache disappears within 1 month after successful treatment or spontaneous remission of the underlying disorder
Neck, cervical spine diagnostic criteria
  A. Pain localized to neck and occipital region; may project to forehead, orbital region, temples, vertex, or ears
  B. Pain is precipitated or aggravated by special neck movements or sustained neck posture
  C. At least one of the following:
    1. Resistance to or limitation of passive neck movements
    2. Changes in neck muscle contour, texture, tone or response to active and passive stretching and contraction
    3. Abnormal tenderness of neck muscles
  D. Radiologic examination reveals at least one of the following:
    1. Movement abnormalities in flexion/extension
    2. Abnormal posture
    3. Fractures, congenital abnormalities, bone tumors, rheumatoid arthritis, or other distinct pathology (not spondylosis or osteochondrosis)

Comment: Cervical headaches are associated with movement abnormalities in cervical intervertebral segments. The disorder may be located in the joints or ligaments. The abnormal movement may occur in any component of intervertebral movement, and is manifest during either active or passive examination of the movement.

of headaches or pain included increased muscle tension in the facial, frontal and jaw/masseter regions in two of four patients (50%) along with worsening dystonia in three of four (75%) of patients. No relationship to menses, sleep, family history, or season was noted.

Blepharospasm

Seventeen patients with a mean age of 54.7 years (range 38–73) were studied. Nine patients (53%) had headaches. All had TTH characteristics as described in Table 43-1. Average age at onset of headaches was 42 years (range 35–40). The average onset of discomfort was 2 years earlier than the onset of blepharospasm. In all patients, the headache worsened when the dystonia worsened. All (100%) found relief after BT therapy. Headache was present on average eight times per month decreasing to none per month after BT therapy, for a 100% improvement rate.

All patients (100%) had their symptoms located in the frontal area and 77% in the temporal region. In addition, one patient (33%) had occipital pain. Most patients (88%) found relief 1 to 7 days after BT therapy, and 11% more than 1 week after therapy. Patients rated themselves at 7 points in the VAS before BT therapy and at 1 point after BT therapy, resulting in an 86% differential improvement rate (Fig. 43-2). Twenty-two percent of patients had no warning signs of impending headaches, 33% complained of pressure around the eyes, and 44% noted reappearance of dystonia as warning signs of impending headache. Patients described themselves as depressed (33%) and stressed (11%).

Cervical Dystonia

Forty-five patients with CD were studied. Twenty-one had TTHs, 16 had cervicogenic headaches, five had migraine headaches without auras, and one had migraine headaches with auras. Forty-three percent of patients localized their pain in the frontal region, 53.5% in the vertex region, 68% bitemporal, 61% occipital, 71% in the cervical/neck area, 18%

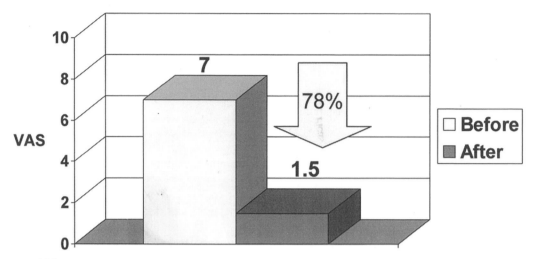

FIG. 43-1. Pain severity in patients with oromandibular dystonia (see text for discussion).

in the shoulder area, 11% around the head, and 50% in the mandibular area.

The patients rated pain using a VAS obtaining 7.42 points before and 1.5 points after BT therapy for an 80% improvement rate. Using the TWSTRS, the patients rated themselves as having 13.24 points before and 1.75 after BT therapy for an improvement of 87% after therapy, in keeping with the findings noted by using the pain VAS (Fig. 43-3).

Blepharospasm
Pain Severity:

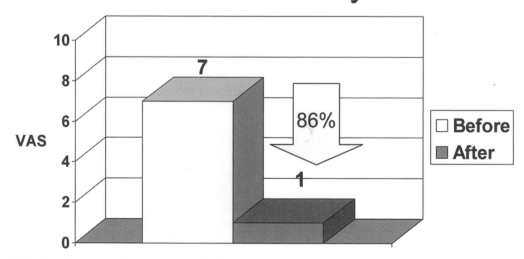

FIG. 43-2. Pain severity in patients with blepharospasm. VAS, Visual analog scale before and after BT treatment.

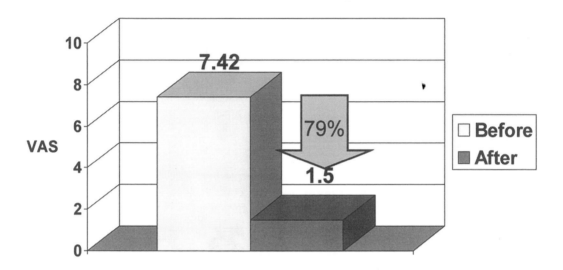

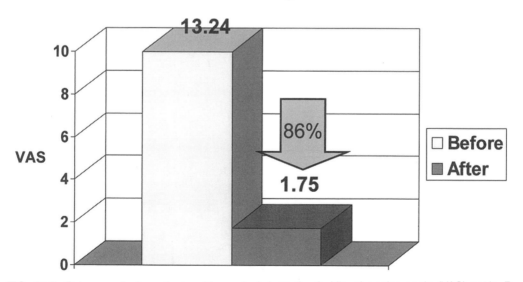

FIG. 43-3. Pain severity in patients with cervical dystonia. **A:** Visual analog scale (VAS) scale. **B:** Toronto Western Spasmodic Torticollis Rating Scale (TWSTRS) pain scale (see text for discussion).

The pain was described as dull pressure in 92% of patients, 53% sharp stabbing, 29% radiating from the neck, 11% throbbing, and 14.2 band-like. Other associated symptoms included neck and shoulder pain in 82% of patients, fatigue in 50%, photophobia in 14.2%, nausea in 3%, and no associated symptoms in 18%. Symptoms of impending headaches included neck tension in 89%, exacerbation of dystonia in 78%, pressure around the eyes and forehead in 18%, visual auras in 3.5%, and no warning signs in 7.1% of patients. Patients with CD had comorbid conditions including anxiety (65%), depression (21%), stress (57%), perfectionist profile (14%), and content and happy (18%).

had pain localized to the frontal regions. In contrast, only 43% of patients with CD had a similar location. Seventy-five percent to 77% of patients with oromandibular dystonia and blepharospasm had discomfort localized to the temporal areas; 68% of those with CD had a similar location. In addition, 61% of patients with CD and 33% of those with blepharospasm had symptoms localized to the occipital area. Patients with CD had pain localized to the neck (71%), shoulder (18%), and band-like around the head in 11% of cases. None of the patients with oromandibular dystonia or blepharospasm had pain in these areas.

Group Comparison

A comparison of the three groups of patients (Fig. 43-4), showed all patients with blepharospasm and oromandibular dystonia

DISCUSSION

Our group was composed of 70 patients with craniofaciocervical dystonias who have in common the presence of pain and discom-

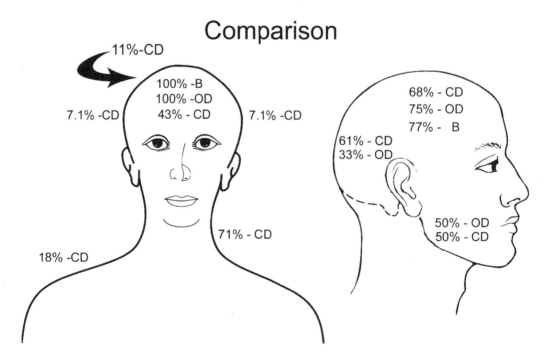

Comparison

11%-CD

7.1% -CD
100% -B
100% -OD
43% - CD
7.1% -CD

68% - CD
75% - OD
77% - B

61% - CD
33% - OD

71% - CD

18% -CD

50% - OD
50% - CD

CD: Cervical Dystonia   OD: Oromandibular Dystonia   B: Blepharospasm

FIG. 43-4. Comparison group. Headache distribution in patients with oromandibular dystonia, blepharospasm, and cervical dystonia. Patients with oromandibular and blepharospasm have pain localized predominantly in the frontal and bitemporal areas, whereas patients with cervical dystonia have pain localized predominantly in the occipital and neck regions (see text for discussion).

fort in the head, neck, and face mimicking cervicogenic headaches, chronic TTH, and atypical facial pain. The striking findings included the presence of frontal (100%) and temporal pressure/tightening like quality of pain (77%), moderate in intensity, bilateral in location without autonomic/migrainous symptoms such as nausea, vomiting, phonophobia, or photophobia in all patients with blepharospasm and oromandibular dystonia. All patients found improvement or resolution of their symptoms with BT therapy. This is in contrast to patients with CD whose complaints were located mostly in the neck, shoulder, and occipital and vertex regions. Only 43% of patients with CD had pain localized to the frontal regions. All patients had resolution of their symptoms with BT therapy.

In reviewing the literature, no studies specifically addressing the issue of pain and headaches in patients with craniocervical dystonia were found. This is in contrast to the common reported complaints of neck pain in patients with CD. In the headache and neurologic literature, the explanation of pain and neck disorders is murky at best. Brain (1) in 1963 stated that headache was an uncommon feature of cervical spondylosis and herniated discs. Lance (9) stated that patients with cervical spondylosis involving the upper cervical spine often report neck and shoulder pain with occasional suboccipital headache, which, when severe, may radiate to the frontal areas, eyes, or temple, occurring usually in the morning, aggravated by neck movements and by coughing and straining. Cervicogenic headache has been defined by Edmeads (10) as a headache caused by diseases or dysfunction of structures in the neck. He proposed that certain features of a headache may suggest its origin from the cervical spine, including (a) persistent, unilateral suboccipital pain; (b) reproduction or alteration of headache with neck motion; (c) abnormal postural attitudes of the head and neck; (d) aggravation or reproduction of headache by deep suboccipital pressure; (e) painful limitation of neck movements; and (f) signs and symptoms referable to cervical nerve roots. Our patients with CD fulfilled many of the

characteristics enunciated by Edmeads, including the suboccipital location of the pain, worsening or reproduction of pain with worsening dystonia and head movements, and Lance's (9) descriptors of severe pain of cervical spine origin such as radiation to the vertex, forehead, eyes, and temple areas, aggravated by neck movements (in our cases with worsening dystonia and head position). In addition, symptoms of impending headaches were those related to the onset or recurrence of CD after BT therapy such as increasing neck tension, exacerbation of dystonia, and pressure around the eyes (referred pain). The role that muscle contraction plays in these cases cannot be excluded, as in our experience many of these patients have trigger or tender points in the neck and shoulder musculature.

In Tarsy and First's (5) questionnaire, specifically developed for their study, 91% of their responders had pain with an overall frequency of 71%. Pain was located in the neck, shoulder, lower and upper back, and arms. The pain was described as pulling, aching, burning, or tightness commonly worse ipsilateral to the side of head deviation. All patients found relief after BT therapy. Twenty-three percent of patients found pain relief more striking than the relief of CD. Jankovic et al. (7) studied 300 patients with CD and found that 68% of them complained of pain, 32% had evidence of a secondary cervical radiculopathy, and 39% had scoliosis. Over 90% of patients found relief of neck pain after BT therapy. Chan et al. (2) found that neck pain was present in 75% of their CD patients and was a source of disability. Furthermore, they found that pain was strongly associated with constant head turning, severity of head turning, and presence of spasm. Chan et al., Dauer et al. (4), and Comella et al. (6) found that pain distinguished CD from all other types of dystonia.

The cause of pain in patients with CD is unknown. Tarsy and First (5) suggested continuous muscle contraction, cervical radiculopathy and spondylosis, and mechanical traction on musculoskeletal structures as potential causes of pain. The mechanism of pain in cervicogenic headache is believed to be due to involvement of the joints and ligaments in the atlantoaxial and occipital joints, C2-C3 zygophyseal joints, the suboccipital, upper posterior neck and prevertebral muscles, vertebral artery, C2-C3 intervertebral disc, and trapezius and sternocleidomastoid muscles sending their nociceptive afferents to the trigeminal-cervical nucleus complex. The trigeminocervical nucleus complex receives multiple convergent collaterals and overlapping afferents from the trigeminal nerve and the first three cervical spinal nerves, accounting for the referred pain experienced by many of these patients. These structures are similar to those believed to be affected in CD (11–14).

Chawda et al. (15) demonstrated that in patients with CD, moderate-to-severe degenerative changes of the cervical spine are seen in 14 of 34 patients most notably at the C2-C3 and C3-C4 levels and most likely to occur on the side of the main direction of the spasmodic torticollis. In their study, pain was present but not found to be related to the degree of arthritis. These findings suggest that pain may originate in the nonbony supporting structure of the cervical spine. Lobbezoo et al. (16) found that pain pressure threshold perception in the trapezius and sternocleidomastoid muscles is decreased in patients with CD. Kutvonen et al. (17) found that two thirds of the 39 patients with CD studied demonstrated pain in the splenius capitis and trapezius muscle with little cervical radicular pain. Seventeen percent of our patients with craniocervical dystonia were depressed. Jahanshanhi et al. (18) reported depression in 24% of 67 patients with cervical dystonia.

Headaches and other facial pain may be common concurrent complaints in patients with craniocervical dystonias. Patient with blepharospasm and oromandibular dystonia may have frontal, bitemporal headaches simulating TTHs responsive to BT therapy, whereas CD patients have symptoms in keeping with cervicogenic headaches in addition to neck and shoulder pain. BT therapy appears to be effective as adjuvant therapy for the treatment of these complaints. In our experience, patients with oromandibular dystonia usually complain of a deep-seated discomfort in the temporomandibular joint area, or in the facial muscles. In our analysis, most patients with oromandibular dystonia have pain in the frontotemporal area, and in one patient, concurrent pain localized to the jaw and facial area. In all patients the pain can be ascribed to the dystonia, as in most patients the pain began with the onset of dystonia and improves after BT therapy.

REFERENCES

1. Brain WR. Some unsolved problems of cervical spondylosis. *Br Med J* 1963;1:771–777.
2. Chan J, Brin MF, Fahn S. Idiopathic cervical dystonia: clinical characteristics. *Mov Disord* 1991;6:119–126.
3. Kutvonen O, Dastidar P, Nurmikko T. Pain in spasmodic torticollis. *Pain* 1997;69:279–286.
4. Dauer WT, Burke RE, Green P, et al. Current concepts on the clinical features, aetiology and management of idiopathic cervical dystonia. *Brain* 1998;121:547–560.
5. Tarsy D, First ER. Painful cervical dystonia: clinical features and response to treatment with botulinum toxin. *Mov Disord* 1999;14(6):1043–1045.
6. Comella CL, Stebbins GT, Millet S. Specific dystonic factors contributing to work limitation and disability in cervical dystonia. *Neurology* 1996;46(2 suppl):A295(abst).
7. Jankovic J, Leder S, Warner D, et al. Cervical dystonia: clinical findings and associated movement disorders. *Neurology* 1991;41:1088–1091.
8. Headache Classification Committee of the International Headache Society. Classification and diagnostic criteria for headache disorders, cranial neuralgias and facial pain. *Cephalalgia* 1988;8:1–96.
9. Lance J. *Mechanism and management of headache.* Oxford: Butterworth-Heinemann, 1993.
10. Edmeads JG. Disorders of the neck: cervicogenic headache. In: Silberstein SD, Lipton RB, Dalessio DJ, eds. *Wolf's headache and other head pains,* 7th ed. Oxford University Press: 2001:447–458.
11. Bogduk N. Headache and the neck. In: Goadsby PJ, Silverstein SD, eds. *Headache.* Oxford: Butterworth-Heinemann, 1997:369–379.
12. Bogduk N. Headaches and the cervical spine. An editorial. *Cephalalgia* 1984;4:7–8.
13. Bogduk N, Corrigan B, Kelly P, et al. Cervical headache. *Med J Aust* 1985;143:202–207.
14. Bogduk N, Lambert G, Duckworth JW. The anatomy and physiology of the vertebral nerve in relation to cervical migraine. *Cephalalgia* 1981;1:11–24.
15. Chawda SJ, Munchau A, Johnson D, et al. Pattern of premature degenerative changes of the cervical spine in patients with spasmodic torticollis and the impact on the outcome of selective peripheral denervation. *J Neurol Neurosurg Psychiatry* 2000;68:465–471.
16. Lobbezoo F, Tanguay R, Thu Thon M, et al. Pain perception in idiopathic cervical dystonia (spasmodic torticollis). *Pain* 1996;67:483–491.
17. Kutvonen O, Dastidar P, Nurmikko T. Pain in spasmodic torticollis. *Pain* 1997;69:279–286.
18. Jahanshahi M, Marion MH, Marsden CD. Natural history of adult-onset idiopathic torticollis. *Arch Neurol* 1990;47:548–552.

Dystonia 4: Advances in Neurology, Vol. 94. Edited by Stanley Fahn, Mark Hallett, and Mahlon R. DeLong. Lippincott Williams & Wilkins, Philadelphia © 2004.

44

Rating Scales for Dystonia: Assessment of Reliability of Three Scales

The Dystonia Study Group[1]

The selection of a rating scale to assess disease severity is one of the crucial elements in designing a clinical trial of a therapeutic intervention. A useful scale is one that is designed to measure a particular disorder, and that demonstrates validity, reliability, and reproducibility. The scale should be sensitive, or responsive, to change in the disorder secondary to intervention. Finally, the rating scale should be efficient and practical in a clinical setting (1,2). The World Health Orga-

[1]The sites and investigators of the Dystonia Study Group are as follows: Barrow Neurological Institute, Phoenix, AZ—M. Stacy; Beth Israel Deaconess Medical Center, Boston, MA—D. Tarsy; Boston Medical Center, Boston, MA—J. Friedman; Colorado Neurological Institute, Englewood, CO—L. Seeberger; Columbia Presbyterian Medical Center, New York, NY—B. Ford; Emory University, Atlanta, GA—M. Evatt; Foothills Hospital, Calgary, Canada—O. Suchowersky; Hospital of Cleveland, Cleveland, OH—D. Riley; London Health Sciences Center, London, Ontario—M. Jog; Long Island Jewish Hospital, New Hyde Park, NY—M. F. Gordon; Mayo Clinic, Scottsdale, AZ—C. Adler; Neuropsychiatric Institute, Chicago, IL—M. Brandabur; National Institute of Neurological Disorders and Stroke, Bethesda, MD—M. Hallett, B. Karp; Parkinson's Disease and Movement Disorders Center of Albany Medical Center, Albany, NY—S. Factor; Rush-Presbyterian-St. Luke's Medical Center, Chicago, IL—C. Comella, S. Leurgans, J. Wuu, G. Stebbins, T. Chmura; The Parkinson's Disease and Movement Disorders Institute, Fountain Valley, CA—D. Truong; Toronto Western Hospital, Toronto, Canada—R. Chen; University Hospital, Vancouver, Canada—J. Tsui; University of Chicago, Chicago, IL—U. Kang; University of Indiana, Indianapolis, IN—A. Brashear; University of Louisville, Louisville, KY—M. Swenson; University of Minnesota, Minneapolis, MN—P. Tuite; University of Southern California, Los Angeles, CA—M. Lew, G. Petzinger; University of Virginia Health Sciences Center, Charlottesville, VA—D. Trugman.

nization (WHO) developed a model to standardize disease outcomes into four categories: pathology, impairment, disability, and handicap (3). Impairment refers to the functional consequence of a disease process, reflecting organ dysfunctions or abnormalities of body structure. Most current dystonia rating scales have been assessed primarily for their clinimetric properties relative to impairment (motor abnormalities) (4,5).

Dystonia is a dynamic disorder manifested by involuntary, abnormal sustained postures that change in severity based on posture and activity (6). This feature of dystonia has made the development of reliable rating scales to evaluate dystonia severity problematic. To capture the fluctuations in dystonia severity occurring from position and movement factors, several scales have incorporated ancillary scales that modify the motor severity ratings. An examination (or videotape protocol) methodology is necessary to ensure consistent and complete assessment of the patients. The primary aim of this study was to assess the internal consistency, interrater agreement, and content validity of the Fahn-Marsden Dystonia Rating Scale (F-M), the Unified Dystonia Rating Scale (UDRS), and the Global Dystonia Rating Scale (GDS).

The F-M was published in 1985 (7). It provides a movement scale that consists of a severity and provoking rating for nine body regions (Fig. 44-1). The severity rating assesses

Region Product	Provoking Facotr		Severity Factor	Weight
Eyes 0-8	0-4	X	0-4	0.5
Mouth 0-8	0-4	X	0-4	0.5
Speech 0-16 Swallow	0-4	X	0-4	1.0
Neck 0-8	0-4	X	0-4	0.5
R arm 0-16	0-4	X	0-4	1.0
L arm 0-16	0-4	X	0-4	1.0
Trunk 0-16	0-4	X	0-4	1.0
R Leg 0-16	0-4	X	0-4	1.0
L leg 0-16	0-4	X	0-4	1.0

Sum:
Maximum=120

I. Provoking Factor
A. General
    0- No dystonia at rest or with action
    1- Dystonia only with particular action
    2- Dystonia with many actions
    3- Dystonia on action of distant part of body or intermittently at rest
    4- Dystonia present at rest
B. Speech and swallowing
    1-Occasional, either or both
    2- Frequent either
    3- Frequent one and occasional other
    4- Frequent both

II. Severity Factors
Eyes
    0- No dystonia

Speech and swallowing
    0- Normal
    1- Slightly involved; speech easily understood or occasional choking
    2- Some difficulty in understanding speech or frequent choking
    3- Marked difficulty in understanding speech or inability to swallow firm foods
    4- Complete or almost complete anarthria, or marked difficulty swallowing soft foods and liquids

Neck
    0- No dystonia present
    1- Slight. Occasional pulling
    2- Obvious torticollis, but mild
    3- Moderate pulling
    4- Extreme pulling

Arm
    0- No dystonia present
    1- Slight dystonia. Clinically insignificant
    2- Mild. Obvious dystonia, but not disabling
    3- Moderate. Able to grasp, with some manual function
    4- Severe. No useful grasp

Trunk
    0- No dystonia present
    1- Slight bending; clinically insignificant
    2- Definite bending, but not interfering with standing or walking
    3- Moderate bending; interfering with standing or walking
    4- Extreme bending of trunk preventing standing or walking

Leg
    0- No dystonia present

FIG. 44-1. The Fahn-Marsden Dystonia Rating Scale.

1- Slight. Occasional blinking
2- Mild. Frequent blinking without prolonged spasms of eye closure
3- Moderate. Prolonged spasms of eyelid closure, but eyes open most of the time
4- Severe. Prolonged spasms of eyelid closure, with eyes closed at least 30% of the time
 	
Mouth
    0- no dystonia present
    1- Slight. Occasional grimacing or other mouth movements (e.g., jaw opened or clenched; tongue movement
    2- Mild. Movement present less than 50% of the time
    3- Moderate dystonic movements or contractions present most of the time
    4- Severe dystonic movements or contractions   present most of the time
	1- Slight dystonia, but not causing impairment; clinically insignificant
	2- Mild dystonia. Walks briskly and unaided
	3- Moderate dystonia. Severely impairs walking or requires assistance
	4- Severe. Unable to stand or walk on involved leg

FIG. 44-1. (*continued*)

the severity of dystonia in the nine regions regardless of the circumstances in which the dystonia appears. The provoking factor rates the circumstance under which the dystonia occurs. Ratings obtained for neck, eyes, and mouth are halved before summing the scores for the body areas. The maximal score of the F-M movement scale is 120. The F-M was shown to have reliability among four raters at a single site in ten dystonia patients. The construct validity of the scale was established by correlations with an overall global dystonia severity scale and a separate dystonia disability scale. The clinometric properties of the F-M were not established in larger multicenter studies.

The UDRS and GDS were developed by a panel of dystonia experts in 1997 (8). The UDRS assesses dystonia in 14 body regions (Fig. 44-2). The UDRS has both a motor severity and duration of dystonia rating. The objective behind the development of the UDRS was to include a more detailed assessment of individual body areas, with separate ratings for proximal and distal limbs; to eliminate the subjective patient rating for speech and swallowing; and to remove the weighting factors for neck, eyes, and mouth that were included in the F-M. The duration rating of the UDRS was based on a duration factor. On the UDRS, the severity rating is specific for each body region assessed and ranges from 0 (no dystonia) to 4 (extreme dystonia). The duration rating is based on the duration factor previously validated in the Toronto Western Spasmodic Torticollis Rating Scale (TWSTRS) (9–11). The UDRS duration rating assesses whether dystonia occurs at rest or with action, and whether it is predominantly at maximal or submaximal intensity during the period of the examination. The total score for the UDRS is the sum of the severity and duration factors. The maximal total score of the UDRS is 112.

The GDS has ratings for dystonia severity in the 14 body areas already described for the

I. Duration Factor

0	none
0.5	occasional (< 25% of the time); predominantly submaximal
1.0	occasional (< 25% of the time); predominantly maximal
1.5	Intermittent (25-50% of the time); predominantly submaximal
2.0	Intermittent (25-50% of the time); predominantly maximal
2.5	Frequent (50-75% of the time); predominantly submaximal
3.0	Frequent (50-75% of the time); predominantly maximal
3.5	Constant (> 75% of the time); predominantly submaximal
4.0	Constant (> 75% of the time); predominantly maximal

2. Motor Severity Factor

EYES AND UPPER FACE

0.	none
1.	mild: increased blinking and/or slight forehead wrinkling (≤ 25% maximal intensity)
2.	moderate: eye closure without squeezing and/or pronounced forehead wrinkling (> 25% but ≤ 50% maximal intensity)
3.	severe: eye closure with squeezing, able to open eyes within 10 seconds and/or marked forehead wrinkling (> 50% but ≤ 75% maximal intensity)
4.	eye closure with squeezing, unable to open eyes within 10 seconds and/ or intense forehead wrinkling (> 75% maximal intensity)

LOWER FACE

0	none
1	mild: grimacing of lower face with minimal distortion of mouth (≤ 25% maximal)

LARYNX

0	none
1	mild: barely detectable hoarseness and/or choked voice and/or occasional voice breaks
2	moderate: obvious hoarseness and/or choked voice and/ or frequent voice breaks
3	severe: marked hoarseness and/or choked voice and/or continuous voice breaks
4	extreme: unable to vocalize

NECK

0	none
1	mild: movement of head from neutral position ≤ 25% of possible normal range
2	moderate:movement of head from neutral position > 25% but ≤ 50% of possible normal range
3	severe:movement of head from neutral position > 50% but ≤ 75% of possible normal range
4	extreme:movement of head from neutral postion > 75% of possible normal range

SHOULDER AND PROXIMAL ARM (Right and Left)

0	none
1	mild: movement of shoulder or upper arm ≤ 25% of possible normal range
2	moderate: movement of shoulder or upper arm 25% but ≤ 50% of possible normal range
3	severe: movement of shoulder or upper arm 50% but ≤ 75% of possible normal range
4	extreme: movement of shoulder or upper arm 75% of possible normal range

DISTAL ARM AND HAND INCLUDING ELBOW (Right and Left)

0	none
1	mild: movement of distal arm or hand ≤ 25% of possible normal range
2	moderate: movement of distal arm or hand 25% but ≤ 50% of possible normal range
3	severe: movement of distal arm or hand 50% but ≤ 75% of possible normal range
4	extreme: movement of distal arm or hand 75% of possible normal range

FIG. 44-2. The Unified Dystonia Rating Scale (UDRS).

2	moderate: grimacing of lower face with moderate distortion of mouth (> 25% but ≤ 50% maximal)	PELVIS AND PROXIMAL LEG (Right and Left)	
3	severe: marked grimacing with severe distortion of mouth (> 50% but ≤ 75% maximal)4 extreme: intense grimacing with extreme distortion of mouth (> 75% maximal)	0	none
		1	mild: tilting of pelvis or movement of proximal leg or hip ≤ 25% of possible normal range
		2	moderate: tilting of pelvis or movement of proximal leg or hip 25% but ≤ 50% of possible normal range
		3	severe: tilting of pelvis or movement of proximal leg or hip 50% but ≤ 75% of possible normal range
JAW AND TONGUE		4.	extreme: tilting of pelvis or movement of proximal leg or hip 75% of possible normal range
0	none	DISTAL LEG AND FOOT INCLUDING KNEE (Right and Left)	
1	mild: jaw opening and/or tongue protrusion ≤ 25% of possible range or forced jaw clenching without bruxism	0	none
		1	mild: movements of distal leg or foot ≤ 25% of possible normal range
2	moderate: jaw opening and/or tongue protrusion > 25% but ≤ 50%of possible range or forced jaw clenching with mild bruxism secondary to dystonia	2	moderate: movements of distal leg or foot 25% but ≤ 50% of possible normal range
		3	severe: movements of distal leg or foot 50% but ≤ 75% of possible normal range
		4	extreme: movements of distal leg or foot 75% of possible
3	severe: jaw opening and /or tongue protrusion > 50% but ≤ 75%of possible range or forced jaw clenching with pronounced bruxism secondary to dystonia		normal range
		TRUNK	
		0	none
		1	mild: bending of trunk ≤ 25% of possible normal range
4	extreme: jaw opening and/or tongue protrusion > 75% of possible range or forced jaw clenching with inability to open mouth	2	moderate: bending of trunk 25% but ≤ 50% of possible normal range
		3	severe: bending of trunk > 50% but ≤ 75% of possible normal range
		4extreme:bending of trunk > 75% of possible normal range	

FIG. 44-2. (*continued*)

UDRS (Fig. 44-3) (8). The GDS is a Likert-type scale with ratings from 0 to 10 (0 = no dystonia, 1 = minimal, 5 = moderate, and 10 = severe dystonia). There are no modifying ratings or weighting factors in the GDS. The total score is the sum of the scores for all the body areas. The maximal total score of the GDS is 140.

METHODS

The F-M, UDRS, and GDS were tested for interrater agreement and reliability in a large, multicenter study. This study included 100 primary dystonia patients with generalized ($n = 24$), segmental ($n = 37$), and focal dystonia ($n = 39$) videotaped using a standardized videotape protocol. Ten master tapes were edited, with ten patients per tape. Each of the 25 investigators rated two master tapes (20 patients) using the F-M, UDRS, and GDS in random order. At the conclusion of the ratings, the investigator completed a questionnaire that assessed their opinion of the clinical utility of the scales. Reliability and interrater agreement were analyzed separately for sever-

Body Area	Severity of Dystonia Rated 0 to 10 0: No dystonia.....10: maximally severe dystonia	
Eyes and upper face		
Lower face		
Jaw and tongue		
Larynx		
Neck		
Shoulder and proximal arm	R	L
Distal arm and hand including elbow	R	L
Pelvis and Upper leg	R	L
Distal leg and foot	R	L
Trunk		

FIG. 44-3. The Global Dystonia Rating Scale (GDS). The global score is an overall score for the body area. The investigator rates the patient in relationship to all patients. If the dystonia changes during the examination, the rating for the maximal dystonia is recorded.

ity and the modifying factors (UDRS duration and F-M provoking factor) ratings.

The internal consistency of each scale was assessed by Cronbach's alpha. Overall interrater agreement was assessed using intraclass correlation (ICC) coefficient. Interrater agreement for body regions was analyzed in two ways: Kendall's coefficient of concordance and generalized weighted kappa.

RESULTS

Each of the three scales was found to have a high level of internal consistency (Cronbach's alpha range 0.89–0.93). The total score of each scale showed a high level of interrater reliability (ICC coefficients range from 0.71 to 0.78). The ancillary ratings for the both the F-M and UDRS showed consistently lower agreement among raters than did the severity ratings. When separate body areas were analyzed, agreement for duration ratings of the UDRS were notably less for upper face and eyes, lower face and jaw, larynx, and arm. The provoking factor ratings of the F-M likewise were less for upper face and eyes and neck (Table 44-1). The total scores for the three scales are highly correlated with each other, with Pearson correlations of 0.983 (UDRS and GDS), 0.977 (F-M and UDRS), and 0.980 (F-M and UDRS).

Of the investigators, 74% felt that the GDS was extremely or very easy to apply and 82% felt that it was useful in an office setting. Interestingly, despite the fact that only 5% found the UDRS easy to apply, 90% of those responding felt that it was useful in multicenter clinical trials. The basis for the discrep-

TABLE 44-1. *Agreement of raters for motor severity ratings of different body regions: generalized weighted kappa*

Body region	UDRS		F-M		GDS
	Severity	Duration	Severity	Provoking factor	
Leg	0.87	0.80	0.91	0.85	0.80
Trunk	0.90	0.75	0.88	0.81	0.86
Arm	0.82	0.44	0.90	0.89	0.83
Neck	0.81	0.74	0.84	0.51	0.82
Larynx/speech	0.66	0.44	0.82	0.77	0.82
Lower face and jaw	0.63	0.49	0.62	0.61	0.73
Upper face and eyes	0.52	0.43	0.52	0.37	0.58

F-M, Fahn-Marsden Dystonia Rating Scale; GDS, Global Dystonia Scale; UDRS, Unified Dystonia Rating Scale.

ancy in usefulness between clinical practice and clinical trials was not determined by the questionnaire (Table 44-2).

DISCUSSION

This study demonstrates that all three dystonia rating scales have acceptable levels of reliability when tested using a large number of dystonia patients across many investigators. The inter-rater agreement for motor severity of dystonia in separate body regions was good to excellent for all three scales (F-M, UDRS, GDS). The ancillary ratings that modify the motor severity scores in the F-M and UDRS scales showed a lower level of agreement and were problematic in several body areas. The ancillary rating scales are complex, combining presence of dystonia in particular situations, and assessment of maximal or submaximal intensity during the examination. The contribution of these ancillary ratings to the reliability of the rating scales is modest, and the complexities of these additional ratings likely reduce the clinical usefulness of both scales as indi-

cated by investigator response to the clinical usefulness questionnaire.

The validity of each scale has been partially addressed through this study. The methodology of development of the UDRS and GDS by means of a panel of dystonia experts provides content validity. The high correlation of the total scores of the F-M, UDRS, and GDS suggests concurrent validity.

Although reliability and agreement appear equivalent among the three scales, the ease of application of the GDS reported by the majority of raters in this study suggests the GDS may be the most practical to implement in multiple research sites. The drawback of the GDS is the lack of definition for each rating, relying on the investigator's experience with dystonia. Revision of the UDRS and the F-M by deleting the ancillary ratings provides a reasonable alternative. Additional studies of all three scales are necessary to examine the factor structure and other areas of validity such as their responsivity to change and discriminant validity (12–14). The parallel development of a teaching tape, demonstrating the range of rating for each body area, espe-

TABLE 44-2. *Investigators' assessments of the ease of application and usefulness of each dystonia rating scale in clinical trials and office settings: percentage of investigators declaring specific characteristics of each scale, among those who replied*

	UDRS	F-M	GDS
Extremely or very easy to apply	1/20 = 5%	8/21 = 38%	14/19 = 74%
Useful in multicenter clinical trials	19/20 = 95%	16/21 = 76%	8/22 = 36%
Useful in an office setting	9/21 = 43%	16/21 = 76%	18/22 = 82%

cially the face and eyes, will increase the interrater agreement for dystonia in these areas.

REFERENCES

1. Herndon RM. Introduction to clinical neurologic scales. In: Herndon RM, ed. *Handbook of neurologic rating scales.* New York: Demos Vermande, 1997:1–6.
2. Hobart JC, Lamping DL, Thompson AJ. Evaluating neurological outcome measures: the bare essentials. *J Neurol Neurosurg Psychiatry* 1996;60:127–130.
3. World Health Organization. *International Classification of Impairments, Disabilities, and Handicaps.* Geneva: World Health Organization, 1980.
4. Fahn S. Assessment of the primary dystonias. In: Munsat TL, ed. *Quantification of neurologic deficit.* London: Butterworth, 1989:241–270.
5. Lindeboom R, Haan RJ, Aramideh M, et al. Treatment outcomes in cervical dystonia: a clinimetric study. *Mov Disord* 1996;11:371–376.
6. Fahn S, Marsden CD, Calne DB. Classification and investigation of dystonia. In: Marsden CD, Fahn S, eds. *Movement disorders 2.* London: Butterworth, 1987: 332–358.
7. Burke RE, Fahn S, Marsden CD, et al. Validity and reliability of a rating scale for the primary torsion dystonias. *Neurology* 1985;35:73–77.
8. Comella C, Luergans S, Wuu J, et al., and the Dystonia Study Group. Rating scales for dystonia: a multicenter assessment. *Mov Disord* 2003;18:303–312.
9. Consky ES, Basinki A, Belle L, et al. The Toronto Western Spasmodic Torticollis Rating Scale (TWSTRS): assessment of the validity and inter-rater reliability. *Neurology* 1990;40(suppl 1):445.
10. Consky ES, Lang AE. Clinical assessments of patients with cervical dystonia. In: Jankovic J, Hallett M, eds. *Therapy with botulinum toxin.* New York: Marcel Dekker, 1994:211–237.
11. Comella CL, Stebbins GT, Goetz CG, et al. Teaching tape for the motor section of the Toronto Western Spasmodic Torticollis Scale. *Mov Disord* 1997;12:570–575.
12. Burke RE, Fahn S, Marsden CD. Torsion dystonia: a double-blind, prospective trial of high-dosage trihexyphenidyl. *Neurology* 1986;36:160–164.
13. Volkman J, Benecke R. Deep stimulation for dystonia: patient selection and evaluation. *Mov Disord* 2002;17 (suppl 3):S112–S115.
14. Vercueil L, Krack P, Pollak P. Results of deep brain stimulation for dystonia: a critical reappraisal. *Mov Disord* 2002;17(suppl 3):S89–S93.

Subject Index